NOURISHING THE HUMANISTIC IN MEDICINE

NOURISHING
THE

William R. Rogers
David Barnard
Editors

HUMANISTIC IN MEDICINE

Interactions with the Social Sciences

UNIVERSITY OF PITTSBURGH PRESS

In cooperation with the

Institute on Human Values in Medicine *of the*

Society for Health and Human Values

Published by the University of Pittsburgh Press, Pittsburgh, Pa. 15260, in cooperation with the Institute on Human Values in Medicine of the Society for Health and Human Values

This is Report #12 of the Institute on Human Values in Medicine, funded by a grant from the National Endowment for the Humanities.

Library of Congress Cataloging in Publication Data

Main entry under title:

Nourishing the humanistic in medicine.

(Contemporary community health series) (Report—Institute on Human Values in Medicine; 12)
Papers based on dialogues held at various U.S. cities for the past 3 years under the sponsorship of the Institute on Human Values in Medicine of the Society for Health and Human Values.
Bibliography: p. 313
Includes index.
1. Medicine—Philosophy. 2. Medicine and the humanities. 3. Medical ethics. 4. Social medicine. 5. Medical education. I. Rogers, William R., 1932– II. Barnard, David, 1948– III. Institute on Human Values in Medicine. IV. Series. V. Series: Institute on Human Values in Medicine. Report—Institute on Human Values in Medicine; 12.
R723.N68   362.1'04'25   78-26222
ISBN 0-8229-3395-0

Chapter 3, "Advocacy and Corruption in the Healing Professions," by Robert Jay Lifton, was reprinted, with stylistic adaptations, from the December 1975 issue of *Connecticut Medicine,* published by the Connecticut State Medical Society. Copyright © 1975 by Robert Jay Lifton. Used by permission.

Chapter 9, "The Uses of a Diagnosis: Doctors, Patients, and Neurasthenia," by Barbara Sicherman, was reprinted, with stylistic adaptations of the notes, from the *Journal of the History of Medicine and Allied Sciences,* 1977, *32,* 33–54, with permission.

Contents

Foreword

Edmund D. Pellegrino

This volume examining the relationships of some of the social sciences to medicine and the health sciences has been prepared under the auspices of the Institute on Human Values in Medicine. It is one of a series of reports emanating from a program of the Institute on Human Values in Medicine that was devoted to clarifying and defining the research and teaching ground between medicine and selected humanistic disciplines.

The Institute on Human Values in Medicine was established almost a decade ago to foster the engagement of the humanities and medicine through the education of health professionals. The Institute hoped in this way to respond to the need of health professional students for a deeper comprehension of the many value questions then emerging as a consequence of the rapid medical progress and its impact on the lives of individuals and society.

The list of pertinent value issues in medicine has grown exponentially over the intervening decade. They are already the subject of intensive professional and public discourse and debate. Some measure of their importance is evident in the number of medical moral dilemmas that have already come before the courts and governmental bodies. One needs mention only the Supreme Court decision on abortion, the rulings of the Supreme Court of New Jersey on the case of Karen Ann Quinlan and of the Supreme Court of Massachusetts on the Saikewicz case, the Del Zio trial in New York, the California natural death act and its counterparts in some forty other states, and the HEW regulation of recombinant DNA research.

These are just a few instances of the ways in which medical decision-making, scientific investigation, and public policy are clustering as fundamental questions of human values. No physician, lawyer, legislator, or educated citizen can respond intelligently to the issues without confronting questions such as the purposes and value of human life, the requirements of a "good" society, and the rights and obligations of the patient and physician. In a democratic and pluralistic society there is no homogeneity of value systems and, indeed, no consensus on what humans are for, and what constitutes the "good life," to which we can turn for resolution.

It has become increasingly obvious, therefore, that there is a need for a better education in those disciplines which have traditionally explored human-values questions, namely the humanities: philosophy, history, literature, language, and theology. These disciplines have, of recent years, lost some of their pristine authority as instruments of a liberal education because they have become overspecialized and overprofessionalized. Nonetheless, it is these disciplines which retain the possibility for providing the cognitive and affective tools requisite to an intelligent formulation of personal and public opinion.

Accordingly, the Institute on Human Values in Medicine, a program of the Society for Health and Human Values, has conducted a threefold program to encourage the education of physicians and other health workers in the humanities as essential instruments for the responsible practice of their professions. One program is dedicated to institutes and seminars to acquaint faculty members at health professional schools with the methodology and content of teaching ethics and the humanities as an integral part of medical education. A second program supports fellowships for students and faculty members from medical fields or the humanities who wish to do research or prepare themselves for careers in the teaching of humanities in medical situations.

The purpose of the third program, of which this volume is a product, is to deepen the intellectual engagement between medicine and specific disciplines. In this way, issues of mutual pedagogic and research interest can be better defined and the interdisciplinary territory described. Under Institute auspices and with National Endowment for the Humanities funding, scholars and teachers from the health professions were provided an opportunity to meet with their counterparts in the humanities for two to three days, five times in a two-year period. In this way it was hoped that the frequent errors of interdisciplinary discourse—covering too many subjects simultaneously, too few and too brief contacts, and lack of a concrete focus for the discussion—would be avoided.

Five task forces between the disciplines have followed this plan and have completed their work—medicine and history, medicine and religious studies, medicine and the social sciences, medicine and literature, and medicine and the visual arts. This volume explores the ground between the humanistic end of the spectrum of the social sciences and medicine.

Obviously a multitude of questions can be raised under this rubric but only a few were selected by this particular task force. These essays represent a variety of points of view, different values, and different recommendations. No attempt at consensus was made since the aim of the task forces was not to issue a manifesto but to encourage academic and intellectual exchange. The essays do provide the physiognomy of research and teaching challenges at the junction of medicine and the social sciences when viewed from the special viewpoint of human-value questions.

There is currently a need to strengthen the intellectual links between medicine and the social sciences. Teaching the social and behavioral sciences in medical schools was introduced in the United States about twenty-five years ago. After an initial period of what can be best called restrained enthusiasm, these programs have experienced a "postsixties" erosion in many schools. The reasons for this decline are many. Prominent among them is the failure to secure a really firm basis of intellectual engagement. In the past, some social scientists have been too willing to identify with medicine and others too prone to offer condescending criticism. Neither stance favors critical yet sincere dialogue based on mutual knowledge in which each discipline can retain its identity yet contribute to the other.

Anyone who has tried to teach or do research in an interdisciplinary program appreciates how tenuous the interrelationships can be. Only too often one encounters romantic overenthusiasm or skeptical noninvolvement. The only really secure footing for such engagements is a mutuality of intellectual interest around authentic conceptual issues. The Institute hopes this and subsequent volumes will enable the participating disciplines to retain their own identity and yet contribute to one another. The effort is of the utmost practical importance to health professionals, to the humanities, and to the society they serve.

INSTITUTE ON HUMAN VALUES IN MEDICINE

Board of Directors

Joseph M. White
President
University of Health Sciences
The Chicago Medical School
Chicago, Illinois

Richard M. Zaner
Easterwood Professor of Philosophy
Chairman, Department of Philosophy
Southern Methodist University
Dallas, Texas

Staff

Ronald W. McNeur
Executive Director of the Institute
Executive Director, Society for Health
  and Human Values

A. Myrvin DeLapp
Fiscal Agent, Society for Health and
  Human Values

Thomas K. McElhinney
Director of Programs
Institute on Human Values in Medicine

Preface

The essays collected here represent a substantive contribution to a growing exchange of ideas between the social sciences and medicine. They not only represent the scholarship of single authors, working from a specific disciplinary base, but demonstrate also the fruitful results of a relaxed and sustained interaction among these people over a period of two years. Sitting down with one another on five separate occasions, for two days at a time, the participants had a chance to identify a broad range of issues and to push hard against the boundaries of knowledge and mutual exchange in a genuine interdisciplinary discussion.

The unusual opportunity for this style of exchange, and for the thoughtful essays stemming from it, was made possible by a special grant from the National Endowment for the Humanities given to the Institute on Human Values in Medicine. The grant provided for an initial cluster of three "dialogue groups": one on literature and medicine, one on history and medicine, and this one on social science and medicine. Two other dialogue groups dealt with medicine and religious studies and with medicine and the visual arts. Such activities, along with interdisciplinary fellowships in the humanities and medicine, and resource services to assist schools in establishing humanistically oriented medical education, are all part of the imaginative program of the Institute. Conceived in 1970, largely under the leadership of Edmund Pellegrino, presently of Catholic University, and established in 1971, the Institute functions as a project coordinator within the larger Society for Health and Human Values.[1]

Both in the initial framing of topics by the dialogue group and in this final selection of essays developed from our work together, we have attempted to address issues that not only are intrinsically interesting and important, but have direct consequences for the style and curriculum of medical education as well as the context of medical practice. Each of the essays in this volume demonstrates the seriousness and commitment of the authors to a significant level of intellectual exchange that should stand in its own right, as well as to a significant exploration of policy implications with direct bearing on educational planning in medical schools and on governmental decisions in relation to medical care.

The audience we seek includes a broad range of professional and lay people. We address ourselves to medical educators who are responsible for framing the policy, the curriculum, the clinical rotations, and the setting of medical colleges. We speak to health care managers and those in various governmental and consumer groups responsible for the establishment of policy concerning the delivery of health services. We speak with particular vigor and expectancy to the upcoming generation of students whose vision may simultaneously comprise both scientific competence and the humane care of those seeking their help. And we speak, most especially, to all intelligent and concerned people who see the need for effective interaction between humanistic understanding of human life and the provision of effective medical services—to those who yearn for a deepening of medical care as both art and science, those who would find more specific ways of understanding and reforming medicine and the social sciences, both in themselves and in exchange with one another.

NOTE

1. The Society for Health and Human Values and the Institute on Human Values in Medicine have their headquarters at 925 Chestnut Street, Philadelphia, PA 19107.

NOURISHING THE HUMANISTIC IN MEDICINE

CHAPTER 1

The Interaction Between Humanistic Social Sciences and Medical Education

William R. Rogers and David Barnard

> There has been a tendency among physicians to study the health and disease of the individual too much from the standpoint of his nervous mechanism. . . . In my opinion, we ought to reverse the process and study the individual as a conscious, self-active, creative force and ought, especially in talking with laymen, to throw the emphasis upon motive and obligation and social environment in the widest sense as influences for health on the one hand, or for disease on the other.   —James Jackson Putnam

Physicians such as James Putnam and Richard Cabot, writing at the turn of the twentieth century, spoke somewhat philosophically and certainly humanistically about the physician's role. Reflecting on their experiences at Harvard Medical School and Massachusetts General Hospital, they recounted case after case where a broadened understanding of the patient's situation led to more effective treatment and helped prevent future illness. Their discussions of medical care as documented in the first essay by Barbara Sicherman (chapter 5) moved beyond technically proficient discussion of physiology and pathology into examination of "the study of character under adversity" and to the importance of an "attempt to interpret to patients the meaning of their illness."

Such concerns with total life context, with character, with preventive care, with a holistic perception of illness and health, and with the dynamics of the doctor-patient relationship, characterize our perspective on the contemporary interaction between social science and medicine. Richard Cabot has indeed been cited as one of the practitioner-theorists who most capably identified the coordinates of art and science in the practice of medicine.

And although Cabot may have attracted some opposition from his medical colleagues for some of his innovations (such as advocating medical insurance), he certainly did not lack support and acclaim both for his prodigious work on cardiac and blood diseases and for his advocacy of humane concerns in the broadened image of medical responsibility. As further evidence in support of this historic tradition of humanism in medicine, we might cite the work of Dr. Bayard Holmes:

Each patient is always and in an overshadowing sense a man, and when he is sick he presents all the possibilities of disease. The only rational treatment that he can receive must come from the physician who is on his side more a man than a doctor, and more a doctor than a surgeon or other specialist. The higher the mountain peak of special professional excellence the greater, the broader and more massive the plateau of general medical skill and human character on which it must necessarily depend. Under no circumstances can the care of the patient be divided up between several independent and unrelated physicians, whatever their special excellence or skill may be. The primitive relation is the only safe one, a sick man on the one side, a conscientious doctor on the other.[1]

In spite of such auspicious visions at the turn of the century, however, most historical and cultural commentary on the priorities in medicine later in the twentieth century points insistently at the triumph of a dedication to science which has had as its corollary an increasing dependence on technological forms of life support and health care. In the eyes of many, the unquestionable benefits of the rapidly expanding basic and applied sciences have often come at considerable cost to the personal and patient caring of the physician on one side and the recognition of the sick person on the other.

The pendulum has swung very far in the direction of a form of medical education that places heavy demands on a student's competence in the scientific disciplines but leaves very little time for reflection, either about the broader human issues of an individual's life when confronted by the stresses of illness, or about the place of medical responsibility in relation to society and history more generally. It is exactly such broadened reflections that define the most general scope of the exchange between humanistic social science and medicine. It is within this scope that the essays in this volume locate themselves, in the hope that richer detail can be added to the discussion and that the consequences for practical decisions in planning medical education and health care policy will be examined and acted upon.

Our underlying question is: How can the social sciences help to illuminate, contribute to, and make operative the "humanization" of medicine through medical education? In this we are attempting to identify, within the general area of social science and medicine, some of those distinctive points at which value commitments become essential and to suggest modes of reforming or deepening the self-understanding of both social science and medicine. Put most succinctly, our effort is to look consciously and consistently at issues in medicine and social science in such a way as to identify *value* motifs. What is involved in the truly humane care of persons?

Although the signs of dehumanization, denial, and distancing—what Robert Jay Lifton calls "technicism" (chapter 3)— may be apt in the critique of many phases of modern medicine, there is also evidence that the pendulum may be swinging back toward a more balanced vision of the humane functions in social science and medicine, as well as in their interaction.

Evidence of this renewed vision, somewhat reminiscent of the hope of those earlier in this century—although apparently less blessed by the luxury of time for the leisurely pursuit of such humane goals—comes from numerous quarters. There is, first of all, the broad professional participation by academicians and physicians in the work of the Society for Health and Human Values, which sponsored the formation of the present work.

There is the report of emerging multidisciplinary medical education in Great Britain given by John Ellis in "Human Values in Medical Education." There is the Millon volume *Medical Behavioral Science,* which includes over fifty articles concerning the teaching of behavioral sciences and humane issues relevant within medical education. There is the Milbank study, "Interdisciplinary Teaching Programs in Social Science and Medicine," with particular attention to developments in Latin America.[2] There is the emergence of a series of in-depth workshops for medical educators provided by the Center for the Study of the Person and organized under the project heading "Human Dimensions in Medical Education," directed by Orienne Strode. Workshops sponsored by this program have been attended by more than 850 medical administrators, faculty, and students over the last five years. Developed under the leadership and encouragement of the dean of the Johns Hopkins University Medical School and others, these sessions have had an intense impact on the understanding of personal relationships in medical care, as well as on the personal life of the participants—so much so as to win the acclaim of Hilliard Jason, director of the Division of Faculty Development in the Association of American Medical Colleges, who said, "I am fully convinced that the Human Dimensions in Medical Education Program is making a most important, and for now unique, contribution to the improvement of the climate and quality of the medical education enterprise. There is a level of readiness for what HDME is doing that exceeds anything that has gone before, much of that being a consequence of the growth of the seeds planted by [the] program in its first several years."[3]

Further evidence of the exciting intellectual exchange that is developing comes in a series of recent publications which have been well received and influential. There is the *Journal of Values and Ethics in Health Care,* published by the College of Physicians and Surgeons at Columbia University. And there is *Social Science and Medicine,* a journal that includes excellent reviews of literature in addition to some very perceptive articles. One of the newest and most thoughtful publications is the *Journal of Medicine and*

Philosophy, which includes philosophical and social scientific essays on concepts such as health and disease. There is also the series of books on philosophy and medicine edited by H. Tristram Engelhardt and Stuart F. Spicker, published by Reidel, including a valuable volume, *Mental Health: Philosophical Perspectives,* which provides psychological and historical, as well as philosophical, treatments of health, mental health, and illness. Also, from the psychological sciences as well as in sociology, there are important essays in the major professional journals related to the interaction between social sciences and medicine.[4]

We should cite four noteworthy professional developments as well. First, there is an emerging professional association for people involved in teaching and research positions bridging the behavioral sciences and medical education: the Association for the Behavioral Sciences and Medical Education. Although not all of the behavioral scientists in this group would identify themselves as humanists, nevertheless a great many humanistic sensibilities define the vision of education that orients the work of members of this association. A great many of them, for instance, are identified with the primary-care movement.[5]

A second development, unfortunately abortive, occurred in the redesigning of the new Medical College Admission Tests. As announced in the 1975–1976 Annual Report of the Association of American Medical Colleges, these new tests were being designed not only to examine preparation in the four major areas of science knowledge, science problems, reading skills, and quantitative analysis, but to identify so-called noncognitive qualities of medical school applicants that would be important to their overall sensitivity as physicians. The Committee on Admissions Assessment was seeking techniques to assess the following qualities: compassion, coping capabilities, decision-making, interprofessional relations, realistic self-appraisal, sensitivity in personal relations, and staying power.[6] Although these measures could not be developed in time for the new MCAT, work in this area continues and may well be included at a later time.

Third, there is the tangible evidence that hospital practices and community health care have themselves been influenced by findings in the social sciences. Coordination of community services, access to knowledge, broadened consultation with family networks, and enhanced accessibility of neighborhood care units might all be cited. One particular instance of such developments occurred in the fall of 1976, when theoretical and research findings from the behavioral sciences regarding the consequences of parental separation from children influenced the Boston Hospital for Women to develop a new policy of letting children of any age visit their mothers following the birth of new children. The rationale is twofold. First, it is thought that the traumatic effects of suddenly acquiring a sibling will be reduced if the child is able to follow closely the course of the mother's pregnancy. Second, it is thought that maintaining contact with the mother while she is hospitalized will address problems of separation and anxiety for the child who otherwise would have to remain at home with surrogate care during this period.[7]

Fourth, a multimillion-dollar financial commitment has recently been announced by the Commonwealth Fund focusing on the redesign of medical education. This foundation is funding programs in a number of colleges to combine what has been liberal arts education and technical medical education into a four-year program beginning in the third college year and combining biomedical sciences with behavioral and social science studies, followed by a final two years of clinical medicine. The clear intent in such a new design would be an early and ongoing integration of humane and social understanding connected with the more technical and scientific analysis of human disorders. According to one report:

The aim of the program is to "humanize" medical education by integrating it more fully into the intellectual life of the university as a whole. A new curriculum will seek to illuminate the biological and ecological consequences of human intervention in the environment and will explore the behavioral, social and ethical aspects of medicine and health care delivery. The program does not lessen the scientific content of medical and biomedical education, but by channeling students into a "core" curriculum of science and liberal arts courses spread over four years, starting in the middle undergraduate years, it provides continuity in the transition from premedical to professional education.[8]

Carleton B. Chapman, the president of the Fund, has commented that in spite of the apparent desire for revisions in medical education, many faculty members in both arts and sciences and medicine believe that change is difficult or impossible. The Fund is trying to challenge universities to make it possible by financially supporting those commitments of time, faculty, and program which would have to go into a redesign that could seriously integrate humanities and social sciences into the total educational preparation for medicine.

It is most likely too early to assess the impact of a swelling interest in humanistic social sciences and medical education. Many of the developments cited here have occurred only in the past year or two. In our judgment, both the theoretical and the practical surfaces have just been scratched. Although there is good will for significant cooperation, the depth and the substance of the interaction have yet to be firmly established. It is fundamentally in an effort to identify some of the significant issues and to trace out some of their policy implications that the essays in this volume have been constructed.

But before homing in on more careful arguments about the importance of this exchange and about the specific foci it may adopt, it might be wise to identify two possible pitfalls. First, in our effort to identify the importance for both the medical profession and the social science community to work in humanized, personalized ways, we must guard against tendencies toward arrogance or self-righteousness. Clearly, no one professional group has any more claim to being the fully humanizing caretakers than other professional groups might have. Indeed, the very notion of professionalism can be distorted if, in its claims to specialized knowledge, social sanction, skilled methods, and privileged information, it begins to construe its prerogatives not ethically but somehow as legitimations of higher status, power, or virtue. Such a perversion would be all the more regrettable if any attempt to understand and advocate a "humanizing" position became a criterion for negative judgments against individuals or institutional practices with punitive disregard for other institutional or educational concerns:

There is a deplorable self-righteousness underlying all attempts at making anyone "more human." Whatever else the humanities may be about, they are not about proselytizing for any single point of view. The goal and the hope are that, by exploring professionally vital issues from a humanistic perspective, and applying the methods and concepts of the humanities to such issues, medical students may become not "more human" (what could that conceivably mean?) but perhaps more circumspect, more reflective about themselves in relation to patients and about the relation of their profession to the larger community.[9]

A second danger could be that, in our enthusiasm for expanding the notion of medical education and medical care by attention to these broader personal and social issues, we might be seduced into grandiose expectations about the omnicompetence of the physician—or be tricked into some sentimental but dilettantish dabbling in a variety of fields beyond the basic sciences related to physical health care. Indeed, in an editorial, F. J. Ingelfinger offers simultaneously the bemused observation that doctors are coming to be considered as the complete factotum of health, the slogan "Care not Cure" being the tiresome motto, and an impassioned plea for a renewed clarity of the physician's dedication to cure.[10] Medical pedagogy, in this argument, should bring its energies to bear on scientifically accurate diagnosis and treatment, with attention to specific disease patterns and modes of specialization in medical science. To pretend to know something about broader social factors influencing health or the role of the physician might be luxuries, and might arouse false expectations. Yet even in this otherwise resistant editorial, Ingelfinger leaves the door somewhat ajar by suggesting that appropriate medical education and knowledge would "include an awareness of the equally important but nevertheless paramedical determinants of health." The real issue here seems to boil down to a question of how extensive, coherent, and relevant that awareness should be, and how carefully it might be integrated into the technical scientific knowledge related to diagnosis and treatment. One real point of tension between this editorial and the essays represented in the present volume is the question of whether or not the sources of illness and the modalities of treatment can be so distinctly defined as within the sphere of the biomedical sciences. The essays by Barbara Sicherman, John Stoeckle, and Paul Pruyser make a strong case for the necessity of more flexible and multidisciplinary attempts to understand and diagnose the difficulties encountered by patients.

The Importance of the Enterprise

Having surveyed several aspects of the scope and intent of the exchange between humanistic social science and medicine, as well as several pitfalls, we would do well to inquire more systematically into some of the arguments for its importance. This may provide an intellectual frame for moving into a discussion of the selection of particular issues for examination. In developing this argument, we hope to demonstrate, among other things, a genuine desire for a true *exchange*. That is, we wish to eschew any reductionistic stance in which, for instance, the aim might be construed simply as social science informing or reforming medical education or, conversely, medicine challenging, testing, and criticizing the obscurities or provincialism of social science.

At its best, an exchange between humanistic social science and medicine assumes give-and-take from both sides. Its central assumption is that both medicine and the social sciences are susceptible to criticism and liable for reform. Just as medicine is provided with the opportunity to see itself more reflectively (as a profession, a body of knowledge, or a set of interpersonal behaviors), the social sciences are able to appreciate a wider range of approaches, assumptions, and applications. Their operational categories are refined and altered as they are called upon to acknowledge the exquisite complexities of clinical judgment, for example, just as clinical judgment is made more sensitive and responsible by virtue of knowledge gained from, say, social ethics, economics, or personality psychology. In other words, the gaze that social science directs at medicine is also reflected inward, and value judgments passed on the medical profession spring from an increased awareness of the moral dimensions and implications of social scientific thought.

This understanding of the nature of the exchange—particularly its constant focus on *values*—distinguishes it from another possible and significant type of interaction between social science and medicine, the investigation of social and behavioral factors in the etiology of disease and the efficacy of treatment programs. In this instance, social science and medicine are predominantly diagnostic partners and, although their collaboration indeed includes mutual influence as to methodology and epistemology, the basic values of the diagnostic and therapeutic tasks are not primarily at issue. To identify and assess these values, while continually examining the norms and principles of that assessment, is the essential *raison d'être* of the essays in this book.

This exchange is also to be distinguished from the fertile but specific discourse between *ethics* and medical practice. The attention that has been given increasingly to methods of decision-making about particular modes of treatment or about the utilization of scarce technological resources (such as hemodialysis machines) should certainly be welcomed. And the systematic understanding of such ethical reasoning has been enhanced by work at places like the Hastings Institute in Hastings-on-Hudson, New York. But that work does not attempt to probe the array of personal, public, and philosophical issues that can and, we believe, should be addressed in the broader interaction of social science and medicine, particularly as it relates to the philosophy, setting, and curriculum of medical education beyond medical ethics.

There are many areas where this exchange seems quite natural, as it brings to the surface issues common to both the social sciences and medicine, concerning which tensions and ambiguities in both fields run parallel and for which the resolution of a conflict in one discipline may be instructive to the other. One such area, in which it would be hard to decide who is the critic and who is being criticized, is the relative status of quantitative data and measurement as compared with intuitive, introspective, or interpretive methods. A closely related issue is the proper role of mechanical technologies in data collection, in social, political, or medical intervention, and in the conferring of status and prestige. Together, these issues raise the question of the difference between "science" and what might be called "scientism," or an ideology of exactness, technical mastery, and professional omniscience. These essays reveal some of the struggles within both social science and medicine with this question.

Another common issue is that of *classification*. In the practice of medicine, it is easy to see the consequences that flow from a person's being assigned the status of "sick" or "well." The first status entitles one (given certain socioeconomic qualifications) to benefit from the entire range of diagnostic and therapeutic skill and resources. The second status either precludes the application of these resources or signals their termination. Beyond this broad differentiation, however, are occasions for far subtler distinctions and discriminations in medicine, either as part of the diagnostic process or in the allocation of resources for research and treatment.[11] Social science is in a position to identify patterns and methods underlying many of these classificatory schemes and to record their social and moral consequences. As it does so, it is inescapably led to reflect on the principles of classification within social science itself.

The critique of medicine, designed to reveal the ways in which medicine impinges on society as a whole, thus occasions a similar confrontation with the effects of many of the fundamental distinctions and categories of social research and policy. These might include classifying processes or conditions as normal or deviant; propositions as facts or values; nations as developed or underdeveloped; even, for that matter, social sciences as humanistic or experimental-behavioral. An important dimension of the dialogue is the opportunity for demonstrating that in neither medicine nor the social sciences are distinctions such as these merely intellectual or heuristic. Rather, human beings' lives and reputations, well-being and destiny, are affected by them.

In reality, however, classification may be only one in a complex of issues concerning the use of language and patterns of communication that is important to both medicine and the social sciences. In an era that celebrates the silent efficacy of drugs and surgical techniques in its healing processes, and the mute reliability of mathematical prediction in its social scientific research, the most fateful and fundamental question may well be the value that is attached to *the word* as a legitimate and respected unit either of comprehension or of intervention. One of the most important products of a sustained interaction between social science and medicine might be the development of means of expression at once adequate to reflect ambiguous, fleeting, even well-nigh ineffable human predicaments, and yet precise enough to permit empathy, guide action, and inform a wider community of what is learned through experience.[12]

Another dimension to this set of problems is the flow of information and the control of knowledge. Once again, the social and behavioral sciences have evolved elaborate theoretical constructs to analyze or recommend medical practices relating to the conveyance—or withholding—of knowledge.[13] These critical perspectives are not always balanced, however, with similarly penetrating assessments of disciplinary jargon, intellectual elitism, relations between researchers and subjects, or interdisciplinary rivalries and their relation to the communication and impact of knowledge gained in these sciences. The exchange between social science and medicine responds to this in two ways. First, the tradition of *service*, which is as deeply embedded in medicine as is the goal of research, presents itself as a challenge and an inspiration to the social scientist, and as a model for an intellectual style steeped in social engagement. Second, the exchange becomes the forum in which to bring to light the fruits of speculation and observation in the social sciences, where they can gain an immediate hearing from those seeking to rest medical practice on an informed, humane value foundation.

This foundation will not be laid all at once. Yet the work exemplified in this volume can provoke and sustain movement in this direction along at least three lines. First, it can further the discovery and clarification of just what is meant by "human values." Participants may avail themselves of theoretical discussions of such organizing conceptions within social science as "optimal human functioning," "wholeness," or "self-determination"; and they may attempt to incorporate value-laden clinical experience in medicine centered on—among other things—the sense of satisfaction, movement free of restriction or pain, and the powers of the human being to adapt to infirmity and loss.

The probing and articulation of values that is supported by this theoretical and clinical collaboration leads to the second area of influence of the exchange between humanistic social science and medicine: the possibility of providing a meaningful value orientation for further research. A perusal of the literature in medical sociology and anthropology, social and institutional psychology, the phenomena of stress and coping, ethics and decision-making, and related fields confirms Ernest Becker's judgment that we are today literally "choking on truth," that "knowledge is in a state of useless over-production, strewn all over the place, spoken in a thousand competitive voices." [14] The focus that this value orientation can provide may alert us to what to look for, what questions to ask, how to proceed, and how to interpret our findings. For example, as suggested by Frank Sloan's work in this collection (chapter 8), research into health services may be patient-oriented, service-oriented, or cost/benefit-oriented. Which view shall predominate, and how may they be balanced? In another example, the recent work of Shelley Taylor and Smadar Levin cited by William Rogers, as well as the work in chapter 2 of this present volume, illustrates how a mass of findings in social science research may be organized and clarified, with significant implications for policy as well as for methodology, when considerations of value and respect for the human person inform scholarship. [15]

Finally, this exchange envisions the process of medical education as a critical opportunity to give potency and clarity to humanistic dimensions in both social sciences and medicine. Fundamental to this hope is the conviction—expressed throughout these essays—that medical education is itself a dynamic, social enterprise, affected by, and affecting, developmental, moral, and intellectual configurations within individual students and teachers, and situated in consequential social, historical, and economic contexts. Increased sensitization to these circumstances is the first step in the evaluation of education. Beyond this is the task of observing how the various factors interact, and serious consideration of the potential for various reforms, not only within educational institutions themselves but also in public attitudes, cultural trends, and political arrangements.

To state such an agenda is to be immediately humbled. In addition to the fantastic complexity of the conceptual and empirical issues that social scientists, physicians, and educators are asked to face, there are important questions of the *will and desire for change* and the nurture of social responsibility. Yet the commitment to human values in social science and medicine may only bring out questions of confidence and vulnerability that are already at the heart of medical practice. The interaction between these disciplines calls attention to many forms of vulnerability, ranging from the relativity and ambiguity of intellectual constructs to medicine's often tenuous grasp of skills and powers for care and cure. Underlying this analysis, however, is the ideal of a true confidence and verve, of an ability to decide and to act, free of enervating preoccupation with the likelihood of failure, but with a realistic appreciation of finitude and limitation.

Renée Fox and Judith Swazey invoke this balance of confidence and vulnerability in the introduction to their study of organ transplantation and dialysis. Their comments may sum up the essential importance of continuing exchange between social science and medicine:

The probability of failure in transplantation and dialysis is high. These therapeutic innovations are in a stage of development characterized by fundamental scientific and medical uncertainties, and they are applied only to patients who are terminally ill with diseases not amenable to more conventional forms of treatment. In this context, the death of the patient is the archetype and pinnacle of failure for all concerned. Confronting this situation with courage is an ultimate value shared by physicians and patients. As they themselves recognize, the supreme form of courage that transplantation and dialysis asks of them is "the courage to fail."

We have chosen our title [*The Courage to Fail*] with full consciousness that it evokes religious associations. (Its relationship to the title of Paul Tillich's renowned theological work, *The Courage To Be,* is apparent.) For we believe that the largest and perhaps most enduring significance of organ transplantation and dialysis lies in the ethical and existential questions they raise. Problems of uncertainty, meaning, life and death, scarcity, justice, equity, solidarity, and intervention in the human condition are all evoked by these therapeutic innovations. . . . [The] growth of interest in these problems that is now observable in our society, and especially the degree to which they are manifesting themselves in medicine, suggests that reformulations of quite fundamental aspects of our societal value system may be under way. A rapprochement seems to be occurring between scientific and religiomoral orientations toward health and illness, life and death. In this regard, *The Courage to Fail* is a case study not only of therapeutic innovation in modern society, but of more general processes of social and cultural change.[16]

Focus and Organization of Topics Within the Dialogue Group

The character of the interaction we are introducing here has both intellectual and tangible, practicable components. The intellectual give-and-take, the mutual informing and reforming, that we have been speaking of occurs in real working groups. One such group was the "dialogue group" out of which the chapters of this particular volume emerged. And insofar as our experience may prove instructive for others interested in these issues, as well as helpful in introducing the essays, it might be useful to review some of the process of that group.

The dialogue group was initiated through the efforts of the Institute on Human Values in Medicine, funded in part through a grant from the National Endowment for the Humanities. This funding enabled us to bring together creative social scientists and physicians from across the country, but similar groups could be organized within local academic and medical communities for personal and professional exchange and for the formation of educational and health service programs.

We found it helpful to select meeting sites and extended meeting times that would take all of us out of the turmoil of our daily responsibilities, somewhat on the pattern of a retreat, so that we could give full attention to the constructive exchange with one another (possible only through careful advance planning!). As a model within education, such serious time together seems necessary for university and medical school people to engage the important issues from their disparate fields in cooperative discourse and planning.

The optimal size for such a group seems to be from six to twelve participants. Fewer than that does not do justice to the range of disciplines and professional problems that should be engaged (although in actual course planning or community-clinic supervision the number typically is smaller). More than twelve leads to problems in group process and efficiency. For all to be genuinely engaged, each must have ample opportunity to be heard and understood, as well as to have group support (including challenge) in puzzling through the meaning of these questions for one's own work.

Despite the real cost of professional time and the urgency of goal orientations in many of our lives (and in the meetings), we found it profoundly important to spend the early part of our time together in reflective sharing concerning our personal lives. In a mode that some characterize as "telling our story," we recounted and assessed aspects of our pilgrimage through important experiences, ideas, professional settings, relationships, and critical incidents that had brought us to our present positions. Naturally, many of these related to our particular interest in themes that we wished to explore further. And, appropriately, a number of the reflections brought back specific memories of our own encounters with illness, tragedy, medical care, and healing. The importance of linking this level of personal discussion with exploration of professional and intellectual issues is attested in all the work that emerged, but most explicitly in the first three chapters that follow (Rogers, Lifton, and Oliver-Smith). Risking this kind of sharing proved to be simultaneously a "humanizing" dimension of our group experience together, and an unexpected source of creative understanding and new ideas.

In a second round of more focused contributions we each identified three or four specific issues that we hoped to address in the group, or that we were working on independently but for which we sought resources or methodological suggestions. This conversation led to a number of lines of crossfertilization, and it helped to shape the character of some specific projects that we felt would be valuable not only to others in the group but to a wide audience concerned wtih humanistic social science and medical education.

Among the issues that emerged were several we did not pursue in detail, but which we list here for their potential utility to other investigators or dialogue groups:

• Medical and social problems emerging in the context of shifting family-life patterns (the changing constellation of the nuclear family, dual-career parenting, single working parents, multiple child care facilities, increased percentages of women in the national work force, experiments in extended family constellations).

• The effects on health and self-image of the cultural loss of dominant hero myths and religiously or civically grounded images for the construing of meaning and experience.

• The analysis of social structure within the professions generally and among health care professionals in particular.

• Problems and implications of recruitment, training, and advancement of minorities in health care professions.

• The sources of human values in medicine and in social sciences (traditional values, dominant cultural values, social-class values, media and popular culture values, academic values, or professional and collegial values as organized and advocated through consortia, associations, or academic and medical faculty promotion standards).

• Problems of the epistemological status of medical and social science knowledge (empirical scientific, received tradition, symbolic authority, "protégé-sponsor," personal authority, intuitive, rational, structural, and so on).

• Problems of diverse claims of accountability and responsibility in medicine and social science (to the patient [person], the family, the community, one's peers, the ethics of the profession, employer standards, the law, third-party insurance, government regulations).

• Problems of health standards and divergent value systems within developing nations.

• Psychohistories of physicians and medical researchers.

• Variables related to the consistency or change in value orientations as they are presented in either medical practice or social science theory.

Before introducing the specific topics we did deal with, a word should be said about our common starting point. One issue that we identified very early as cutting across understanding of medical values, as well as across social science investigation, was the character of implicit and explicit ideas of *optimal human functioning*. Normative ideas about optimal forms of personal development appear in social sciences under topics like maturation, the goals of therapy, the quality of life, and higher stages in developmental paradigms. The notion of optimal human functioning also informs medicine at the point of identifying those norms which can realistically be hoped for in a positive theory of health that moves beyond the mere absence of pathogens. Potentially, each discipline could contribute to the other in its quest to understand its underlying presuppositions about what goals are being sought in its various patterns of treatment and investigation. In addition, such a dialogue might move our vision forward to goals more worthy of our seeking.

This initial identification of an area of exchange does not appear consistently through the essays presented here, although it remains a silent partner in nearly all of them. Insofar as each is concerned with "the humanizing dimension" of social science and medical practice, it implies the norm for what is humane or, put differently, for what generates optimal qualities of personhood. The investigation of the doctor-patient relationship, the nature of the diagnostic functions, the pilgrimage of the medical student and of the physician in training, the economic analysis of the rights of equal access and the basic ethical grounding in a notion of respect for persons, all imply some normative assessment of what is most fundamentally and, one might say, optimally human.

The topics to which we addressed these normative concerns can be seen reflected in the present chapter headings. What needs emphasis here is the procedure by which these topics came to be developed. Having identified a range of issues that we agreed were significant, we spent time together developing some of the complexity of the problem. Then each of us took responsibility for preparing material for a later group session. At that session the group engaged the presenter in debate and elaboration. Only after this were the final papers drawn up. Consequently, the essays as they appear here carry the *joint* responsibility of author and group in a fashion seldom found in books edited from invited autonomous pieces.

Each of the following chapters is introduced by some bridging comments of the editors, reflecting the themes woven through the essays. There is no essential sequence of chapter arrangement; however, there are some identifiable clusters. The essays of Rogers, Lifton, and Oliver-Smith all give some indication of the tone of the dialogue as it addresses specific concepts and methods in social science coupled with important dimensions of the ethos of medical education—agency, control, accountability, numbing, self-identity, limitation, responsibility. They also demonstrate the link between personal experience and professional sensibilities, and they move directly to implications of a clinical and educational order.

The middle essays by Sicherman, Wallwork, McElhinney, and

Sloan address broader historical, philosophical, and public policy questions. They call our attention to the ramifications of a view of medicine as art and science concerned with persons. They define directly the meaning of "humanization" and suggest what this implies both for medical research (especially in genetics) and for health care. They detail the ethical themes of information control and equity in access to medical services.

The final essays by Sicherman, Pruyser, Stoeckle, and Banks apply the value discussions to special policy subareas in medicine and medical education. They examine in particular the formation and functions of diagnosis, the character of the doctor-patient relationship, the importance of primary care, and the strategies of medical curricula, training sites, and educational policy responsive to needs for humane care. The concluding chapter summarizes a series of policy recommendations growing from the entire process.

Throughout, our attempt is to illustrate ways in which this interaction between social science and medicine can nourish humane values, as well as be nourished by them.

NOTES

1. "The Hospital Problem," *Journal of the American Medical Association*, 47, no. 5 (August 4, 1906):320.

2. Ellis Oration of the Society for Health and Human Values, Philadelphia, 1976; Theodore Millon, ed., *Medical Behavioral Science* (Philadelphia: W. B. Saunders, 1975); *Milbank Memorial Fund Quarterly*, 44, no. 2, pt. 2 (1966):187–237.

3. For further comment and details of programming in the Human Dimensions in Medical Education project, contact Orienne Strode, Project Director, Human Dimensions in Medical Education, 1125 Torrey Pines Road, La Jolla, Calif. 92037.

4. See, for instance, Murray Wexler, "The Behavioral Sciences in Medical Education," *American Psychologist*, 31, no. 4 (April 1976):275–83.

5. Further information about the Association for the Behavioral Sciences and Medical Education may be obtained from Dr. Donald Kennedy, Assistant Dean for Behavioral Sciences, College of Human Medicine, University of Wyoming.

6. *Annual Report:1975–1976,* Association of American Medical Colleges, One Dupont Circle, N.W., Washington, D.C. 20036, p. 15.

7. As reported in the *Boston Globe,* October 19, 1976, p. 3.

8. For a full report of this foundation program, see the Commonwealth Fund's *Annual Report* for 1976. For synopses, see the *New York Times,* November 23, 1975, p. 28, or publications from participating universities such as the University of Rochester or the University of Chicago.

9. Richard C. Reynolds and Ronald A. Carson, "Editorial: The Place of Humanities in Medical Education," *Journal of Medical Education,* 51, no. 2 (February 1976):142–43.

10. "The Physician's Contribution to the Health System," *New England Journal of Medicine,* 295, no. 10 (September 2, 1976):565–66.

11. Obviously medical treatment is frequently terminated for those at the "sick" end of the spectrum as well, and issues surrounding the decision to suspend treatment of hopelessly ill patients have occasioned a very recent example of medical classification: a "patient-care classification system" for all critically ill patients ("Optimum Care for Hopelessly Ill Patients: A Report of the Critical Care Committee of the Massachusetts General Hospital," *New England Journal of Medicine,* 295, no. 7 [August 12, 1976]:362–64). In this system, a patient who is critically ill is assigned to one of four classes: *Class A,* "maximal therapeutic effort without reservation"; *Class B,* "maximal therapeutic effort without reservation, but with daily evaluation because probability of survival is questionable"; *Class C,* "selective limitation of therapeutic measures . . . [and] particular attention . . . given to resuscitation measures of all kinds"; or *Class D,* "all therapy can be discontinued. Any measures which are indicated to insure maximum comfort of the patient may be continued or instituted" (p. 362).

It is of particular interest, in the light of many of the values to be discussed later in this volume, that this system, together with the formation of an "Optimum Care Committee" to advise in difficult or questionable cases, was designed above all to encourage the informed participation and unity of purpose in these decisions of patients, families, nurses, supporting staff, and physicians, and to "maximize support for the responsible physician who makes the medical decision to intensify, maintain, or limit effort at reversing illness" (p. 364).

12. An approach that may be of considerable promise for this endeavor is Eric J. Cassell's distinction between "analytic thought" and "valuational thought" in what he calls "the medical paradigm." Cassell argues that analytic thought, most suitable for technical and scientific communication, has largely overshadowed—and is on the verge of entirely displacing—valuational thought, which is addressed to personal and moral concerns, in the physician's mind set. He calls for a greater recognition of the complementarity of these modes of thinking, and for an enriched medical paradigm that can enhance the human dimensions of medical training, practice, and research. ("Preliminary Explorations of Thinking in Medicine," *Ethics in Science and Medicine,* 2, no. 1 [May

1975]: 1–13). We should also call attention to the work done by the Institute for Human Values in Medicine dialogue group on literature and medicine, which addresses this question intensively and imaginatively.

13. See, for example, Anselm Strauss and Barney Glaser, *Awareness of Dying* (Chicago: Aldine, 1965), for a detailed description of the strategies for avoiding communication of "terminality" to a patient; also Howard Leventhal, "The Consequences of Depersonalization During Illness and Treatment: An Information-Processing Model," in *Humanizing Health Care,* ed. Jan Howard and Anselm Strauss (New York: John Wiley, 1975).

14. *The Denial of Death* (New York: Free Press, 1973), p. x.

15. Taylor and Levin, "The Psychological Impact of Breast Cancer: Theory and Practice," in *Psychological Aspects of Breast Cancer,* ed. A. Enelow (London: Oxford University Press, 1977). A wide-ranging discussion of the potential for value-oriented social science research in medicine is provided by Sol Levine in *Humanizing Health Care,* ed. Jan Howard and Anselm Strauss (New York: John Wiley, 1975), chap. 17, "A Sociologist's Perspective."

16. *The Courage to Fail: A Social View of Organ Transplants and Dialysis* (Chicago: University of Chicago Press, 1974), pp. xv–xvi.

CHAPTER 2

Helplessness and Agency in the Healing Process

William R. Rogers

Each of the chapters in this book presses for a deeper understanding of specific issues that are of common concern to social science and medicine. Helplessness and agency (individual experiences of self-control and potency) are two such issues. It is suggested in this chapter that a more comprehensive recognition of the dynamic tension and interaction of these experiences will increase our understanding of both patients and doctors, and may bear explicitly on the character of medical education.

This chapter begins with a very personal account, showing something of the interaction between experience and theory. Although such connections are always seen more clearly in retrospect, they remind us that what we think is shaped by what we see and feel, as well as by what we read in research reviews. And, similarly, the findings of research and the formation of policy (especially regarding health services and medical education) have an obvious bearing on human life and motivation. Consequently, it seems fitting to keep a balance among rigorous research, constructive theory, human sensitivities, and our grounding amid at least glimpses of what is ultimately worthwhile. That, after all, is what lies at the heart of work that espouses human values. The basis and content of those values should become clear as we move along.

This essay is an attempt to identify a special constellation of factors in the system of patient care and physicians' self-image that can be elaborated in psychodynamic and interactional analyses, and can serve as an instructive point for reflection on medical training and practice. Such reflection will give rise to both descriptive assessment of values implicit in health services delivery systems (including specific patient care) and normative judgment concerning some optimal values that could (and, I will argue, should) serve as guidelines in medical practice.

Among the various areas of social science research and theory that can contribute to the concerns of medicine are the concepts of *helplessness* and *agency*. Helplessness is the fear of impotence in effecting change or control. It is experienced by both patient and physician—in some cases generating healthy acknowledgment of limits and, in others, elaborate defensive schemes. Agency carries the sense of empowerment, potency, internal force, or confidence in initiating change or control. Although helplessness and agency appear mutually exclusive, even polar, I will argue that in some important aspects they actually complement or augment each other. Primarily I will argue that they shed light on important dynamics in the patient-doctor interaction and that an understanding of them generates policy implications for medical education.

A Personal Account

Allow me to start very personally with an account of myself as patient. In 1954–55 I was hospitalized with tuberculosis for ten months in a major university medical center. I had been married only two months and had just begun graduate studies. Everything seemed new and hopeful—I was in a new city, at a new university, in my first apartment, had a substantial graduate fellowship, and was (and am) with a delightful and intelligent woman.

I had spent the summer working outdoors and in the proshop of a country club. I felt in great health, was well tanned, had new athletic competence, and was raring to go. Early in the fall I experienced considerable tiredness, though, and within two weeks I felt so drained that I had to go to the hospital one evening (the emergency room, since the student health service was closed). The immediate diagnosis was mononucleosis, but it seemed severe enough that I was admitted to the hospital—weak, tired, and apprehensive. Within a day or two, further tests confirmed that I had TB, and I was isolated in a room for contagious patients on the chest service where I was to remain for the better part of a year.

As a patient, especially with TB, adjusting to the hospital routine is almost too easy. It is comforting to be totally cared for.

Nurses can be signaled by the press of a button, baths and meals are brought regularly, pain and discomfort are ameliorated as much as possible. Doctors appear seriatim, taking the same professional-sounding medical histories, and then in groups with the chief of service and a full entourage on rounds. There is mindless piped music and the possibility of incessant television.

From week to week there was the gnawing anxiety as to whether there would be surgery, finally resolved in the negative, as chemotherapy for TB had just started coming into its own. But even more discomforting was the dawning awareness of my "existential numbness." Everything was decided for me: wake-up time, medication, visiting hours, ward containment, bed clothing, even the issue of where I could go to the bathroom (in a urinal or bedpan for four months). More disconcertingly, the life-and-death questions of diagnosis and treatment were out of my hands completely, as were the economically (and psychologically) debilitating issues of financial charges. My career, my marriage, my strong self-image, my sports, my reading, my mobility—all seemed to stagnate as I lay helplessly in bed, routinized by decisions over which I had no control. My only free act seemed to be choosing among two or three items on the daily menu that I was given ritualistically each morning by the grace of the dietitian, under the direction of the physician.

I suppose the sense of deprivation within such a helpless posture was exaggerated in my case by the additional prohibition against *seeing* real people. Infectious diseases necessitate masks, gowns, and physical distance. Everyone who entered the room was in a real sense hidden. The normal facial expressions and gestures we rely on for communication were muted and disguised. Verbal communication was most often brief and problem-specific. And there were those long periods when no one would enter. All I would see was the detail of the closed door, its stainless-steel hardware, and the vacant shafts of light from above and below. This separation, added to the feeling of emotional distance in the professional procedures, left me feeling isolated, useless, and sterile in a lonely world.

There was not even a window onto the shimmering world outside. All I could see beyond my room was the black apparatus of the smokestack from the boiler room that came up past my seventh-floor "light" (a bit puzzling as I think about it, considering the vulnerability of chest patients).

The most humane aspects of my stay were the humorous conversations with one attendant who would occasionally be assigned for my bath, and the evening visits with my wife who brought both her own love and support, and precious reports of the events of work, culture, and friends. Furthermore, it is no small matter that I owe my life, in one sense, to the medical judgment involved in the diagnosis and treatment in my case.

Also on the positive side, I increasingly felt a sense of my own agency even in the midst of considerable real helplessness. In fact, I found it possible to be helpful to people who obviously were feeling uncomfortable in not knowing how to be helpful to me. Visitors, new friends and neighbors, would come to call but would hardly know what to say, how to comfort, how to deal with the unfamiliar and vaguely threatening precautions of the infectious ward. And somehow this aroused in me the stirrings of empathy, understanding, curiosity, verbal initiative, and wit that later would become more developed as part of my agency as a therapist. Ironically, the one who was helpless was becoming the helper.[1]

What I discovered only later is that I am also indebted to that experience for the roots of some of my present research interests. It was in 1968 that, by an ostensibly independent route, I came to what I thought was a breakthrough in understanding the dynamics of psychopathology and the psychotherapeutic relationship. In reflecting on a series of cases, several of which involved transition into intensive psychotic periods, I became increasingly convinced that one of the most fearsome internal processes of consciousness is the apprehension of helplessness—the overwhelming awareness of psychic onslaughts over which the person feels no control. The collapse, not only of "will" or a sense of self-determination, but also of every shred of rudimentary confidence that one can even understand where thoughts or impulses are coming from, or what they mean—that is a terrifying brink, and consequently one of the most critical for the understanding and effective work of the psychotherapist.

To avoid the terror of that brink of loss of internal control, people take up many strategies. They baffle themselves with intellectual obfuscations and rationalized ambivalences. They melt into passive docility. They fly into a melee of frantic but purposeless activity. They absolve their anxiety in the potency of transcendental dependency on "transference" gods. They collapse into fragmented and disoriented ideation. They abandon hope of internal integrity and self-direction. They capitulate to the demagogues of political tyranny, whether in the marketplace, the state house, or the hospital.

Only after writing about the psychodynamics and social psychology of such mechanisms[2] did I begin to wonder how such an investigation was located in my own interests. Having lectured on scholars like Dilthey and Polanyi, I had agreed with the claim that nearly all intellectual interests can be traced to threads of concern emerging from, and important to, the fabric of the investigator's own life experience. Gradually I recognized that in this case my own history was indeed instructive. And only then was I able to name the tyranny of the helplessness to which I had so docilely capitulated. In writing, I thought the strong and compassionate social scientist–philosopher was doing the searching. In reality, it was as much the weak and bewildered patient.

On the other side of helplessness, I had meanwhile become interested in *agency* and self-actualization as important dimensions of optimal human development, in a way parallel to my experience of agency in the hospital. The movement toward increasingly autonomous self-direction as characterized conceptually by Erich Fromm, the "agentic" aspects of self-initiated action characterized by David Bakan, the autonomous person as characterized by David Riesman, and the independent self-concept of the fully functioning person characterized by Carl Rogers all congealed in a compelling image of maturity.[3] Obviously, this image had to be qualified with the important recognition of our social and communal functioning—our interpersonal interdependence—and our more profound participation in ontological processes. To ignore this would be to fall into the conceit of what Paul Tillich calls "self-sufficient finitude." [4] Yet, given that context, the possibilities of responsible decision and self-initiated action in the "agentic" mode certainly mark a cornerstone of the social scientific view of normative (valued) human development.

As sketchy as this account is, I trust it will reveal something of both the personal and intellectual roots of my interest in helplessness and agency as important categories in understanding human experience. It is further my view that these categories identify broader human issues in the realm of medical practice and in the self-understanding of the physician as healer.

Although I must guard against the arrogance of imposing categories that are solely of self-reference, I am strengthened in this analysis by the ample research and theory in personality and social psychology that likewise attest to the significance of these categories. In the following sections, I will detail some of the major findings of this research, directly in conjunction with their implications for an understanding of the patient and the physician.

The Patient

At least three distinguishable lines of investigation and theory in the social sciences bear on the question of helplessness and agency: the clinical and theoretical material within psychoanalysis and ego psychology; studies of "learned helplessness" and locus of control within learning theory; and material on the character and effects of "total institutions" in social psychological theory. Each of these can be seen as driving toward some similar conclusions with regard to the effects of institutional practices that generate feelings of helplessness and loss of control. After examining what these lines of reasoning entail, we can look more carefully at the effects of particular hospital and treatment contingencies that have a bearing on the well-being of persons as patients.

In psychoanalytic thinking, particularly as it pertains to the psychosexual development of individuals, explicit attention is given to the psychodynamic impact of patterns of helplessness and dependency in childhood. In the discussions of Freud, particularly *Civilization and Its Discontents, The Ego and the Id,* and *The Future of an Illusion,* there is an attempt to trace both individual psychopathology and cultural-institutional (especially religious) "pathology" to an etiology marked by the ubiquitousness and power of experiences of infantile dependency. Freud cites the helplessness of a child as a condition that only gradually diminishes with the emergence of a mature ego. He also cites the cultural dangers of early dependency (herd instinct and crowd behavior) in *Group Psychology and the Analysis of the Ego.* Yet even with an apparently successful migration through the tortuous routes of the psychosexual stages, there is always a certain precariousness in that, under situations of stress or crisis, one may regress to infantile forms, including the posture of helplessness and dependency. With that posture, in Freud's view, is also a deep yearning or "wish" for authority—that is, for the safety and reassurance of a figure who could guard our welfare, bring wisdom and comfort in distress, answer our deepest yearnings, misgivings, unspoken questions, and bring our ways to a more secure end.

In its furthest extension, this argument of Freud's is applied to his analysis of a neurotic need for God. "A terrifying impression of helplessness in childhood aroused the need for protection—for protection through love—which was provided by the father; and the recognition that this helplessness lasts throughout life made it necessary to cling to the existence of a father, but this time a much more powerful one." [5] Although the concern of physicians and medical educators focuses less on the need for God and divine comfort, it is possible to suggest that, in clinical settings, patients under stress and with the substrate of such historic feelings of helplessness might and often do turn to the physician as "the more powerful one" who could easily be invested with the infantile wishes for complete protection and security.

It would be irresponsible to leave the argument at this point, however, casting the taint of neuroticism on most desires for security, either from God or from the physician. In a perceptive and illuminating interpretation of Freud, Peter Homans has attempted to differentiate between the "transference God" of the anxious and displacing neurotic and the more mature affirmations of faith in which incompleteness as well as authority, judgment as well as compassion, are understood to characterize God—a conception which, in finite humility, we must always acknowledge as beyond the limitation of human perception.[6] A similar differentiation should be made between the neurotic desires for an all-wise and omnicompetent physician representative of unconscious wishes for absolute protection, versus mature patient awareness of the strength and necessity of wise clinical judgments and simultaneously of the limits of medical knowledge and practice. It would appear, however, that even such attempts at mature and balanced judgment on the part of the patient are confounded in a double way: both by the residual apprehensions of helplessness, particularly in relation to the mysteries of one's own body and the dynamics of recovery or death; and by the propensities of physicians who know full well the psychological importance of patient confidence and trust in the physician as part of the healing process, and who therefore tend to accentuate the relatively nonporous image of authority, exactness, and control in patient management.[7]

Important extensions of psychoanalytic perspective on this issue can also be traced in some of the writing of the ego psychologists. For instance, in John Bowlby's work on attachment and loss, as well as in the work of W. R. D. Fairbairn, Harry Guntrip, and Paul Bohanann, attention is given to the emotional reactions to loss and separation.[8] Such reactions involve especially feelings of bewilderment, anger, sometimes guilt, loneliness, and fear, as well as helplessness—which, depending on the severity of the situation, may also involve despair or depression. Both Fairbairn and Guntrip are also helpful in differentiating components of regressive helplessness and dependence from forms of mature dependence.

Obviously the dynamics of loss relate to a patient's period of hospitalization in at least two respects. First, patient care often involves removal from loved persons, one's family or friends. Second, medical procedures may in some instances involve removal or restructuring of either physiological or biochemical aspects of the patient's body, sometimes generating feelings of alienation or loss (most conspicuous perhaps in the celebrated cases of "phantom" limbs or organs following surgery).

Ego psychologists like Anna Freud, Heinz Hartmann, and Norma Haan have all attempted to differentiate healthy functions of the ego and adaptive mechanisms from maladaptive defense mechanisms.[9] Clearly maladaptive mechanisms of regression, rationalization, projection, dissociation, fixation, repetition compulsion, and the like all involve attempts to preserve the intactness of a vulnerable ego by mechanisms that repeat more infantile procedures for dealing with stress. Consequently, they can be seen as driven in part by the anxiety of helplessness to which there is a threat of succumbing were the mechanisms to fail. But even in the more adaptive mechanisms of the ego under stress—mechanisms that involve flexibility, empathy, logical analysis, and even what Hartmann and Haan call "regression in the service of the ego"—there is still at least the threat of a form of helplessness that functions in this case as a more characteristically constructive anxiety actually motivating agency in the sense of desire for control, at least of the contents of one's own consciousness, even when it may be impossible to manipulate the influence of outside factors.

This is to suggest that in clinical settings, particularly hospitals, a patient's adaptive capabilities are considerably strained and may very well be led to the brink of maladaption if circumstances of control, decision-making, and knowledge containment are kept as the prerogative solely of external agencies—specifically, operating procedures or therapeutic decisions extrinsic to the patient. It also suggests some constructive possibilities for mature adaptations, especially when the therapeutic milieu supports the patient's agentic possibilities.

A second line of reasoning that leads to somewhat similar con-

clusions from quite different (and often antithetical) presuppositions in methodology comes out of behaviorism and learning
theory. Learning theorists pay little attention, except in negative
critique, to unconscious psychodynamic forces. But clearly they,
like the analytic theorists, are interested in the influence of childhood learning (although modified by later contingencies). The
behaviorists have emphasized a form of agency in their attention
to issues of self-management and self-reinforcement, despite the
frequent charge that their view of human life is simply that of a
"response" agent. Also, studies of the array of learned responses
have recently included attention to helplessness. Such attention
started, typically enough, with research on animals in which a
phenomenon was isolated and characterized as *"learned helplessness."* Martin E. P. Seligman and Steven Maier first identified this
phenomenon when working with dogs who had previously been
strapped in Pavlovian harnesses and given traumatic but not physically damaging electric shock.[10] These same dogs, when unhar-
nessed and put in experimental boxes also delivering shock, but
with the possibility of escape over a barrier (a strategy quickly
learned by naive dogs put in the same experimental situation),
would remain passively taking the shock through yowling or
whimpering. The experimenters realized that the degree of initiative or agency taken by animals under such experimental conditions was directly related to prior experiences of having no control over traumatic events occurring to them. Only those animals
who had received uncontrollable shock in the past gave up the
struggle. "The experience in the harness had taught the dog that
its responses did not pay, that its actions did not matter. We
concluded that the dogs in our experiments had learned that they
were helpless."[11]

Similar experiments have been done with rats who were trained
to jump from a platform through a choice of three openings, one
of which contained food pellets. Although that learning could be
accomplished quickly and retained through periods of intermit-
tent reinforcement, when the opening containing the food pellets
was *randomly* varied, the degree of apparent frustration and

helplessness intensified so greatly that a number of rats simply refused to jump at all, even though that eventually meant protracted hunger, even to starvation.[12]

Studies of learned helplessness have also been done with human subjects.[13] Again, the conclusions are similar: When a person does not experience a sense of control or mastery in events or, put in behavioral terms, when people find no connection between their behavior and a consistent enforcement pattern such that there are no learned connections between activity and effective feedback, they learn helplessness and passivity that in some cases move toward depression.[14] The importance of this research bears not only on understanding of education and psychopathology but also on social and political matters. One of the effective researchers who has dealt with that extrapolation is Julian Rotter, who developed instruments that differentiate internal and external "locus of control." [15] The issue of whether or not one experiences oneself or one's community as having agency in the sense of being a locus of control was seen to have a direct bearing, not only on self-esteem and the degree of individual initiative, but also on the entire sense of well-being, socialization, and community development in the social matrix (obviously social and individual dynamics always must be understood as mutual influences).[16]

The importance of the *community* context of experience of internal locus of control has a direct bearing on health services insofar as it marks one of the important features of community health programs. Easily accessible neighborhood or community health facilities tend to enhance feelings of familiarity and initiative on the part of the patient, increasing the sense of control or agency. This stands out clearly against the experience of loss of control represented by removal from the community into an institution remote from the typical life space of the individual. Such experience can be characterized more by what Rotter would call "external locus of control."

This leads to the third line of reasoning regarding helplessness and agency coming from social psychology, particularly the work of Erving Goffman, who has attempted to characterize the dimensions of both "total institutions" and "stigmatization." [17] Although Goffman started out to study mental hospitals, his work has been extended into analyzing the characteristics of prisons, educational institutions, and hospitals, all of which provide services designed for the complete life support and rehabilitation or reeducation of its participant community—read "inmates." Endemic to Goffman's characterization is the priority the institutions typically place on decisions and procedures that ensure the maintenance and smooth running of the institution itself. I suppose it should be noted that this does not always mean efficiency, for sometimes the bureaucratic mechanisms are immensely complex. The point usually is that the complexity has to do with administrative procedures and safeguards which themselves often function under the pressure of external loci of control (such as government regulations and surveys, professional questionnaires, and insurance requirements) but which leave patients or inmates all the more baffled as to the forces determining their fate. Other characteristics of routinization of daily life, maintenance of an authoritarian system of policy formation, punishment or isolation for aberrant behavior, maintenance of confinement, the control of information, and the maintenance of a system of professional secrecy relatively inaccessible to public scrutiny or censorship—all of these can be seen as perpetuating a situation in which the helplessness or loss of control of residents, including patients, is exacerbated.

Again in Goffman's studies there is attention to the kind of "learning" that goes on within "total institutions." The evidence is very clear that people who remain in such institutions for even a short time quickly adapt to the routinization of the procedure and in effect *learn to be "patient"* (with both meanings). In the case of mental hospitals, it can be demonstrated that many patients learn crazy behavior because the institution in one sense rewards that behavior with special attention (read "reinforcement"). In medical hospitals, too, patients learn their role fairly quickly. And it is unfortunately true that this role too often is construed as one of passive waiting and compliance rather than as one of effective agency and knowledge in the active role of healing itself.

Current research on this problem has drawn on role theory and pays special attention to the learning of the *sick role*. Alexander Segall has documented the research demonstrating the pervasiveness of components of the sick role originally conceptualized by Talcott Parsons.[18] In Parsons' view, the sick person has two major rights and two related duties. The rights are exemption from responsibility for incapacity (as the illness is construed to be beyond one's control), and exemption from all other normal social role obligations. The legitimation of this withdrawal, however, is accompanied by the dual duties of recognizing the inherently undesirable character of sickness and the obligation to "try and get well," and the obligation to seek technically competent help (a physician) and to cooperate in the processes prescribed.[19] In practice, the two obligations tend to merge; and, as Segall's findings indicate, even in the mode of trying to get well, "the medical patient is expected to cooperate by being *passive, submissive* and generally *dependent* upon the doctor." [20]

Further empirical research on the styles and pervasiveness of systems that encourage patient passivity and dependence is reported by Gerald Gordon, Daisy L. Tagliacozzo, and Hans O. Mauksch.[21] And in an examination of what might be thought of as a form of agency, namely "self-reliance," D. L. Phillips has found that many people see such strength as *antithetical* to the "sick role" and, by implication, inappropriate to the process of recovery.[22]

This brings us to a more direct citation of the particular characteristics in medical settings that may contribute to the patient's sense of helplessness. Most conspicuous among these are the experiences of an external locus of control in the sense of management of information, conduct of the diagnostic process, the direction of treatment procedures, the extent and duration of direct medical intervention, submission and adaptation to technological apparatus, and ward and room confinement. What I am suggesting is that, particularly under conditions of hospitalization, the very procedures intended to enhance health and well-being may turn out to accentuate precisely those feelings of helplessness that reside in everyone as a substrate of the processes of development and learning. Furthermore, the desire for security, protection, and healing may in fact welcome or extend the compliance in a system of operation that exacerbates helplessness. There is, from this perspective, both willed and unwilled consent that could easily be misconstrued by those in authority as giving license for the kind of practices that generate "reassurance" to those longings for external power in healing.

What our analysis should suggest, however, is that both those longings and the practices of institutions that play into them in fact generate conditions of passivity and detachment, or perhaps their opposite—anger, struggle, and resentment—neither of which facilitates the healing process. To be genuinely engaged in healing, I believe we must reassess the way in which both we as professional caretakers and the institutions for which we work can develop greater sensitivity to the possibilities of self-initiation and internal locus of control for the patient.

In our best moments, we know that we stand by more as facilitators and expediters of the internal healing capabilities of the organism itself. The agency for healing and for development is indeed an internal matter to which we can give aid but which we do not command. The urgency of that humility is essential, for although we cannot command, we can destroy. Our own agency in aiding the healing process must always be synchronous with the agency of the patient. Without confidence in such shared agency, we may both fall into helplessness.

The Physician

This brings us to the importance of examining ways in which medical practitioners and medical education may be involved in the dynamics of helplessness and agency. It has frequently been observed that one of the strongest assets of the physician is a sense of confidence and responsibility. Such professional confidence is not cheaply won but is rather the product of years of study, laboratory work, patient care, and accrued knowledge that generates significant competence. True confidence always is directly correlated to true competence.

But what is sometimes ignored in the education of competent physicians is what I would call the covert "crisis of helplessness." Having endured the hard-fought battles for adequate undergraduate preparation, high grade-point averages, the endorsements of knowledgeable mentors, and the prize of medical school admission, the young medical student usually is initially expectant and eager. It may well be that much of the motivation for a career in medicine has been stimulated by a vision of personal and social *agency*—from the simple account ("When Mother was sick, no one could help, until the doctor came. I decided then . . .") to more philosophical or social articulations of the virtue of a caring profession. Medical training is envisioned as leading not only to personal satisfaction and material success but, more important for many, toward the tangible actualization of valuing human life and well-being through minimizing pain, disease, and dysfunction.

But right on the heels of that expectancy, some rather discomforting things happen. For one thing, first-year medical and laboratory courses may seem disconnected, irrelevant, or overwhelming in their demands. For another thing, the callousness, political infighting, and materialism of some colleagues and mentors may be shocking. But more than anything, the young medical student is bombarded with an awareness of pain, of blood, of agony, of personal and familial chaos, and finally of death that is extremely difficult to cope with. The adaptive mechanisms discussed earlier normally come into play. A certain distancing is learned in relation to patients and, to some extent, in relation to colleagues. There is a kind of "psychic numbing" that Robert Jay Lifton speaks of elsewhere in this book that is typical of a psychological reaction to disaster. There also may be elements of the "guilt of survivorship" when surrounded by so much suffering and constant reminders of the precariousness of life in others. The overloading of our sensibilities is almost too severe, and to survive in the face of that overloading there is the doubling of brutalization in the sense that we brutalize our own responses into numbness, in part as a response to having been brutalized by the overwhelming awareness of disease, deformity, and death.

Death itself has to be encountered—with a sense of respect and meaningfulness, it is hoped. But more often it is treated with still other forms of distancing and brutalization. Many medical students experience for the first time the *killing* of an experimental animal for dissection and the study of anatomy, an experience intended to be an important lesson in itself: The power and finality of a surgeon's knife is awesome and quick. Our control is over life and death. Then there is the ritual of the cadaver. One receives and proceeds to dismember and dissect what was a human being. The shock of this act is ameliorated by a hundred jokes and frequently by the nicknaming of the corpse itself, as though to invest it with an artificial personality totally under the control of the imagination of the dissector. The integrity of the dead person as person is almost utterly disguised. Again, the potency is totally with the medical student; the compliance of the human cadaver is absolute. And finally, even with increased public awareness of the process of dying, it is still rare to find within the medical school a course dealing humanely with this process and the medical responsibilities to the bereaved.

The questions such observations raise have to do with the learning process at its most fundamental core. I am suggesting that medical students learn simultaneously the depth of their own helplessness and the ideal of an absoluteness of medical agency. The helplessness lies in the apprehension that human suffering is too much. It is so widespread, so debilitating, so repeated, and so final that at best we can assuage fate for only brief moments on the vast horizon of time. Death in the end is victorious, and to deny that is to deny our own humanity. To deny that is to capitulate to the arrogance of a godlike virtuosity in which the possibility of self-deceit is all too tempting. For at the same time that our most serious reflections put us in awe of the final helplessness of the human condition in its inability to control the barrier of death, we are engaged in the preparation of whatever skills are available to preserve and enhance life.

It should certainly be acknowledged that the experiences of

helplessness for the physician may frequently be exacerbated by the behavior and attitude of the patient. Some patients are not only misleading and uncooperative, but whiny, manipulative, malingering, and bitchy. They put pills down the sink and confound the most rigorously worked-out treatment regimen; they complain about services and prices; they act mistrustfully and try to set one physician against another.

Perhaps one of the most serious current forms of patient infringement on the agency of the physician, however, is the threat of *malpractice suits*. Aside from the legal and financial dimensions of this problem, the threat of malpractice litigation ironically redoubles in compounding the forms of helplessness for both physician and patient. The threat of lawsuits adds to the pressures that constrain and sometimes paralyze the physician's ability to act quickly and effectively in treatment. And the physician's response is typically and predictably one of caution, demonstrated always in more conservative decisions, more protracted tests and consultations, and more guardedness in sharing information with the patient. Under such psychological conditions, when the medical work is slowed or stalled, clearly the patient also becomes a victim of the very procedures that may initially have appeared as a form of his or her internal agency. That is, the possibility of such agentic acts by the patient may result in the further manipulation of the patient.

What emerges here is an awareness that the patient-physician relationship has the potential for each to exacerbate the other's tendencies toward defensiveness, counterassertion, and reciprocal maneuvers. While examining these dynamics in terms of helplessness and agency, we can see a possible (and perhaps unexamined) struggle for control. Furthermore, this struggle may be unconsciously driven by deep-seated psychological associations to the specific areas in which the struggle often occurs: cleanliness, manipulation of objects, control of body functions (especially eating and excretion), and autonomy and shame. Consider, for instance, the importance to physicians of procedures related to asepsis and sterility; manipulation of surgical instruments, numerical data, patients-as-objects, information; control and management of the patient's organ systems; professional pride regarding outside regulation; resistance to consultation (especially psychiatric); and attention to patient "management." It is also interesting how often a patient attempts to reassert control in any of these areas: self-soiling and exaggeration of physical decay to gain attention; attempts to manipulate staff (bell-pulling, delay of bathing); attempts to control mobility (extreme forms: escaping from wards) and bodily functions such as eating and fluid intake; and the struggles to assert autonomy at various stages of illness in self-care, dressing, and so on. Exaggeration of any one of these is likely to call up a counterassertion in the same area or a closely related one. Success in one may compensate for failure in another. For example, when a doctor fails to control a patient's bodily functions—that is, when the patient is going to die—the doctor may substitute control of information by not telling the patient the truth. Barney G. Glaser and Anselm L. Strauss, in *Awareness of Dying,* describe the elaborate strategies used by medical staff to exert this information control.[23] Notice, too, incidentally, on the subject of the dovetailing effect, how often patients who seek second, third, and fourth medical opinions may be reacting to hit the doctor at the level of the doctor's autonomy, just as patients attempt to act with autonomy themselves.

The possibility of a physician's self-learning as well as understanding of the dynamics of these reciprocal transactions could be helpful. It would be useful to have a situation in which some aspects of motivation and emotional response patterns could be explored sympathetically. Then, if a doctor found himself or herself entering this circle of assertiveness and defensiveness, even with unconscious conflicts, the circle could perhaps be broken by insight and awareness. In this context, self-learning groups would have meaning from the *intrapsychic* standpoint analogous to Lifton's and Barnard's recommendations elsewhere that student "rap groups" could bring to light *ethical* and *political* issues.[24]

There are also aspects of the medical environment that limit the physician's sense of agency: problems in securing sufficient support services, complexities in maintaining current pharmaceutical supplies, problems in obtaining and maintaining various complex forms of technical apparatus, regulations and space alterations mandated by hospital administrators and community citizens' boards; records, paperwork, and complicated regulations pertaining to third-party payments; and the necessity of governmental diagnostic and statistical reports as well as financial reports.

It may seem ironic to some that such attention would be given here to the ways in which the agency of physicians is inhibited, when one could argue that other hospital personnel have even more limited power. Certainly attendants and housekeeping staff, for instance, as well as others within the care-giving system, live under regulations that routinize existence to a large degree and certainly limit the range within which effective decisions can be made. Their occasional envy of the status and apparent agency of physicians, however, may tend to obscure in the hospital routine as well as in the mind of the public the main point being emphasized here: the severe limits—even to a certain point of helplessness—of physicians themselves.

In response to these forms of potential helplessness on the part of the physician, particularly in respect to the ultimate limitations and frustrations in relation to death itself, a number of adaptive moves may be employed. Some of these may be psychologically damaging and others may be constructive and ego-adaptive. Among the unconstructive responses, it is striking that a number of physicians fall into the traps of psychological denial and escape that have been discovered as strategies incorporated in broader samples of people under more severe situations of helplessness.[25]

One strategy may be the overdetermined compulsion to identify with symbols of power. Such identification, whether it be with material or social power, and whether or not it is expressed through ownership of conspicuous properties or through membership and decision-making on significant institutional boards, may obscure those realms of limited agency, especially in health care and life-and-death issues to which one's primary commitment has been given.

Another strategy may simply be overwork. The good of one's

seriousness, dedication, and responsiveness to the myriad forms of suffering may easily turn into its demonic opposite: a tyranny of drivenness that conceals a refusal to accept limits of time, responsibility, and energy as part of the human condition.

A third strategy could be called *distantiation*. Distantiation comprises those emotional distancing processes by which one insulates oneself from the deeply personal, disturbing as well as joyous, dimensions of genuine participation in the human realities of one's associates. Although such characteristics may start as a way of maintaining professional distance from patients, they can generalize into a mode of insulation characteristic of the emotional quality of many relationships, even those presumably most "intimate."

Finally, there is the strategy of surrounding oneself with technology to disguise some forms of anxiety about helplessness in the interpersonal context. Overattention to the detailing of health-monitoring systems and life-support systems may both intrigue and absorb the physician's creative technical genius, but it may also occasionally represent forms of overreliance that suggest psychological denial of the importance of human engagement in effective medical involvement with individuals and families.

The constructive responses to limitations on our agency involve in part recognizing the valuable components in the forms of reaction just mentioned, but without the excesses of overdetermination. There are certainly constructive uses of power that make possible effective patient-care procedures, but that also acknowledge the limits or side effects of those procedures. There is value in hard work, and in the protection of a professional stance that does not become overinvolved in emotional identification with each patient. And there is the constructive utilization of technology in human care. The point is that one must be cautious about the self-deception that can occur when those values and strategies become so dominating that they obscure the real limits of one's effectiveness in giving medical care. It is the good gone wrong, when the effective possibilities of these responses become obsessive and self-deceptive, that would lead me to call the unconstructive responses "demonic."

The most constructive response to the limits of agency and the real possibilities of helplessness may be the acknowledgment of the *real limits* we face and, within that, of the potential areas where we *can* do effective work. Try as we will to extend life, we cannot control death. Try as we will to provide the most effective treatment for specific dysfunctions, we cannot control the regenerative processes, the hope, or the will to live of the patient. Try as we will to develop a particular medical specialty, there are many, many other problems we cannot treat. If the temptation in the rebound from the medical student's crisis of helplessness is the delusion of omnipotence, then the recovery of a mature physician is related to the humility and humanness that come with the full awareness of our finitude.

Furthermore, it should be clear that the awareness of helplessness leads to a form of agency; and conversely, the awareness of agency leads to a form of helplessness. As we acknowledge the real limits of our time, training, disposition, and context, we may less anxiously and more effectively work with dedication in those areas where we are skillful. And as we agentically do more and know more, we inevitably run into limits, we come to the boundary, we raise the new questions, we find that realm in which we cannot yet help.[26] It is at this point that I believe helplessness and agency may be seen, not as contradictory, but as mutually engaged in the self-understanding of the physician. For although they certainly stand in tension as polar categories, what we have come to see is the importance of differentiating real helplessness and professional limits from obsessive and worrisome forms of imagined helplessness. Standing in the face of our existential finitude—that is, in the face of death—we must acknowledge the realities of time and of human life that we cannot change. But I want to suggest at the same time that such an acknowledgment may actually free us to engage all the more energetically in affirming our capabilities to endow life with meaning and sustenance, and to celebrate the precious uniqueness and autonomy of other human beings who stand beside us as time-limited creatures. We are in this sense very much companions, sharing the fate of our patients, although we are also the agents of knowledge and care, extending for a time the possibilities of life.

Policy

Having looked at a number of the dynamics of helplessness and agency in both patient and physician, I would like to suggest some policy implications that stem from these observations. I will make six suggestions here, but I expect that other thoughtful recommendations could be added. Suggestions 1, 3, 4, 5, and 6 may be especially relevant to doctors, 2, 3, 4, 5, and 6 to medical educators, and 2 and 3 to hospital administrators and social planners.

1. *Access to knowledge.* One of the most effective ways to increase patients' sense of agency would be to involve them more (where possible) in the discussion of symptoms, treatment alternatives, expected outcomes, side effects, and medical implications. This would imply increased patient access to knowledge relevant to both the illness and treatment patterns—and especially knowledge about the patient's own level of dysfunction. While this might involve physicians or other medical staff in educational functions and take some time, it is the clearest way of resisting the all-too-easy capitulation by the patient into the regressive or learned posture of helplessness and dependence. It would be a vivid way of attesting to the centrality of the patient as decision maker and agentic person, finally responsible for her or his own life and recovery.[27]

2. *Flexible treatment settings.* Although in many cases there are a number of obvious advantages to centralized hospital treatment, we are beginning to see the harmonizing effect of community health clinics and home care. Certainly, the process of displacement from one's home into a strange and highly regulated envi-

ronment tends to exaggerate the forms of learned helplessness and institutionalized behavior reviewed earlier. The sense of agency and responsibility on the part of the patient can remain more intact when treatment is *in situ*. Familiar people, objects, schedules, aromas, and vistas may enhance the sense of internal locus of control while facilitating acknowledgment of mature dependence on necessary modes of medical expertise.

3. *Empowerment.* The first two items consider the specific process and location of medical treatment. Beyond that, I would argue that the medical community should be concerned about the political and social processes through which greater agentic empowerment might be actualized—especially for people whose economic or social status has led to forms of entrapment that must exaggerate the experience of social helplessness. For we can see direct connections between the helplessness that comes from victimization and unjust social discrimination, and the helplessness that experientially defeats patients in medical settings and simultaneously frustrates the physicians trying to be of service to them. Empowerment in political access, jobs, housing, and education is directly related to empowerment in health care access and the financial coverage of health insurance. The changes that would be experienced with such empowerment would be directly congruent with attitudes of hope, cooperation, and potency that are so important in the medical processes of healing.[28]

4. *Awareness of limits.* In addition to the excellent training that medical schools may provide in the life sciences and clinical techniques, our discussion here suggests that attention should also be paid to the limits of medicine—in particular, to the realities of death and dying and to the physician's response to these realities. Perhaps courses on death and bereavement or on the philosophy of medicine would be helpful, or courses on the social psychological context of illness and treatment giving attention to dynamics such as those of helplessness and agency.

5. *Self-learning.* Ways might also be found in medical schools, through a system of advisors, mentors, or small groups, to facilitate self-learning. Such learning seems important in at least two

respects related to the issues in this essay. First, it would be useful in working through feelings of professional identity and the onslaught of suffering, tragedy, and disillusionment so often present in the students' first year—feelings related to the forms of helplessness experienced. Second, they could be useful in sorting out individual motives in one's medical career and in identifying the focus of specialization to be pursued (agentic center) and the real boundaries of training, time, and so on. In short, self-conscious attention should be given to learning one's own configuration of skills and limits for reasons of personal maturity that include the disavowing of pretenses of either helplessness or omnicompetence.

6. *Team healing.* In relation to the awareness of specialization and limits, considerable progress has been made in the cooperative interaction of healing teams representing intraprofessional specialties in medicine as well as crossprofessional skills in the realms of other physical sciences, social science, psychology, economics, and religion—an acknowledgment that help can be increased with a broadening of perspectives. To increase this sharing of agency farther, and to take into account the danger of forms of helplessness in both patient and physician, the concept of the "team" could be broadened to include the patient as well as other specialists—which returns us to the first recommendation.

What is being argued here is the importance of both agentic medical specialization and broad human concern. We need to give attention simultaneously to the ways in which we can minimize the dehumanizing dangers of practices that allow regressive or learned helplessness in the patient and to the ways in which dysfunctional denial and overcompensation against potential helplessness may be guarded against in both patient and physician, emphasizing instead the mature adaptation and competence that can be fostered in medical education and practice.

Toward these ends, the contributions of social science may in the short run increase complexity and perhaps even anxiety; but, in the long run, they can yield greater agency and control, both in human experience generally and in the medical profession particularly.

NOTES

1. Some of the further reaches of the therapeutic truth of this irony have been beautifully spelled out by Henri Nouwen in *The Wounded Healer* (Garden City, N.Y: Doubleday, 1972).

2. William Rogers, "The Phenomenology of Helplessness," *Soundings*, 52, no. 3 (Fall 1969):334–49.

3. Fromm, *Man for Himself* (New York: Rinehart, 1947); Bakan, *The Duality of Human Existence* (Boston: Beacon Press, 1971); Riesman, Reuel Denney, and Nathan Glazer, *The Lonely Crowd* (New Haven: Yale University Press, 1950); Rogers, *Client-Centered Therapy* (Boston: Houghton Mifflin Co., 1951).

4. *The Courage to Be* (New Haven: Yale University Press, 1952).

5. Sigmund Freud, *The Future of an Illusion* (Garden City, N.Y.: Doubleday, 1927), p. 47.

6. *Theology After Freud* (New York: Bobbs-Merrill, 1970).

7. It is important to point out that the overly paternalistic and, many would say, sexist imagery of Freud's argument about the need for a father protector does not fundamentally discredit the dynamics he identified. Indeed, Erik Erikson has developed a similar dynamic discussion, particularly in relation to child-mother relationships, that treats the residual effects of infantile awareness of "smallness" or helplessness as a substrate of the mind coupled with the frequent intensification of feelings of inability to control the mother—similar to dynamics dealt with in Freud's analysis in *Beyond the Pleasure Principle*. It is that experience of physical smallness and ineffectiveness in control of others that may return under conditions such as hospitalization, leading to feelings of bewilderment and helplessness—again in relation to the caretaker, the physician, who could just as easily and perhaps more appropriately (if we trust psychoanalytic studies of the dynamics of physicians) be understood as a "mothering" figure.

8. Bowlby, *Attachment and Loss* (New York: Basic Books, 1973); Fairbairn, *Psychoanalytic Studies of the Personality* (London: Tavistock Publications, 1952); Guntrip, *Schizoid Phenomena: Object Relations and the Self* (New York: International Universities Press, 1969); and Paul Bohanann, *Divorce and After* (Garden City, N.Y.: Doubleday, 1971).

9. Freud, *The Ego and the Mechanisms of Defense* (New York: International Universities Press, 1967); Hartmann, *Ego Psychology and the Problem of Adaptation* (New York: International Universities Press, 1958); and Haan, "Proposed Model of Ego Functioning," *Psychological Monographs*, 77, no. 8 (1963):1–23.

10. Martin E. P. Seligman and S. F. Maier, "Failure to Escape Traumatic Shock," *Journal of Experimental Psychology,* 74, no. 1 (1967):1–9.

11. Martin E. P. Seligman, "Fall Into Helplessness," *Psychology Today,* 7, no. 1 (June 1973):44.

12. Martin E. P. Seligman and Gwyneth Beagley, "Learned Helplessness in the Rat," *Journal of Comparative and Physiological Psychology,* 88, no. 2 (1975):534–41.

13. See especially the work of Jerry W. Thornton and Paul D. Jacobs, "Learned Helplessness in Human Subjects," *Journal of Experimental Psychology,* 87, no. 3 (March 1971):367–72.

14. The symptoms of learned helplessness in Seligman's studies have also included depression, passivity, difficulty in learning which responses produce relief, lack of aggression, weight loss and undereating (in some cases anorexia), sexual deficits, norepinephrine depletion, and so on. See especially M. E. P. Seligman, *Helplessness: On Depression, Development and Death* (San Francisco: W. H. Freeman, 1975).

15. *Social Learning and Clinical Psychology* (Englewood Cliffs, N.J.: Prentice-Hall, 1954).

16. Learned helplessness is also very poignantly illustrated by Aleksandr Solzhenitsyn. He writes with unflinching detail about a 1949 revolt in one of the Siberian prison camps. It went off like clockwork: " 'Escort soldiers disarmed, the seizure of six to eight machine guns, the camp attacked from the exterior, the wardens liquidated, the telephone wires cut, the freeing of the prisoners.' But when they were liberated the prisoners would not flee: 'The camp contained only men with numbers, hopelessly scarred by their life there, dedicated to dying, deprived of all hope.' " (*Gulag Archipelago, III,* tr. Harry Willetts (New York: Harper and Row, 1977), p. 183.

17. *Asylums: Essays on the Social Situation of Medical Patients and Other Inmates* (Garden City, N.Y.: Anchor Books, 1961); *Stigma: Notes on the Management of Spoiled Identity* (Englewood Cliffs, N.J.: Prentice-Hall, 1963).

18. Segall, "The Sick Role Concept: Understanding Illness Behavior," *Journal of Health and Social Behavior,* 17 (June 1976):163–70.

19. Parsons, *The Social System* (New York: Free Press, 1951).

20. Segall, "Sick Role Concept." p. 164, italics added.

21. Gordon, *Role Theory and Illness: A Sociological Perspective* (esp. chap. 5, "Behavioral Expectations Related to Illness") (New Haven: College and University Press, 1966); Tagliacozzo and Mauksch, "The Patient's View of the Patient's Role," in *Patients, Physicians, and Illness: A Sourcebook in Behavioral Science and Health,* ed. E. Gartly Jaco (New York: Free Press, 1972).

22. D. L. Phillips, "Self-reliance and the Inclination to Adopt the Sick Role," *Social Forces,* 43 (1965):555–63. Another fascinating essay dealing with the rituals of admission to hospitals is also worthy of note. William May interprets the loss of identity and autonomy in such admission rites as a form of "institutional death by

devouring" in "Institutions as Symbols of Death," *Journal of the American Academy of Religion*, 44, no. 2 (1976):211–23.
23. (Chicago: Aldine, 1965).
24. David Barnard has indeed been helpful in also illuminating many forms of these personal and interpersonal conflicts which exacerbate reciprocal helplessness. For an excellent sociological account of patient and doctor strategies for mutual control, with frequent aggravation of each other's sense of helplessness, see Gerry Stimson and Barbara Webb, *Going to See the Doctor: The Consultation Process in General Practice* (London: Routledge and Kegan Paul, 1975), esp. chaps. 6 and 7.
25. Rogers, "Phenomenology of Helplessness."
26. The real dimensions of this reality, particularly in the realm of community health services, are portrayed beautifully by Ernest Becker in *Angel in Armor* (New York: Braziller, 1969).
27. Parallel support for such a recommendation has also been carefully developed by Shelley Taylor at Harvard. She has recently completed an extensive, very insightful review of the literature on breast cancer, particularly its psychological impact in all phases of symptomatology, diagnosis, treatment, and postmastectomy recovery. Her goals in this work are policy formulation and advancement of social science research methodology. Her central theme is the elaboration of what she calls the "patient participation model":

> The course of events in breast cancer often involves loss of control by the woman over her own body and life. Several studies, of high methodological quality, show that returning to patients some sense of control actually enhances coping with surgical pain and treatment of discomfort, lowering the need for medications and speeding recovery rates. This sense of control is most effectively achieved through *informed participation*, whereby the patient is informed of the medical procedures and accruing physical sensations and is permitted to take part in the decision-making concerning her various treatments. In this way, the patient is neither a passive recipient of services nor fully in charge of medical decisions. Rather she is an informed, active member of the team that is responsible for her health. (S. E. Taylor and S. Levin, "The Psychological Impact of Breast Cancer: Theory and Practice," in *Psychological Aspects of Breast Cancer*, ed. A. Enelow [London: Oxford University Press, 1976])

28. Further constructive recommendations that address this connection between patient helplessness and sociopolitical powerlessness are available in H. Jack Geiger, "The Causes of Dehumanization in Health Care and Prospects for Humanization" (esp. the section on "Sources in the Social Order") in *Humanizing Health Care*, ed. Jan Howard and Anselm Strauss (New York: Wiley Interscience, 1975).

CHAPTER 3

Advocacy and Corruption in the Healing Professions

Robert Jay Lifton

The confrontation with helplessness and death is not only an intensely personal and complicated experience shared by medical students, physicians, and patients, but also a metaphor for the struggle to maintain the ethical integrity of the medical profession as a whole. Robert Jay Lifton sees a close connection between the personal encounter with death and the tendency for the professional ideals of scientific and technical competence to be interpreted to avoid social and political responsibility. "Psychic numbing," a protective response to the overwhelming presence and power of death, can envelop moral perception, too. The result is a professional self-understanding that celebrates not only emotional stoicism, but the claim of ethical neutrality as well, and disengagement from historical and cultural conflict.

Lifton's essay suggests that medical professionals must balance loyalties that are pulled in several directions. There are loyalties to patients, whose sufferings have an immediacy that at times is nearly intolerable. There are loyalties to scientific integrity, with its demands and promises of intellectual fulfillment that can seem more alluring than the details of daily life in the clinic. And there are loyalties to society, whose investment in medical institutions is great, and yet whose inequities are apparent in the services those institutions provide. The tensions of these very conflicts can be prematurely resolved by forms of numbing. To counter this tendency, Lifton delves into the meaning of professionalism for sources of self-criticism and moral commitment that do not conflict with a dedication to mastery of technical knowledge and skills. His essay calls attention to some possibly hidden meanings of "scientific medicine," and to the potential moral implications of the use of this term as the sole criterion of educational policy. His suggestions for medical education point to the value of honest attention to those moments when medicine's scientific limits are reached.

1

In looking at the professions, one does well to hold to the old religious distinction between the ministerial and the prophetic. One should not assume, as many do, a simple polarity in which the sciences are inherently radical or revolutionary and the healing professions intrinsically conservative. The professions must minister to people, take care of them, and that is a relatively conservative process. But there are prophets who emerge from the healing ministrations of the professions—Freud is a notable example—with radical critiques and revolutionary messages. Moreover, even "pure scientists" (in biology or physics, for example) spend most of their time ministering to the existing paradigm, doing what Thomas Kuhn calls "normal science,"[1] and strongly resist the breakthrough that is inevitably charted by the prophets among them. There are ministerial and prophetic elements in both the healing professions and the sciences.

But one must also distinguish between the professions, which have profound value in their capacity for continuity and renewal, and professional*ism*, the ideology of professional omniscience, which in our era inevitably leads to technicism and the model of the machine. The necessity for such a distinction becomes painfully clear if one looks at the situation that prevailed for psychiatrists in Vietnam, where the professional may have been no better able than his soldier-patient to sort out the nuances of care and professional commitment on the one hand, and moral (or immoral) action on the other. I want to take that extreme situation as a starting point for a broader discussion of these dilemmas and their moral and conceptual ramifications.

Central to my view of the present predicament of the professions is the psychology and spirit of the survivor. The concept of the survivor derives in my work from the study I did in Hiroshima a little more than ten years ago,[2] and has been fundamental to my subsequent thought. I define a survivor as one who has touched, witnessed, encountered, or been immersed in death in a literal or symbolic way and has himself remained alive.

There are five patterns to this concept, which I found Hiroshima survivors to share to a rather striking degree with survivors of Nazi death camps, the plagues of the Middle Ages, natural disasters, and what Kurt Vonnegut calls "plain old death." The first pattern has to do with the survivor's indelible death image and death anxiety. This "death imprint" often involves the loss of a sense of invulnerability. The second, that of death guilt, is revealed in the survivor's classic question, "Why did I stay alive when he or she or they died?" The question itself has to do with a sense of organic social balance: "If I had died, he or she would have lived." That image of exchange of one life for another is perhaps the survivor's greatest psychological burden. A third pattern is that of desensitization or what I call psychic numbing, the breakdown of symbolic connectedness with one's environment. Numbing is a necessary protective mechanism in holocaust, but it can become self-perpetuating and express itself in sustained depression, despair, and apathy or withdrawal. A fourth survivor pattern has to do with the "death taint," as experienced by others toward survivors and by survivors themselves, resulting in discrimination against them and mutual suspicion and mistrust. Central to this pattern is the survivor's "suspicion of counterfeit nurturance," his combination of feeling in need of help and resenting help offered as a reminder of weakness. (This kind of suspicion occurs not only in holocaust but in any situation in which "help" is offered by the privileged to the downtrodden or oppressed, as in white-black relations; and one can readily find models for this pained interaction in parent-child relationships.)

The fifth pattern is fundamental to all survivor psychology and encompasses the other four. It is the struggle toward "formulation" (following Susanne Langer)[3]—in order to be able to find form and significance in one's remaining life experience. This formulative struggle is equally visible in more symbolic experiences of holocaust, those of surviving ways of life one perceives to be "dying." Thus, rapid social change makes survivors of us all.

More particularly, however, medical professionals are survivors in many respects. In the literal way, the profession is directly engaged with those who suffer disease, disfigurement, and death. For the medical student, especially, leaving the laboratory and the classroom for the clinic and the hospital ward can be a thorough-going death immersion. Questions of judgment and responsibility for the failure of life-saving procedures are frequently colored by guilt over real or imagined errors and omissions. There is the unavoidable, glaring contrast between the vigor and optimism of medical personnel, filled with enthusiasm for their own life prospects, and the shrunken, uncertain horizons of those whom they accompany toward death.

To these direct encounters with death must be added significant symbolic survivals. Perhaps the most important is the loss of innocence: the abrupt awakening to the finitude and limitation of medical science and practice in its attempts to alleviate suffering and ensure well-being. This entails the awareness of scarcity of resources, and the knowledge that many who require help must be denied; the experience of accidental miscarriage of treatment, of lethal errors in judgment or technique; the encounter with the frustrating boundaries of knowledge; and the perpetual discovery that one's personal intentions and energies will always be spent before the tasks of care are completed.

In examining our healing professions in relation to these survivals, we should keep in mind two general survivor alternatives. One can retreat from the issues raised by the death immersion and thereby remain bound to it in a condition of stasis (or numbing). Or one can confront the death immersion and derive insight, illumination, and change from the overall survivor experience.[4] The latter response to some kind of experience of survival has probably been the source of most great religious and political movements. In professional life, it has stimulated many breakthroughs, whereas the first response frequently manifests itself in technicism and dehumanization.

A related issue is that of advocacy, which in our profession applies both to investigation and therapy, and is crucial to issues of professional renewal. In my work with Vietnam veterans, I sought to combine detachment sufficient to enable me to make psychological evaluations (which I had to do at every step) with involvement that expressed my own antiwar commitments and moral passions. I believe that we always function within this dialectic between ethical involvement and intellectual rigor, and that bringing our advocacy "out front," and articulating it, makes us more, rather than less, scientific. Indeed, our scientific accuracy is likely to suffer when we hide our ethical beliefs behind the claim of neutrality, the assertion that we are nothing but "neutral screens." The Vietnam war constituted an extreme situation, in which the need for an ethical response was very clear. But we have a tradition of great importance in depth psychology, much evident in Freud, of studying extremes in order to illuminate the (more obscure) ordinary.

2

I want to use my experience of over three years with "rap groups" of antiwar veterans as basis for generalizing about certain issues central to the professions generally and to the medical profession in particular. These issues include aspects of the relationships between healers and clients, doctors and patients, and medical students and their instructors; the nature of technicism as it relates to the human values in medical care and education; and the possibility for a renewed image of the healing professions that can incorporate both our shared human survivorship and a posture of ethical advocacy that is consistent with scientific integrity.

The veterans' rap groups came into being because the veterans sensed that they had more psychological work to do in connection with the war.[5] Yet although they knew they were in psychological pain, they did not consider themselves patients. They wanted to understand what they had been through, to begin to heal themselves, and at the same time to make known to the American public the human costs of the war. These two aspects of the veterans' aspirations in forming the groups—healing themselves while finding a mode of political expression—paralleled the professional dialectic of rigor and advocacy mentioned earlier. Without using those words, the veterans had that combination very much in mind when they asked me to work with them, and from the beginning the therapeutic and political aspects of our work developed simultaneously.

There was an assumption, at first unspoken and later articulated, that everybody's life was at issue; professionals had no special podium from which to avoid self-examination. We, too, could be challenged, questioned about anything—all of which seemed natural enough to the veterans but a bit more problematic for the professionals. As people used to interpreting others' motivations, we at first found it a bit jarring to be confronted with hard questions about our own, and with challenges about the way we lived. Yet we were required to join with our soldier-clients in a common self-examination that did not exempt medicine or psychiatry from accountability and the liability for change. Although the question in the groups was usually framed in terms of the moral dilemma of psychiatry in Vietnam, the essential lesson was that the medical and other healing professions cannot restrict their responsibilities to the immediate care-giving task, but must address themselves to the social and moral climate within which those tasks are being performed.

Before long, I came to recognize three principles that seemed important in our work. The first was that of *affinity*, the coming together of people who share a particular historical or personal experience, along with a basic perspective on that experience, in order to make some sense of it. The second principle was that of *presence*, a kind of being-there or full engagement and openness to mutual impact—no one ever being simply a therapist against whom things were rebounding. The third was that of *self-generation*, the need on the part of those seeking help, change, or insight of any kind to initiate their own process and to conduct it largely on their own terms so that, even when calling in others with expert knowledge, they retain major responsibility for the shape and direction of the enterprise. These principles seem to be necessary ingredients for making a transition between old and new images and values. To the extent that they are included in the basic structure of the relationship between physicians and their patients, the medical profession may contribute significantly to the increased autonomy and self-determination of those whom it serves. As Paul Pruyser argues later in this volume, the guiding spirit of such a relationship is one of genuine collaboration.

The rap group experience showed, however, that attempting to uphold the values of affinity, presence, and self-generation within a context of therapeutic professionalism can create genuine tensions. For example, there was a real conflict between two views of what we were doing. In the beginning, a majority of the professionals felt that the essential model for our sessions was group therapy. They argued that the men were "hurting" and needed help, and that if we as therapists offered anything less than group therapy we were cheating the men of what they most needed. On one level, the veterans tended to favor a second model: a sustained dialogue between professionals and veterans based on a common stance of opposition to the war in which both groups drew upon their own special knowledge, experience, and needs. This model did not abolish role definitions—the veterans were essentially there to be helped and the professionals to help—but it placed more stress on mutuality and shared commitment. On another level, though, the veterans did not want to be shortchanged in terms of the help they wanted and needed. Their conflicting expectations and demands say much about the ambivalence that underlies the negotiations between physicians and patients trying to arrive at a satisfying helping relationship (even when these negotiations are only implicit or unspoken). In the first place, it makes any simple contrast between the "impersonal expert" and the "caring friend" unrealistic and dangerous. Responsible and responsive caring in the rap groups had to find a genuine mixture of human equality (especially with respect to our common survivorship) and helpful professional expertise. Similarly, medical professionals must retain real pride in the knowledge and skills of their craft, while at the same time not reflexively offering and applying techniques and interpretations that fail to respond to the patient's psychological, physical, and historical actuality. The result of respect for the patient's self-generation and autonomy is not, then, the relinquishing of special knowledge and the prerogatives of expertise, but it is the ability to discover— without predetermination or intimidation—just what the person is seeking.

3

Considered historically, the attempt to bring these ambivalent demands and values into some kind of balance carries on the competition between views of medicine as primarily art or primarily science. The work of Barbara Sicherman in this volume illustrates this tension in earlier periods, in which physicians' loyalties were divided between more traditional reliance on social and psychological observation and intuition, and the emerging methodologies of scientific laboratory investigation. Central to the view of medicine as art is the recognition that both physician and patient are enmeshed in social, political, and economic realities that impinge on the ultimate possibilities for well-being, the availability of expert care, and the direction and outcome of treatment. Although not necessarily formulated in these words, this was the implicit view of the second model for the rap group sessions just described.

Considered *psycho*historically, the current conflict between these views manifests the themes of survivorship and technicism. The technicist model in medicine and psychiatry works something like this: A machine, the mind-body function of the patient, has broken down; another machine, more scientifically sophisticated— the physician-psychiatrist—is called upon to "treat" the first machine; and the treatment process itself, being technical, has nothing to do with time, place, or individual idiosyncrasy. It is merely a matter of being a technical-medical antagonist of a "syndrome" or "disease." Within the healing professions, the problem is not so much the medical model as such— which is here admittedly overdrawn—as it is the technicism operating within that model.[6]

Technicism feeds on—and is fed by—a denial of acting within and upon history. In medicine, this denial may take the form of a refusal to notice the complex moral and social implications of decisions such as whom to treat, when to stop treatment, and the use of patients for experimental purposes. Each of these issues has ramifications beyond the immediate diagnostic and therapeutic intervention, and rightfully involves a network of people in the decision-making process. The actions and procedures indicated by specifically scientific and technical considerations may not exhaust the significant options in a particular case, even though seeking counsel and judgment from other sources exposes the professional to a more complicated, no longer omniscient, and less autonomous view of medical practice.[7]

Denial may also insulate the healer from the bewildering and frightening aspects of suffering and death. In this sense, technicism is directly related to the psychology of the survivor, particularly to psychic numbing. Once again, it is a refusal of full engagement in the personal and social realities of the healing situation. The use of technologically sophisticated instruments and machinery in the hospital can serve the process of psychic numbing in many ways that are similar to the process observed among Hiroshima survivors. By cutting off communication, for example, as with continuous mechanical ventilation, or by immobilizing and confining patients during extensive diagnostic procedures such as endoscopy, radiologic examination, or cardiac catheterization, the physician is distanced from the immediate human experience of the patient. This distancing may interrupt the potential identification process of the survivor-physician with the victim-patient, as in the Hiroshima survivor's unconscious equation, "I see you dying, but I am not related to you or your death." Similarly, these procedures may protect the physician from feelings of helplessness and impotence in the face of intractable disease and pain.

All of these results can be genuinely adaptive responses on the part of the medical staff as a whole, not unlike those of survivors in disasters of many kinds.[8] At the same time, they can contribute

substantially to the isolation of the profession from empathic respect for the autonomy and actuality of its clients, and from the
legitimate interests of other sectors of society in the patterns,
methods, and values of medical care. These trends are reinforced
and solidified, then, by the fact that technicism as a model of
professional competence and expertise links up with internal,
psychological mechanisms called into play by the circumstances of
actual care-giving.

Technicism further isolates the professional from what might
be called "animating guilt." In contrast to static (neurotic) forms
of guilt and immobilizing self-condemnation, animating guilt can
provide energy toward change via the capacity to examine the
roots of that guilt in both social and individual terms.[9] The rap
group experiences raised questions about the extent to which
everyday work in our profession, and the professions in general,
tends to wash away rather than pursue fundamental struggles
around integrity—the extent to which the special armor of professionals' technicism blocks free exchange between them and the
people they intend to serve. One of the principal values of this
free exchange is the opportunity it affords for self-criticism.

The type of self-criticism that emerged for psychiatrists dealing
with Vietnam veterans centered around the veterans' special
anger toward chaplains and "shrinks" who blessed the troops,
their mission, and their killing, or "helped" them to remain on
duty and (in many cases) to carry on with the daily commission of
war crimes. In a sense, the chaplains and psychiatrists formed an
unholy alliance, not only with the military command, but also with
the more corruptible elements in the soldier's psyche, corruptible
elements available to all of us, whether soldier, chaplain, or psychiatrist.[10]

The same kind of self-criticism and willingness to pursue feelings of guilt and responsibility is required by the nature and
organization of current medical practice, even in more ordinary
situations. For example, how is the physician's impact on the state
of public health affected by the concentration of medical expertise, sophistication, and education in major hospital centers? To

what extent do the prestige and stimulation attached to medical research and the treatment of certain complex and challenging pathologies tend to denigrate the less spectacular—and often more psychologically demanding—maintenance of patients with chronic conditions, which often requires extensive knowledge of and sympathy with a patient's life-style, occupation, and family structure? How often are decisions as to which patients to treat, and to what extent, affected by the point of intersection of a patient's moment of need with the trajectory of the physician's career?

A spirit of free exchange would encourage self-criticism on the part of the patient, as well as the collaboration and partnership that can at least potentially inform physician-patient relations and allow questioning of the way social or legislative trends victimize both professionals and clients. Central to the issue of malpractice, for example, are deep questions of public expectations of the medical profession that stem both from ignorance of the complexity of the medical art and from a fear of dying. In this case, the physician could attempt to complement the pervasive quantitative measurement of the good life in our society—with its consequent insistence that the doctor extend life under almost all circumstances and with almost any effects—with a traditional medical concern for the overall quality of life, for the well-being of the individual as an autonomous and dignified person. By educating people to the rhythms and cycles of vigor and decline, by being realistic in assessing infirmity without appearing to lose interest, enthusiasm, or patience, and by carefully evaluating the possibilities of various resuscitative measures, physicians might become resources for human understanding and courage, rather than, as is frequently the case, first agents of delusion and false hope, and then sudden bearers of devastating news.

To introduce these concerns into the medical encounter requires that the physician assume a measure of responsibility to values and norms that surpass the dictates of "state-of-the-art" techniques and therapies. And this in turn implies the recognition that past standards of professional excellence and advancement

may have ignored or subverted these values. Animating guilt—
the awareness of error and shortcoming coupled with insight into
the social and personal factors contributing to that shortcoming
—thus initiates for the professional important struggles around
living and working that have to do with intactness and wholeness,
with what we have called integrity. And because these struggles
emerge out of relations of mutuality and sharing, the fruits of
insight and commitment to change extend beyond the profession
to those whom it serves.

4

The medical student in search of professional integrity is thus
pulled in two directions. On the one hand there is the drive toward integration with peers and colleagues, toward the assumption of a professional identity. This requires the acquisition of
knowledge, skills, and techniques, and the result is a sense of
connection to the profession as a whole. This sense of connection
is vital to all psychic life, and it is one of the first victims of a literal
or symbolic death immersion.[11] In fact, the student's sense of
connection is threatened by the many forms of guilt and isolation
discussed earlier, as, for example, when technical skill thrusts the
student into circumstances where that skill is frequently inadequate to maintain life, or where sophisticated but costly procedures must be withheld from many people who would benefit
from them. Technicism and psychic numbing often come into
play to preserve professional integrity from these threats. On the
other hand, the student may attempt to confront his or her
animating guilt, and to face the issues of survivorship and loss of
innocence that attend the acquisition of expertise and competence. Therewith begins the struggle for another kind of integrity
that is preserved, not by the denials and isolation of the technicist
image of the profession, but by a renewed image that emerges
from that very struggle.

One source of perspective on that struggle is a return to the
root ideas of profession, the idea of what it means to profess.
Indeed, an examination of the evolution of these two words could

provide something close to a cultural history of the West. The Latin prefix *pro* means forward, toward the front, forth, out, or into a public position. *Fess* derives from the Latin *fateri* or *fass,* meaning to confess, own, acknowledge. To profess (or be professed), then, originally meant a personal form of out-front public acknowledgment. And that which was acknowledged or "confessed" always (until the sixteenth century) had to do with religion, with taking vows of a religious order or declaring one's religious faith. But as society became secularized, the word came to mean "to make claim to have knowledge of an art or science" or "to declare oneself expert or proficient in" an enterprise of any kind. The noun form, *profession,* came to suggest not only the act of professing but also the ordering, collectivization, and transmission of the whole process. The sequence was from "profession" of religious conviction (from the twelfth century) to a particular order of "professed persons," such as monks or nuns (fourteenth century) to "the occupation which one professes to be skilled in and follow," especially "the three learned professions of divinity, law, and medicine" along with the "military profession." So quickly did the connotations of specialization and application take hold that as early as 1605 Francis Bacon could complain: "Amongst so many great foundations of colleges in Europe, I find strange that they are all dedicated to professions, and none left free to Art and Sciences at large."[12]

Thus the poles of meaning around the image of profession shifted from the proclamation of personal dedication to transcendent principles to mastery of a specialized form of socially applicable knowledge and skill and membership in a group that possessed such mastery. In either case, the profession is immortalizing—the one through the religious mode, the other through works and social-intellectual tradition. And the principles of public proclamation and personal discipline carry over from the one meaning to the other—the former taking the shape of study, training, and dedication, the latter of examination and licensing. Overall, the change was from advocacy based on faith to technique devoid of advocacy.

One can observe this process in the modern separation of *profes-*

sion from *vocation*. Vocation also has a religious origin in the sense of being "called by God" to a "particular function or station." The secular equivalent became the idea of a personal "calling" in the sense of overwhelming inclination, commitment, and even destiny. But the Latin root, *vocare*, "to call," includes among its meanings and derivatives vocable, vocation, vouch, advocate, advocation, convoke, evoke, invoke, provoke, and revoke. Advocacy is thus built into the original root and continuing feel of the word *vocation;* and vocation in turn is increasingly less employed in connection with the work a man or woman does.

To be sure, contemporary professions do contain general forms of advocacy: in law, of a body of suprapersonal rules applicable to everyone; in medicine, of healing; and in psychiatry, of humane principles of well-being and growth. But immediate issues of value-centered advocacy and choice (involving groups and causes served and consequences thereof) are mostly ignored. In breaking out of the premodern trap of immortalization by personal surrender to faith, the "professional" has fallen into the modern trap of pseudo-neutrality and covert immortalization through technique. As a result, our professions are all too ready to offer their techniques to anyone and anything. I am not advocating a return to pure faith as a replacement for the contemporary idea of what profession means. But I am suggesting that the notion of profession needs to include these issues of advocacy and ethical commitment. One must distinguish, among other things, between group integration and integrity—the latter including moral and psychological elements that connect one to social and historical contexts beyond the immediate. Group integration can undermine integrity, as, for instance, in Vietnam, where both soldier and psychiatrist had to grapple with the struggles to adapt to institutions and goals seen as absurd and evil. The clear implication here is that the psychiatrist, no less than the combat soldier, was confronted with the important question of the group he was to serve and, above all, the nature and the consequences of its immediate and long-range mission. Facing that question, and such questions embedded in medical practice as those alluded to earlier, requires that we overcome the technicist assumption that we fall into all too easily, namely: "Because I am a healer, anything I do, anywhere, is good." It may not be.

Nor does embracing this heritage of advocacy imply a renunciation of scientific rigor and competence. For the profession of medicine in particular, it has been cogently argued that complete knowledge of the particular individual to be treated, although unattainable absolutely, would have to include knowledge of the *good* of that individual, and all the factors that contribute to maintaining that good. Rigorous diagnosis and treatment, then, implies advocacy on behalf of values that enable life not only to continue, but to prosper.[13]

The image of the healing profession and the concept of professional integrity that appear from this perspective would view people undergoing discomfort or incapacity, and the "healers" or "professionals" of any kind from whom they sought assistance, as coming together at a particular historical moment during which a culture tends to promote certain styles or types of disturbance (or deformation) and certain kinds of "treatment." The understanding that their approach is only one among many sociohistorical possibilities could foster, among "healers" (not only medically oriented, but also teachers, clergymen, and in many cases social and political activists, too), crucial restraints against technicism and claims to omniscience. With that knowledge also conveyed to those who seek help or change, choices are possible for everyone: "Seekers" may select healers sympathetic to the forms and goals they wish to cultivate (whether having to do with modes of therapy, directions of change, or forms of clinician-patient interaction); and even if their quest for health and personal integration should lead them to modify or abandon these forms, they would be active agents in those decisions rather than becoming passively entrapped in someone else's expertise. Healers, in turn, would make conscious decisions about where to apply their capacities, according to the personal and professional forms they seek to investigate or cultivate. Professionals could thus combine the technical knowledge and skill associated with the profession with ethical and political decisions concerning what they do, to what effect, and for whose benefit. And these decisions would involve not only people with whom they seek to work, but also institutions and groups with whom they become affiliated and the overall question of the extent to which they lend their talents to perpetuating—as opposed to significantly changing—existing social and political arrangements. What I am suggesting is that the healer, no less than the seeker, functions intellectually and ethically from a particular formative place, and from a particular relationship to history.

5

This view of the profession draws special attention to the process of medical education. Much of what has been said here reflects a concern for a recovery of the broad range of "caring tasks" discussed elsewhere in this volume by John Stoeckle in connection with educational reform. In addition, however, the experience in the rap groups suggests certain elements of that reform along the lines of a model for change I have elaborated in earlier work, based on a sequence of confrontation, reordering, and renewal.[14] Indeed, the rap groups may represent the type of forum in which medical students and their instructors could work together on the issues of common survivorship, moral conflict, and hierarchical distancing that emerge in clinical practice and in the educational process itself.

Specifically, confrontation in medical education would involve taking seriously the ancient paradigm of death and the continuity of life. This in turn could relate living and dying to larger historical processes, and help physicians cast off their death- and life-denying image of themselves as technicians of the human body, or even of being itself. Genuine confrontation would require combining intellectual recognition of death with critical examination of one's own (and one's patients') life and death, and probing, not once, but continuously, our own modes of symbolic immortality —the ways in which our ultimate concerns enter our lives and work. This in turn would call forth risk, make it conscious and legitimate, and raise fundamental questions not only about man's own mortality but about the mortality of ideas, techniques, and institutions. Always at issue would be the many forms of collective psychic numbing that now desensitize the profession to critical ethical questions.

Reordering would entail the joint (student-instructor) examination of various forms of professional guilt, whether associated with technicist transgressions (mechanical, institutional, or chemical—as, for instance, in the wide prescriptive use of tranquilizers or antibiotics) or exploitative arrangements of any kind—ultimately with a critical examination of the present ethical-historical "place" of the profession. This continuing pursuit of integrity and wholeness, once initiated in the reordering process, could become self-energizing, in the true sense ecstatic, as one experiences a new level of harmony around being both a professional and a person. But such integrity and harmony in turn depend upon altered institutional and group arrangements in the direction of more human professional sensitivities at all levels of medical education, including the truly humble participation of "experts" and instructors in this very enterprise.

Renewal in the medical profession, and in medical education, would center upon desperately needed breaking out from technicism and numbing, and especially the social extension of the capacity to feel. The crucial process might well be the rediscovery of professional play. "Being professional" has too long stood for the antithesis of being playful, thereby narrowing professional function to rules and responsibilities and eliminating the very qualities of imagination and spontaneity that would render professional work more sensitive and humane. Involved here are the joyful possibilities of the marriage of professional discipline to this imaginative spontaneity, the coming together of ethic and technique, the playful freedom from denial, isolation, and claimed omniscience that can live with the demands of ultimate concern and the ambiguity of unpredictable change.

Finally, this view requires that the process of medical education

itself be seen in its own social and historical context. To a great
extent, the professional image just described is not so much new
as old. As this essay has tried to show, notions of advocacy, historical and ethical consciousness, and reliance on empathic sharing of
patients' actuality are rooted in the history of the medical art. Yet
these values, like all the dominant symbols of order and meaning
in contemporary life, have been radically confused by a combination of forces: the breakdown of commonly shared symbolic
systems, the flooding of new imagery provided by the com-
munications revolution, and the overarching dangers of nuclear
annihilation and environmental poisoning which threaten to
make all purposeful striving appear absurd. In addition,
medicine's successive epochs of technical and scientific transformation have created new issues, sources of professional pride and
of intellectual and personal fulfillment that compete for attention
and devotion. This loss of permanent structures of order and
meaning, which I have elsewhere called our "metaphorical survivorship," stimulates a continual quest for new possibilities and
combinations of meaning and value, accompanied, however, by
considerable distrust of permanence, stability, and commitment.[15]
This would seem to be an important consideration in connection
with the institutionalization of curricular reforms. That is, the
renewal of professional advocacy and sensitivity cannot be imposed as one dogma in place of another. Rather, it is an important
task of medical education to bring into fresh relief the heritage of
value advocacy and personal openness that endures in the midst
of this continual novelty and transformation—both societal and
professional—and among countertendencies toward freezing
oneself defensively in constricted, rigidly held images of professional purity and omniscience.

I want to conclude with two quotations. The first is from Stanley Milgram, who performed controversial experiments on the
willingness of people to cause pain and even endanger the lives of
others, when authoritatively requested to do so. Whatever one's
views of the scientific and moral aspects of these "Eichmann experiments," one of Milgram's own conclusions is worth thinking

about: "Men are doomed if they act only within the alternatives handed down to them."[16] And finally, Joseph Campbell, the distinguished American student of mythology: "A god outgrown becomes immediately a life-destroying demon. The form has to be broken and the energies released."[17]

NOTES

1. *The Structure of Scientific Revolutions* (Chicago: University of Chicago Press, 1962).

2. *Death in Life: Survivors of Hiroshima* (New York: Random House, 1967). See esp. chap. 12, "The Survivor."

3. *Philosophy in a New Key* (Cambridge: Harvard University Press, 1942); *Feeling and Form* (New York: Scribners, 1953); *Philosophical Sketches* (Baltimore: Johns Hopkins Press, 1962); and *Mind: An Essay on Human Feeling,* 2 vols. (Baltimore; Johns Hopkins Press, 1967, 1972). See also Ernst Cassirer, *An Essay on Man* (New York: Doubleday Anchor, 1944); *The Myth of the State* (New York: Doubleday Anchor, 1946); and *The Philosophy of Symbolic Forms,* 3 vols. (New Haven: Yale University Press, 1953–57).

4. See Robert Jay Lifton, *Home from the War* (New York: Simon and Schuster, 1973), chap. 13, "On Change."

5. For a detailed description of the rap group experience, see *Home from the War,* chap. 3, "Rap Groups."

6. In this sense I am in sympathy with Thomas Szasz and Ronald Laing in their stress on the repressive uses of the medical model, but also with Humphrey Osmond's defense of the enduring, human core of the medical model, which has "stood the test of the millennia" and still contains untapped resources for us, although requiring liberation from its technicist fetters. Szasz, *The Myth of Mental Illness* (New York: Harper and Row, 1961); Laing, *The Divided Self* (London: Penguin, 1960) and *The Politics of Experience* (New York: Ballantine, 1967); Osmond, "The Medical Model in Psychiatry: Love It or Leave It," *Medical Annals of the District of Columbia,* 41 (1972):171-75.

7. See Jay Katz and Alexander Capron, *Catastrophic Diseases: Who Decides What?* (New York: Russell Sage Foundation, 1975).

8. Lifton, *Death in Life,* pp. 500 *ff.*

9. Robert Jay Lifton, "Questions of Guilt" (presentation and exchange of views with Leslie H. Farber), *Partisan Review,* 39 (Fall 1972): 514–30.

10. The October 1971 issue of *The American Journal of Psychiatry* contains a description by Douglas R. Bey, Jr., and Walter E. Smith of their "workable method of organizational consultation developed and employed in a combat

division in Vietnam" ("Organizational Consultation in a Combat Unit," vol. 128, 401–06). They acknowledge that commanders "were far better prepared to work out solutions to their problems than we, since their area of expertise was in administration and fighting whereas ours was in the area of helping them to see where their feelings might be interfering with their use of these skills." To back up their position they quote, appropriately enough, from an article by General W. C. Westmoreland recommending that the psychiatrist assume a "personnel management consultation type role." The title of Westmoreland's article— "Mental Health—An Aspect of Command"—makes quite clear just whom psychiatry in the military is supposed to serve. The authors' combination of easy optimism and concern for everyone's feelings and for the group as a whole makes one almost forget the kinds of activities the members of that group were engaged in. Reading that lead article in the official journal of the national organization of U.S. psychiatrists gave me a disturbing sense of how far this kind of managerial technicism could take a profession, and its reasonably decent practitioners, into ethical corruption. I do not exempt myself from this critique, for I served as a military psychiatrist in the Korean War under conditions at least somewhat parallel to those discussed here.

11. Robert Jay Lifton, "The Sense of Immortality: On Death and the Continuity of Life," *American Journal of Psychoanalysis*, 33, no. 1 (1973): 3–15.

12. Quotations and etymological sequences are from the *Oxford English Dictionary* and the *American Heritage Dictionary*.

13. Samuel Gorovitz and Alasdair MacIntyre, "Toward a Theory of Medical Fallibility," *The Journal of Medicine and Philosophy*, 1, no. 1 (March 1976): 51–71.

14. Robert Jay Lifton, *Thought Reform and the Psychology of Totalism* (New York: Norton, 1961), pp. 462–72; and *Home from the War*, chaps. 13 and 14.

15. Robert Jay Lifton, *History and Human Survival* (New York: Random House, 1970), chap. 15, "Protean Man."

16. "Behavioral Study of Obedience," *Journal of Abnormal and Social Psychology*, 67 (1963): 371–78; "The Compulsion to Do Evil," *Patterns of Prejudice* (London), 1 (November–December 1967); and *Obedience to Authority* (New York: Harper and Row, 1974).

17. *The Hero with a Thousand Faces* (New York: Meridian, 1956).

CHAPTER 4

The Crisis Dyad: Meaning and Culture in Anthropology and Medicine

Anthony Oliver-Smith

Once again, a critical experience in the life of a social scientist provides the point of departure for a discussion that affirms important values in both social science and medicine. Indeed, nowhere is it more apparent than in Anthony Oliver-Smith's essay that exchange between these two disciplines fosters the type of mutual self-criticism advocated by Robert Jay Lifton. In this case, the probing investigation of a person's life, the imparting of information, and the task of formulating contexts of meaning are seen as essential features of both anthropological research and patient care. The connection becomes more apparent—and the implications more profound—in the case of research into surviving natural disaster and relating to dying patients.

Underlying both the anthropologist's and the physician's situations is the question, What is the proper "scientific" attitude toward one's subject—or patient—and where do personal and scientific responsibilities begin and end? Oliver-Smith identifies one particular responsibility that binds the scientific and personal dimensions together. It is the commitment to assist subjects or patients to formulate a meaning for critical events that allows them to remain human, in the richest sense of that term, embracing the full range of cultural and symbolic adaptive powers, throughout the personality-threatening chaos of intense suffering or impending death. The real test of this commitment arises in the actual attempt to construct meaning. Here, the professional—anthropologist or physician—must enter into a genuine negotiation with the subject or patient to discover a language and set of meaningful symbols compatible with traditions for understanding that are already part of the life experience of each. This negotiation is complicated by a fact discussed by Rogers and Lifton: Professionals' structures of meaning are often as vulnerable as those of their clients. Oliver-Smith's own encounter with this issue forms the basis for his appreciation of intimate acquaintance and sharing in the crisis dyad as helping both partners fashion a meaningful sense of themselves and their world.

The extent to which Oliver-Smith advocates a mutual disclosure of world views by patient and physician, and the completeness of fit between the anthropological and medical situations, may provoke honest debate. Yet two points are clear. First, the construction of shared meaning is not a casual afterthought to either social research or clinical medicine, but is central to the humanistic performance of each. Second, the many examples within medicine of faithful and sensitive care of the dying are models with much to teach other disciplines, including those from which medicine, too, can learn.

> A tremendous gap surrounded man: he did not know how to justify, explain or affirm himself, he suffered from the problem of his meaning. He suffered in other ways too; he was in the main a sickly animal; yet suffering as such was not his problem; but that the answer was lacking to the cry of the question, "Why suffer?" Man, as the animal that is most courageous, most accustomed to suffering, does not negate suffering as such; he wants it, even seeks it out, provided one shows him some meaning in it, some wherefore of suffering. The meaninglessness of suffering, not suffering itself, was the curse which hitherto lay spread out over mankind.
> —Friedrich Nietzsche, "Toward a Genealogy of Morals"

For most human beings, the problem of meaning becomes acute only in extreme circumstances. Otherwise, we are remarkably unquestioning. Indeed, we have a ready set of culturally acceptable answers to most of the questions that arise from the events of normal existence. Culture provides us all with a context for extracting meaning from experience. Culture, as a set of rules and meanings, constitutes the primary adaptive mechanism human beings use to cope with the problems presented by their total environment.

The varieties of cultural forms of adaptation developed by human beings to the myriad environments in which they live constitute the prime focus of anthropological inquiry. To pursue this interest, the anthropologist becomes involved in the lives of the people with whom the research is undertaken. The anthropologist must live their reality, must share their experience as much as possible, to gain an accurate and profound understanding of a people and their culture. The critical examination of the anthropologist's own "self" and values, as well as the significant relationships with informants, are crucial in evaluating scientific observation and analysis.[1] When this examination of self and other in crosscultural interaction takes place in a context of extreme individual or societal stress, insights from such anthropological research may suggest fruitful perspectives on health care and medical education.

Because human beings are prismatic creatures existing in a number of different orders of reality (physical, biological, social, and psychological), human adaptation is exceptionally complex, occurring on a multiplicity of levels. It is a truism that human life must survive symbolically as well as physically. Human adaptation is far more complex than that of other animals primarily because human beings are aware not only of themselves as unique individuals, but also of their own mortality.[2] Ernest Becker, a cultural anthropologist developing certain psychoanalytic themes, principally of Freud, Rank, and Adler, posits that the anxiety from this awareness is the basic condition of the human species.[3] The individual must counter this anxiety at his own finitude with an affirmation of primary and lasting worth, a sense of self-esteem founded in the fulfillment of cultural norms. Self-esteem is constituted in the statement, "I am significant, meaningful in the cosmos." Culture therefore becomes the context in which one measures one's primary worth and thereby denies the anxiety engendered by the awareness of death.

Part of human culture, then, is an adaptation to the self, to one's ability to conceive of one's own death, to the human condition. Culture erects a symbolic screen of meanings to shield us from despair at the inevitability of our fate. The essentially thin veil that culture spreads between us and despair, giving us the illusion of control and meaning in our lives and destinies, can be rent by historical accident, exposing us for agonizing moments to stare our fate in the face. Such a naked encounter cannot be endured for very long without the cushioning of culturally viable meanings. It is accident that causes us to question, to embark on quests for new ways to impose meaning on new events. The non-recurrent chance happenings of history must be explained, must be assigned meanings consistent with a culture's systems of belief. Culture prepares us for process, not for history; and people are unwilling "to leave events to themselves." [4] Events must be made coherent with some system of belief and meaning that integrates and supports the involved individual's view of himself or herself as significant in the cosmos. When tragedy strikes an individual or a society, our psychological adaptive powers enable us to mend the torn veil of our culture and restore to our condition, now perhaps altered, a meaning for the event that is congruent with the context of our culture, thereby preserving us from despair and disintegration. Meaning, then, is basic to human survival.

The need to explain, to find meanings in the casual events of nature, involves not only those immediately affected, but also, particularly in catastrophic events, those who witness and those who help. Interaction under these conditions often involves an asymmetrical professional-client relationship that I call the "crisis dyad." This relationship involves two individuals focusing for a variety of reasons on the extreme stress experienced by one of them. For present purposes, the essential element of the crisis dyad is the need for both parties either to extract from or to impose on the experiences of suffering and death a structure of meaning.

The crisis dyad is a formulation that issued from experiences in anthropological field work over five years in a community in the Peruvian Andes ravaged by a natural disaster. In May 1970, an earthquake devastated a large area in the north-central Andes and coastal regions of Peru. It was the worst natural disaster in the history of the Western Hemisphere, killing over 65,000 people and destroying over 80 percent of the structures in an area larger than Belgium and Holland combined. The center of this great destruction was the Andean city of Yungay. The earthquake dislodged a massive section of a glacier on Mt. Huascaran that overlooked the city, and more than 50 million cubic meters of mud, rock, and ice careened down the mountainside and in minutes entirely destroyed Yungay.[5] Approximately 300 people survived out of an estimated predisaster population of 4,500. Essentially, then, we are dealing with people who, to use Lifton's phrase, have had a "permanent encounter with death."[6] The ultimate life crisis has become a permanent, constant fixture in their lives.

An encampment of the survivors was organized less than a kilometer north of the avalanche scar. There, in the midst of their tragedy and destruction, the Yungainos set about the task of building a new town, a new society, and new meaning for their lives. In October 1970, I began a study of social change and disaster in the growing settlement, concentrating on the issues of social-structural change. In the four years after that initial research, I realized that my earlier studies left unanswered a number of profound questions about human adaptation to radical alteration of the social and physical environment. My initial study dealt with the way individuals and institutions adapted to the massive changes in social, political, economic, and demographic patterns brought about by the disaster. It left relatively unexplored the whole question of world view and ethos—that is, the nature of individual psychological adaptation to catastrophe and its ultimate relationship to changes in overall cultural patterns.

I decided to develop a research project that probed the questions of meaning and modes of adaptation of the Yungay survivors. A questionnaire was constructed that focused on the activities of the individual before and after the disaster, recollections of the day of impact and the immediate aftermath, personal loss and current feelings, values and beliefs relating to the relationship with the personal community, the community at large, the environment, the nation, and the world. These issues had all been very common topics of conversation in the survivors' camp in the immediate aftermath of the catastrophe. I felt that it would be relatively simple to conduct the interviews while I lived in the community for a few months and continued research with the more traditional anthropological methods of participant observa-

tion. Perhaps in more normal forms of research such an optimistic viewpoint might be justified. However, there are issues in research on human adaptation to suffering and catastrophe that
carry one to the cutting edge of professional ethics, and beyond
that to questions of simple human decency.

Conducting the initial interviews demonstrated more than
amply the difficulties involved in research through the crisis dyad.
Indeed, after approximately a half-dozen interviews, it became
apparent that structured interviews of the type traditionally used
by social scientists involve severe ethical compromises for the anthropological researcher in issues of human tragedy. Because of
the traditional participant-observation methods, anthropologists
often find themselves studying their friends, people to whom they
have not only a professional responsibility but also one based on
friendship and other cultural values. When subjects of research
are victims of catastrophe, direct, impersonal interviews querying
them on the nature of their loss and pain, as well as on their
efforts, possibly unsuccessful, toward rehabilitation in the aftermath, may bring to the surface emotions and recollections that
cause considerable anguish. Many of the questions rekindled in
the minds of the survivors scenes of hideous destruction and
agonizing grief. The avalanche and the immediate aftermath had
been a descent into hell for these people. Their entire social reality had been utterly destroyed before their eyes in less than four
minutes. Most of the survivors were left totally alone, completely
bereft of all the significant people in their lives. In the days following the avalanche, the mud began to settle, giving forth a grisly
harvest of mutilated and dismembered corpses. Contingents of
police watched over the burial of the dead in order to shoot the
wild dogs that were scavenging the bodies as they emerged
grotesquely on the viscous surface of the avalanche. The desperate search for relatives brought people face to face with indescrib-
able horrors. Many of the survivors still bear the imprint of those
first nightmarish weeks. Some will never recover.

Unwittingly, we had designed the questionnaire in such a way
as to probe mercilessly the most agonizing experiences of these

people's lives. The most intense personal suffering was to be examined through a coldly impersonal instrument. The questionnaire converted human suffering into check marks and human beings into interviews, data resources. In many ways, the questionnaire converted the process from an I-Thou relationship to an I-It relationship, in Martin Buber's terms.[7]

This is not a proper role for an anthropologist. Research in the crisis dyad places special requirements on the investigator. In undertaking research with people under long-term severe stress, the researcher acquires a heavy obligation to the informants and ultimately to science to provide as clear a meaning as possible for the subjects' experience of the research. In the case of disaster, the researcher cannot restore meaning structures assaulted by natural accident. However, a disaster (and, for that matter, most severe crisis experiences) involves more than simply impact. The post-impact experience includes further stages of isolation, rescue, and rehabilitation, which may often be as chaotic as the impact itself. Consequently, the researcher must assume a responsibility to assist the victim in formulating an understanding of the research process, for it is an integral part of the total disaster experience. In this context, the social scientist has inescapably pierced the (albeit mythical) shell of objectivity and has obligations to subjects that extend professional ethics into moral considerations based on shared experience and knowledge, as well as common humanity.

I would maintain that, although no exact parallel is present, similar obligations exist for health care professionals dealing with people afflicted with terminal illness and with the significant others of those afflicted. Just as it is insufficient, and ultimately unethical, to undertake research through the crisis dyad without regard for the psychic costs to a willing informant, so is it equally derelict to treat the dying patient solely on a medical basis, without regard for the emotional ordeal through which she or he is passing. Responsible involvement does not end at the completion of those functions most often associated with one's title. One must enter the crisis dyad not only as professional, but also as human being, at the very least to function as a presence with whom the search for new meanings can be undertaken. Put simply, professionals are challenged to facilitate acquisition by the patient or subject of a context of meaning for the experience, not only of the relevant aspects of their tragedy, but of the research or treatment as well. Ultimately, there seem to be no easy entrances or exits to the crisis dyad for either party.

The solution to the ethical and methodological dilemma I had inadvertently created lay in restructuring the engagement. The Yungainos were my friends and, thus, an interview schedule impersonally querying their tragedy was not only ethically compromising, but totally inappropriate. The formal questionnaire was abandoned in favor of a more loosely structured approach that would allow the individual to tell as much or as little as she or he pleased. The interview could then be transformed into a conversation initiated by a few general questions about postdisaster life.

In addition, although I had explained the purposes of my research before conducting interviews, I subsequently elaborated much more on what I felt to be the significance of the disaster and the research effort to me. I attempted to express some of my own doubts about the project, and I asked for my subjects' opinions of what I was doing. In essence, while actually doing the research, in most cases I attempted to involve the person in a mutual effort at extracting some sort of meaning from the research experience. It was very much a desperate effort on my part to create a sense of meaningful engagement for myself as well as for the Yungainos. It seemed that only through dialogue and meaning formation by both parties could the project become ethically tenable. It was also only through this process that true knowledge of the person's processes of adaptation could be gained. Methodologically, an impersonal questionnaire stultifies the freedom of expression that is vital to a full elaboration of such a process and encounter.

In essence, shared meanings had to be reached; and it was incumbent on me to facilitate this process by initiating an exchange. For both my subjects and myself, a meaning congruent with the values of each of our cultures had to be formulated, not only for the disaster itself, but also for the research experience. The Yungainos ethically should never have been forced into the role of passive research subjects. Their right and ability to participate in structuring the content of the interaction should have been preserved. Indeed, this was perhaps my primary responsibility. To undergo the research experience as initially constructed constituted another passage through the painful experiences of the past without a sufficient context. The Yungainos could not be asked to relive their pain and suffering again for reasons they did not understand and in a situation in which they had little control. Once the issues had been aired, they were able to exercise a measure of control over their participation and to derive some sense of meaning from the experience. In addition, the hyperobjectivity that had proved so pernicious to both informant and investigator was abandoned, enabling me to return to a more appropriate interaction with my friends and to view the project with a greater understanding of the self as a research instrument and the nature of social research.[8]

To return to the question of meaning, and to apply this perspective to the Western field of medicine, it is necessary to view medicine as a human invention and part of human culture. Like every other aspect of culture, medicine is concerned with the survival and adaptation of human beings to their circumstances and environment, processes that are always incomplete in human beings without the added element of a sense of meaning. Life-threatening or terminal illness, particularly (although not exclusively) in Western concepts of disease, may assault not only the physical integrity of the individual, but also the sense of logic and proportion, and the sense of right and justice. It may force the individual to look beyond the veil of cultural "truths" and to confront our ultimate destiny as human beings. In such a confrontation, the emotional support provided by a particular set of cultural truths may collapse. Indeed, catastrophic illness, like massive natural disaster, may demonstrate that one's culture, context for meaning, and protection from and denial of death have been rendered useless. Catastrophic illness is destruction of self, and of meaning. In a very real sense, culture in the guise of medicine in that context may be rendered helpless and desert the individual. Consequently, as in the case of the anthropologist involved in research with a disaster-stricken population, the health care professional's role in dealing with patients with catastrophic illness extends beyond the physical treatment of symptoms into an area where medical expertise may be useful, but not sufficient. Health care professionals face the challenge of assisting patients to reach a state where they may recover their adaptive faculties for structuring significant meanings for the experiences of illness and treatment. In the same sense, where illness is terminal, medicine (read culture, particularly Western culture, and its attendant meanings of death denial) has also deserted the physician. Indeed, it would seem that both patient and physician, much like the anthropologist and informant in high-stress conditions, must cope with the same realities, albeit from vastly different perspectives, and must extract meanings from a situation in which both parties are rendered ultimately helpless in the face of inevitability. The mutual formulation of meaning through professional-client dialogue would seem to offer a fruitful approach to this difficult process.

The patient faced with life-threatening illness must cope with a number of elements. The symptoms of the disease and their effects on the individual's physical and psychological state are among the most immediate sources of stress. In addition— particularly in modern Western culture, in which much disease is chronic rather than acute—the patient must come to terms with the treatment and new regimen. The survivor of Yungay was similarly faced with new realities, one of which was a heightened realization of the precarious nature of life. The research on their adaptation to the disaster was also a unique experience and became a new element to understand in their altered life-style.

In the hospital, the problems of physical symptoms and altered life-style are further compounded by another set of problems that may be considered as extensions of the status and role of patienthood. Patienthood is characterized in the literature by "dependency," "captivity," and a lack of sovereignty. Talcott Parsons considers illness to be "a socially institutionalized role type" characterized by an inability to perform the normally expected tasks or roles associated with the individual when healthy.[9] In other words, although it is socially recognized that the individual is not responsible for the ailment, he or she is no longer performing those functions which have meaning and provide a sense of worth and self-esteem in his or her own eyes or in the eyes of culture and society. Consequently, the personal and cultural bases for the sense of the self as a "meaningful object of primary value" may be assaulted by illness; and the more grave the illness, the more severe may be the erosion of a sense of worth in terms of personal and cultural value structures. Meaning retreats as self-esteem is eroded. The consequent loss of self may hasten the total disintegration of the person both physically and psychologically.[10] In Yungay, the sense of helplessness in the face of disaster, compounded by the extreme dependency of the survivors on outside aid, made the maintenance of a sense of self-worth extremely difficult and severely inhibited the process of rehabilitation in many individuals. In general, the year following the disaster in Yungay was characterized by a high consumption of alcohol, general intragroup violence, a variety of psychosomatic ailments, anxiety, and depression.

Another aspect of patienthood is the lack of equilibrium in social interaction. On becoming ill, a person has stepped outside not only traditional statuses and roles but also the traditional culture. The realm of the physician, the hospital, is a different cultural system with different symbols and different behaviors, all open to widely varying interpretation by the unacculturated patient. Patients entering the hospital for care are frequently under severe stress and are often extremely suggestible and open to influence.[11] The multiplicity of new roles and statuses (including his or her own), the unfamiliar and highly complex technology, and the "mystery and ritual" of modern medical procedure make the patient almost immediately abjectly dependent upon the physician for an accurate understanding of the new surroundings. Although power differential is a structural characteristic of all relationships, rarely is there as much asymmetry as in the patient-physician crisis dyad.[12] As physicians deal with greater power as well as freedom, the burden of ethical responsibility in the interaction falls to them. Power is the crucial variable that assigns primary responsibility for one's values and actions in any relationship. In terms of understanding the context and meaning of the situation, the patient may have only a vague understanding, not only of the disease, but also of the rationale of the therapeutic program. It is therefore incumbent upon the physician to act as guide for the patient who is a stranger as well as the director of the therapeutic regimen.

As the sophistication of medical procedures and technology increases, the obligation to assist patients at meaning formulation becomes more acute. When culture fails, as it inevitably must, to protect us from our fate (whether disease or disaster, it is always an accident!), we look increasingly to medicine first for salvation and ultimately for a context of meaning for what is happening to us. In our present culture, with its scientific world view and technological emphasis, it is most natural that meaning provision should fall to those who, for better or for worse, are seen by laymen as occupying the vanguard of these trends.

The professional may not initiate the crisis-dyad interaction, or control its outcome, but he or she may be the key individual in structuring the process of meaning formation for the events on which the relationship is focused. In the crisis dyad involving a terminally ill patient, both patient and doctor must come to terms with failure—one, the failure to survive, the other, the failure to save. Both must formulate from their own perspectives, in a mutual process, a structure of meaning for the patient's condition, treatment, and fate. Each becomes crucial to the other in the resolution of the crisis event.

Most seriously or incurably ill patients respond best to honesty.[13] In the past ten years, extensive research has shown that most dying people, if given a chance, are willing to discuss their problem. Indeed, even in cases of severe denial, some aspect of the truth is already realized.[14] For the physician to engage in a charade with a patient seeking the truth is to endanger the compact of trust between the two. The difference between a healthy dependency and a sick victim rests on the nature and degree of trust between patient and physician.[15] Such a relationship must be predicated on more than a physician's reputation for technical expertise. It must evolve in the crisis dyad through mutual attempts to understand what is happening and what must be faced. It involves a mutual disclosure of not only "medically relevant" information, but also of each individual's personal perspectives on the problems of human life.

The manner and content of what the physician communicates should be based on as extensive a knowledge of the patient and his or her life situation as possible.[16] Indeed, it is incumbent on physicians to have acquainted themselves as profoundly as possible not only with the patient's medical history, but with the patient's cultural values and world view as well. One of the difficulties in this aspect of the interaction is that patients often expect very scientific explanations, which become the "meaning" of the symptoms for them. Yet it is crucial that the person be able to assimilate even this type of explanation. This means that cultural background, religion, intelligence, and family structure all become relevant in deciding how to convey information. Without a sensitivity to the importance of these factors, the physician cannot know just what the patient can assimilate.

The need for accurate description of the scientific "facts of the case" must be balanced with the understanding that the patient is not an empty vessel, without any capacity for meaning-making at all. In fact, the patient has a responsibility for making a final "fit" between the new life experience as communicated by the physician and all previous experience and traditions. To help the patient accomplish this fit, though, the doctor must be aware of these individual variables, and the doctor and patient should negotiate a balance between the scientific explanation and the patient's legitimate resources for meaning-making. However, there is very little in clinical medicine that cannot be explained to both patient and family in lay language and "demystified" medical terms.[17] It should also be appreciated that "religious" and scientific explanations do not preclude each other. Meaning formulation tends to be a mosaic of many elements.[18] Scientific knowledge should be respected but should not overwhelm the patient's own capacities and symbol systems, since in the long run these personal and cultural resources must be the foundation upon which a meaning is based. Physicians must attempt to provide contexts of meaning that can merge with the patient's own powers and traditions.

It is obvious that a complex, scientifically oriented explanation of the etiology and prognosis of a condition does little to prepare patients for what is to come if their educational and cultural backgrounds are posited on different assumptions than the modern scientific world view. It is equally obvious that an explanation founded on a simplistic, mystical, or childlike interpretation of a disease's course may be ineffective with patients whose world view and culture in general place them squarely within the scientific model. Even worse, perhaps, such an explanation may also endanger trust, respect, and self-esteem in the patient who feels the physician does not respect him or her sufficiently to deal in a straightforward fashion.

This need for sensitivity to the patient's total life situation implies that the physician be more than "truthteller." Still within the role of physician, she or he must also become more than healer, in many senses functioning as much or more as a companion in the ordeal as the patient's family members. Particularly when family members become too threatened by their own fear of annihilation, by the sights and smells of disease, or by the atmosphere of helplessness and despair, it is crucial that the physician become a "significant other," an ally when others have abandoned the patient in the final struggle. In the final stages of terminal illness, when coping with finality may become most difficult, the presence or absence of significant others may be crucial in a final resolution before death.[19] However, at this stage the physician, regardless of a role as significant other, may acknowledge defeat and retreat, precisely when "presence," as opposed to medical skill, is most needed by the patient. The physician's role as friend and listener continues after all therapeutic alternatives have been exhausted. The physician must be "with" the patient.

The importance of being "with" the sufferer was particularly impressed upon me when I returned to Yungay several years after the disaster. During the year following the avalanche, when the Yungainos experienced their most intense grief and suffering, I was unaware that my presence had acquired any symbolic importance to the community at large. It was a year of incredible hardship and pain for the people of Yungay who, because of a number of rehabilitation-administration decisions, had felt abandoned to their misery. When I returned some years later, I was introduced to newcomers in the community simply: "This is Tony. He was with us." In the crisis dyad, the power of sharing an experience becomes immeasurably important. Presence becomes meaning. In this context, to be present means to share; and to share means to acquire a measure of knowledge of another's experience through dialogue.

Physicians, even as they become members of the patient's group of significant others, should take great care to avoid the anticipatory grief that will be experienced by the patient and members of his or her family. As a surrogate mourner, the physician only displays helplessness in the face of the inevitable.[20] The physician must remain a source of hope, becoming a symbol of order, structure, and control in the face of chaos and the unknown. Helplessness to save the patient can be mitigated by abilities to ease discomfort, to render a sense of order and dignity to the patient's passage through the crisis.[21] The physician serves a valuable purpose simply by being "with" the patient, not as mourner, but as ally and companion. Solitude is terrifying, for it is the loss of self before the fact. The loss of self is the loss of meaning.[22] The physician, perhaps even more than others, can forestall the loss of self and meaning through the preservation of self-esteem and self-recognition, both by allowing and requiring the patient to participate meaningfully in the decisions that remain in his or her life.[23]

The health care professional involved in treating a patient with a life-threatening ailment is also confronted with an assault on culturally formulated meaning structures. Indeed, the cultural cushioning that protects most of us in modern Western society from facing the ultimate realities of life is under constant pressure in medical people from the context and environment of their chosen professions. Critical events are more frequent in medical life, but they do not lend themselves any more easily to interpretation for their familiarity. The physician and other health care professionals are not immune to the need to formulate some meaning for the critical experiences of life.

Many of the fears with which the patient must cope on the most immediate levels also oppress the physician, albeit from a different perspective. The patient with a terminal illness must cope physically and psychologically with suffering and approaching death, ideally and ultimately becoming able to perceive it within a satisfactory structure of meaning. Physicians, in treatment and contact with the patient, are constantly reminded of their own vulnerability.[24] Dying patients force doctors to recognize their own mortality and confront unresolved feelings about death, experiences most of us are loath to undertake. The physician must come to terms with this experience and reality much more often in a lifetime than the rest of us. Small wonder that doctors have been known to avoid or deal perfunctorily with dying patients. The death immersion requires either a resolved or formulated meaning for death in one's own life, or the psychic numbing of those stimuli of death anxiety that would eventually be immobilizing.[25]

"As physicians we accept commitment to the lifelong conflict. Every instinct, drive and desire—every intellectual and emotional sinew has been trained to defeat death."[26] The physician's goal, like the goal of culture in general, is doomed to failure. The physician, as physician, can only postpone. Culture can protect only temporarily with denials and illusions of control. Not only is the physician unable to give patients anything more than a postponement, but his or her own existence, which is chartered in the struggle to defeat death, is also finite. The finiteness of life may be an even heavier burden for the physician than for the rest of us. Indeed, unless they have arrived at a formulation of the concept and meaning of death in their own lives, health care professionals are at the mercy of its constant presence. They are denied the distance that most of us in the Western world are able to maintain through the death-denying aspects of our culture. Nonetheless, although neither culture nor the physician, as a part and member of a culture, can defy or defeat death, both can help the afflicted meet it with a sense of meaning, which in human terms becomes a mode of overcoming it.

Consequently, the physician's role in caring for the dying involves severe emotional risks. The human fears of contagion, endangerment, and death, to which the physician is not immune, may prevent a productive dialogue between physician and patient from ever occurring.[27] The physician may take refuge from the death anxiety inherent in the relationship through denial, dissimulation, or hyperobjectivity (psychic numbing), all reflecting a deep-seated desire to dissociate oneself from death. Such behavior not only is fraught with negative consequences for the physician's own emotional health, but also cruelly demonstrates to patients their own separateness from others, forcing them perhaps into detrimental defensive postures of their own.[28]

The physician may also be threatened by the nature of the care demanded by the dying patient, a form of care he or she may feel singularly unprepared to deliver. Indeed, until ten years ago, a few lectures on the importance of emotional and social factors were all the training in these sensitive areas that a medical student could expect. When physicians are called upon for emotional support, to be friend and counselor to the dying patient, they may feel awkward and useless in the realization that their training has stopped short of a positive therapeutic program.[29] In many ways, they are caught between society's (and in part their own) image of the healer and their awareness of the limitations of medicine and of their own knowledge and skills. If self-esteem is eroded by the anticipated failure to combat death, inevitable though it may be, the meaningfulness of their activities and their own sense of self as objects of primary value are thrown into question. When self-image and meaning become threatened, physicians may tend to avoid anything more than minimal contact with patients in their own efforts to deny problems that threaten their self-confidence.[30]

In these contexts, the empathy and affect that may arise from self-disclosure and dialogue between physician and patient can benefit both. Jan Howard states that, although physicians cannot die psychologically with each lost patient, it may be highly functional for the physician to grieve as family members grieve. "The physician gets to know patients and allows himself to feel affect for adults as well as children. If his patient succumbs on the table, he suffers more than if he tried to remain neutral, but his grief helps relieve the guilt he also experiences."[31]

The physician's capacity to be empathetically and affectively (as well as physically) "with" the dying patient may become a positive factor not only in the patient's passage through the crisis, but also in the physician's own passage and resolution of a crisis from which she or he will emerge alive, but altered. If physicians refuse to participate in a mutual effort to formulate meanings and understandings of the crisis with dying patients, they risk the necessity of psychically numbing themselves to the undeniable anxiety-producing aspects of the interaction, thereby occasioning in themselves further dimensions of unresolved conflict and potential emotional anguish. Ultimate questions in such instances often come to be framed in terms of human relationships. It is primarily in terms of human relationships and the values that govern them that human beings can formulate significant meanings for events. We are all creatures within our cultures, the anthropologist, the disaster victim, the physician, the patient. We all suffer from the problem of meaning. We must all either extract meaning from experience or impose meaning on it. When experience is cruel, the need is all the more crucial. In the crisis dyad, neither party's meaning can be complete without including the other, both as experienced self and meaningful self. The achievement of such a process is found in humanistic dialogue.

NOTES

This paper is the product of field research in the Peruvian Andes in 1975 and my participation in the dialogue group on the social sciences and medicine of the Institute on Human Values in Medicine of the Society for Health and Human Values. Institute support for these activities is gratefully acknowledged. Many of the ideas in this paper were born of discussions with the other members of the group who appear in this volume. They will recognize many of their ideas and words in these pages. Their suggestions and criticisms have been most helpful and are greatly appreciated. Particularly valuable in the discussion were the efforts of David Barnard. I would also like to thank Lynda Kapsch, R.N., Robert Lawless, and Dennis Owen for critical readings of the manuscript in its various stages of development.

1. Dennison Nash and Ronald Wintrob, "The Emergence of Self-Consciousness in Ethnography," *Current Anthropology* 13, no. 5 (December 1972):527–42.
2. Ernest Becker, *The Birth and Death of Meaning* (New York: Free Press, 1971).
3. The complete crosscultural validity of this formulation may be a matter of substantial debate. Many anthropologists, such as Malinowski, Roheim, and Benedict, have interpreted culture as being in part a defense against anxiety. However, like many formulations based on a psychoanalytic model, the denial-of-death hypothesis seems vulnerable to the charge that it is not amenable to verification. As Becker himself states:

> The argument of those who believe in the universality of the innate terror of death rests its case mostly on what we know about how effective repression is. The argument can probably never be cleanly decided: if you claim that a concept is not present because it is repressed, you can't lose; it is not a fair game, intellectually, because you always hold the trump card. This type of argument makes psychoanalysis seem unscientific to many people, the fact that its proponents can claim that someone denies one of their concepts because he represses his consciousness of its truth. (*The Denial of Death* [New York: Free Press, 1973], p. 20)

Consequently, if a people does not fear death, it is because their culture has allowed them to repress such fear, which is exactly what Becker maintains culture does. If they have an overwhelming fear of death, then Becker would maintain that their culture is not performing adequately. The only apparent way to test such an idea would be to work with "precultural" humans. The closest we can come are probably newborn infants who, lacking symbolic language and the ability to communicate abstract thought, are singularly difficult to interpret. Robert Jay Lifton reports on work along these lines with infants in *The Life of the Self* (New York: Simon and Schuster, 1976), pp. 36–37. Notwithstanding the difficulty in asserting crosscultural validity, I consider the denial-of-death hypothesis to be extremely powerful in interpreting Western culture and modern medicine.

4. Clifford Geertz, "Religion as a Cultural System," in *Anthropological Approaches to the Study of Religion,* ed. Michael Banton (New York: Frederick A. Praeger, 1966), p. 16.

5. George E. Erickson, George Plafker, and Jaime Fernandez Concha, *Preliminary Report on the Geologic Events Associated with the May 31, 1970 Peru Earthquake* (Washington, D.C.: U.S. Department of the Interior, 1970), pp. 1–12.

6. Robert Jay Lifton, *History and Human Survival* (New York: Vintage, 1971), p. 123.

7. *I and Thou* (New York: Scribner's, 1958), p. 3.

8. Unfortunately, even the restructuring of the encounter did not in all cases nullify its negative elements for all informants or for the researcher. I am now convinced that anthropological research involving relationships predating and extending beyond the research engagement ethically and methodologically preclude the use of short-term formal questionnaires in the crisis dyad. However, research in these issues can be successfully and ethically undertaken, by altering either the methodology or the relationship between researcher and informant. For example, Barbara Bode, an anthropologist, has carried out an exceptionally fine study of meaning formulation with the survivors of the 1970 Peruvian earthquake in the city of Huaraz. She combined extensive interviews with long-term, sustained interaction and personal relationships with her informants. Robert Jay Lifton's now classic study of the survivors of Hiroshima avoided ethical pitfalls by dealing with informants who were unknown to the researcher before the study and who therefore were under little moral obligation, such as that based on friendship, to participate. His informants all participated totally voluntarily, with no constraints placed on them by previous relationships. See Barbara Bode, *Explanation in the 1970 Earthquake in the Peruvian Andes* (Ann Arbor, Mich.: Xerox University Microfilms, 1974); and Robert Jay Lifton, *Death in Life* (New York: Random House, 1967).

9. "Definitions of Health and Illness in the Light of American Values and Social Structure," in *Patients, Physicians and Illness,* ed. E. Gartly Jaco (New York: Free Press, 1972), p. 102.

10. Edward Henderson, "The Approach to the Patient with an Incurable Illness," in *Psychosocial Aspects of Terminal Care,* ed. Bernard Schoenberg, Arthur C. Carr, David Peretz, and Austin H. Kutscher (New York: Columbia University Press, 1972), p. 58.

10. David Mechanic, "Response Factors in Illness: The Study of Illness Behavior," in *Patients, Physicians and Illness,* ed. E. Gartly Jaco (New York: Free Press, 1972), pp. 128–29.

12. Richard N. Adams, "Power and Power Domains," *America Latina,* 9, no. 2 (1966): 3–21.

13. Frederic P. Herter, "A Surgeon Looks at Terminal Illness," in *Psychosocial Aspects of Terminal Care,* ed. Bernard Schoenberg, Arthur C. Carr, David Peretz, and Austin H. Kutscher (New York: Columbia University Press, 1972), p. 83.

14. Avery D. Weissman, "Psychosocial Considerations in Terminal Care," in *Psychosocial Aspects of Terminal Care,* ed. Bernard Schoenberg, Arthur C. Carr, David Peretz, and Austin H. Kutscher (New York: Columbia University Press, 1972), p. 169.

15. Herter, "A Surgeon," p. 82.

16. Ibid.

17. Morton M. Klingerman, "A Radiotherapist's View of the Management of the Cancer Patient," in *Psychosocial Aspects of Terminal Care,* ed. Bernard Schoenberg, Arthur C. Carr, David Peretz, and Austin H. Kutscher (New York: Columbia University Press, 1972), p. 102.

18. Bode, *Explanation in the 1970 Earthquake,* p. 60.

19. The importance of significant others in coping and adaptation is emphasized throughout the literature. The best source on this point is George V. Coelho, David A. Hamburg, and John E. Adams, ed., *Coping and Adaptation* (New York: Basic Books, 1974). The importance of significant others in the resolution before death is stressed in Elizabeth Kübler-Ross, *On Death and Dying* (New York: Macmillan, 1969), p. 276. The physician as significant other is also a major element in Herter, "A Surgeon," and Henderson, "Approach to the Patient."

20. Weissman, "Psychosocial Considerations," p. 171.

21. Herter, "A Surgeon," p. 81.

22. Becker, *Birth and Death of Meaning,* pp. 99–100.

23. Henderson, "Approach to the Patient," p. 61.

24. Bernard C. Meyer, "Truth and the Physician," in *Ethical Issues in Medicine,* ed. E. Fuller Torrey (Boston: Little, Brown, 1968), p. 165.

25. Robert Jay Lifton, "Advocacy and Corruption in the Healing Professions," in this volume.

26. Robert H. Moser, "The New Ethics," in *Psychosocial Aspects of Terminal Care,* ed. Bernard Schoenberg, Arthur C. Carr, David Peretz, and Austin H. Kutscher (New York: Columbia University Press, 1972), p. 43.

27. Weissman, "Psychological Considerations," pp. 170–71.

28. Henderson, "Approach to the Patients," p. 60.

29. Emily Mumford, *Interns: From Students to Physicians* (Cambridge: Harvard University Press, 1970), p. 197.

30. Ibid.

31. "Humanization and Dehumanization of Health Care: A Conceptual View," in *Humanizing Health Care,* ed. Jan Howard and Anselm Strauss (New York: John Wiley, 1975), p. 84.

CHAPTER 5

The New Mission of the Doctor: Redefining Health and Health Care in the Progressive Era, 1900–1917

Barbara Sicherman

So many factors are woven together to produce a professional ethos, or value orientation, that no single perspective can capture them all. Much less can a single perspective reveal how value orientations are modified or reformed to embody new, or rediscovered, values. Thus, it would be unfairly reductionistic to claim that any essay in this volume does more than try to deepen understanding or prompt further questioning from its own vantage point among the social sciences. At the same time, however, one role of the historian is to savor complexity, to hold several dimensions of a problem or period together long enough to suggest the most fruitful and realistic framework for cooperation among these more specific approaches. Here, Barbara Sicherman's work on health and health care in the Progressive era uncovers many of the layers built into the question, How may the art and science of medicine be brought into balance?

Sicherman's essay does have its own special focus. Rather than attempting a picture of the entire period, she emphasizes the figures of Richard Cabot and James Putnam, and their work at the Massachusetts General Hospital. Other figures, such as William Osler at Johns Hopkins University, would certainly belong in a wider treatment of humanistic perspectives in medicine at this time. But it is especially valuable to have a close look at these two men, and at the progress of their work in psychological and social medicine, in order to appreciate the many issues at stake for innovators and reformers in the medical profession.

Among these issues are:

1. The interaction and relative importance of educational curricula, on the one hand, and the organization of health care institutions, on the other, in affecting physicians' sensitivity to the various determinants of illness and health;

2. The influence of individual character on the values and practices of institutions or historical periods, and the significance of support systems and reference groups to nourish risk-taking, initiative, and idealism;

3. The impact of underlying philosophical commitments regarding the nature

of the person and the definition of health on physicians' attitudes and behavior,
and on the organization of the healing professions;

4. The presence of ambiguities and tensions within medicine, such as those
between cure and prophylaxis, patients' and physicians' independence and de-
pendency, peer criticism and individual innovation, the image of the physician as
servant and the prestige of his or her social role; and

5. The interplay between each of the foregoing issues and other forces in the
culture at particular historical moments, including the state of democratic institu-
tions, economic conditions, and the degree to which individuals in society are
willing and able to assume responsibility for their own health and well-being.

Like many other people Cabot and Putnam addressed themselves imaginatively
to these and other questions. Problems such as these still call for careful analysis
from many disciplines and will continue to do so.

"The world is gradually awakening to the fact of its own improva-
bility," declared Irving Fisher, a Yale economist, in his *Report on*
National Vitality: Its Wastes and Conservation, prepared for the National Conservation Commission in 1909. "Hygiene, the youngest
of the biological studies, has repudiated the outworn doctrine that
mortality is fatality, and must exact a regular and inevitable sacrifice at its present rate year after year. Instead of this fatalistic
creed we now have the assurance of Pasteur that 'It is within the
power of man to rid himself of every parasitic disease.' " Fisher's
report, with its optimistic view that disease could be eradicated,
reflected the changing sensibilities of Americans in the early years
of the twentieth century. Concerned with expanding the scope as
well as the length of life, Fisher looked forward to the elimination
of such minor illnesses as the common cold, tonsillitis, and the
psychoneuroses, which caused both economic loss and personal
discomfort. He also foretold "biological engineering," which he
defined as the study of the conditions under which men and
women could attain their "highest efficiency." [1]

René Dubos has claimed that hygiene "never captured the
hearts of men." [2] But it would be difficult to exaggerate the impact that the idea of preventable death had on Americans during

the Progressive era. In fact, preventing disease was more than an idea; by 1920 it had become a reality. Smallpox, yellow fever, typhoid, typhus, and cholera had virtually disappeared from the Western world, and deaths from tuberculosis had fallen sharply. Most striking of all was the reduction in infant mortality. Variously estimated at one in every four or five live births in the 1880s, infant deaths had declined greatly by 1915, as diphtheria, croup, enteritis, diarrhea, and scarlet fever yielded to medical control. During the same period, life expectancy at birth increased by almost thirteen years for males, slightly more for females.[3]

Scientific medicine was not solely responsible for these advances, but the dramatic new discoveries in bacteriology, immunology, and entomology did much to elevate the profession's standing with the public. They also raised unrealistic expectations that the conquest of other diseases would soon follow along similar lines. After 1900 the most thoughtful physicians recognized that further reductions in mortality and morbidity rates would require new tactics and that, even where a definite etiology had been established, science alone was powerless to prevent infection. It was one thing to identify the cause of tuberculosis or syphilis; in the absence of reliable cures, it was quite another to know how to eliminate them.

Tuberculosis provided the model for imaginative new approaches to prophylaxis and treatment in the Progressive era. Despite the discovery of the tubercle bacillus in 1882, experimentation with tuberculin therapy, and the availability of public health laboratories to test sputum, by 1900 it was clear that there would be no easy triumph over the disease. Tuberculosis was the leading cause of mortality, responsible for anywhere from 10 to 15 percent of all deaths. It was also a "disease of the people," as social reformers discovered during their campaigns to improve the wretched housing of the urban poor.

The most promising developments for treatment and prophylaxis of tuberculosis had less to do with medicine than with hygiene. E. L. Trudeau's success with open-air treatment in the 1880s not only overturned conventional medical wisdom, but sparked the sanatorium movement and drugless healing. In 1905, Massachusetts General Hospital (MGH) started a class for tenement dwellers with advanced tuberculosis. Patients camped out in tents on roofs and fire escapes, attended to diet and rest, kept diaries, and received hygienic instruction in class—with good results. Although physicians welcomed public registration of tubercular patients, regulations against spitting, and laboratory analysis as important adjuncts for controlling the disease, they agreed that only a broad educational campaign would reduce the incidence of tuberculosis. To this end they cooperated with lay men and women in founding the Association for the Study and Prevention of Tuberculosis in 1904. The idea of the voluntary health organization, a U.S. contribution to public health, caught on; in the next few years organizations to fight infant mortality, mental illness, cancer, and venereal disease came into being.[4]

Recognition that successful treatment and prophylaxis called for intelligent cooperation from the patient or public had much to do with physicians' willingness to enter the public arena. Traditionally they had opposed publicity, which they associated with quacks, and had been reluctant as well to share professional "secrets" with the public. The open discussion of cancer, syphilis, and mental illness in the decade before the United States entered World War I marked a major advance over the earlier "conspiracy of silence" that so often surrounded disturbing diseases.[5]

As the infectious diseases came under partial control, physicians gave greater attention to less dramatic ills—the chronic diseases of an aging population, minor diseases that sapped vitality, and those caused by environmental pollution. Agreeing that individual hygienic precautions usually constituted the first line of defense, they also considered assistance from public agencies indispensable for lasting change. The school, once regarded as injurious to the well-being of youthful scholars, became a "superhealth organization," where diseased tonsils and adenoids, eye defects, and glandular deficiencies could be detected by a public health nurse and corrected by a physician. Studies sponsored by state and federal agencies often disclosed that industrial diseases and maternal and child mortality could be reduced by relatively simple environmental changes. An editorial in the *Bulletin of the Department of Health of New York City* captured the optimism engendered by such conclusions:

Disease is largely a removable evil. It continues to afflict humanity, not only because of incomplete knowledge of its causes and lack of adequate individual and public hygiene, but also because it is extensively fostered by harsh economic and industrial conditions and by wretched housing in congested communities. These conditions and consequently the diseases which spring from them can be removed by better social organization. . . . Public health is purchasable.[6]

1

Despite their optimism about prophylaxis, physicians were often "dogged by a sense of futility" in the matter of therapeutics. There were few specific remedies available; Richard Cabot of the Massachusetts General Hospital often pointed out that drugs and surgery cured only 8 or 9 of some 215 diseases. William H. Welch, dean of the Johns Hopkins Medical School and the most influential physician in the United States, maintained that nursing outranked science in its contribution to patient care:

There is no improvement in modern medicine which outranks in importance, in its value in the prevention and cure of disease, the introduction of the system of trained nurses. One can put one's finger on great discoveries in medicine, the relation of bacteria, we will say, to the causation of disease, which is of the greatest interest in the progress of medicine, but so far as the treatment of disease is concerned the application of the system of trained nursing counts for as much, if not more than any scientific discovery in medicine.[7]

Caught between the therapeutic nihilism of some professional leaders and the unrealistic hopes raised by the dispensers of nostrums, practicing physicians found themselves in a quandary about how best to help the patients who consulted them about problems for which there were no cures. Among the techniques they found useful were hygienic regimens, hydrotherapy, physiotherapy, and, most surprising, psychotherapy.

Nothing better illustrates the new trends in medicine than the interest in psychotherapy that swept the profession in the years after 1905. Stimulated in part by a desire to counteract the popularity of Christian Science, New Thought, and other forms of mind cure, physicians and even surgeons sometimes made large claims for "scientific" psychotherapy. Morton Prince, the leading U.S. investigator of the subconscious, believed that fully 75 percent of all neurological ills were of the functional sort that could be helped by psychotherapy. Internists claimed that as many as half the conditions they treated, including constipation and insomnia, could be helped by psychic means. Some even urged that psychotherapy be used in treating serious illnesses like cancer to help patients meet their fate courageously. So many claims were made for psychotherapy that sympathetic physicians warned against overselling a useful, but not infallible, technique.[8]

Medical endorsement of psychotherapy, formerly considered taboo, also reflected the shift away from nineteenth-century somatic medicine, best exemplified by Rudolf Virchow's famous dictum that "there are no general diseases, there are only diseases of the cell." By the turn of the century, physicians had come to understand that mere exposure to germs was not sufficient to explain the presence or absence of disease in a given individual. Walter B. Cannon's laboratory demonstration of the effects of fear and rage on digestion and other bodily processes and research on the relationships between hormones and moods also modified the earlier somaticism. The new emphasis on the close relationship between mind and body not only seemed to confirm the central hypothesis of pioneer psychopathologists like Sigmund Freud and Pierre Janet—that emotions could induce physical illness—but also suggested new opportunities for the practicing therapist.

James Jackson Putnam and Richard C. Cabot were among those who thought most seriously about the physician's role as healer. Cousins and members of Boston's socially conscious elite, both were dedicated healers willing to defy medical orthodoxy if they thought it would help their patients. Influenced by Harvard's tradition of philosophical idealism, both had strong philosophical interests and identified with the highest ethical tradition in medicine. Both inspired extraordinary gratitude and affection in patients and friends. Men of almost opposite temperament—Putnam was shy and personally cautious, Cabot bold and energetic—they ended up on opposite sides of such controversial issues as psychoanalysis and the psychotherapeutic role of the clergy. But their similarities outweighed their differences, and they cooperated closely in improving the medical services available to the impoverished patients who visited the outpatient department of MGH, where they both worked.

Putnam, born in 1846, came from a family with a strong medical tradition.[9] His father and older brother were physicians, and his maternal grandfather, James Jackson, had been the acknowledged leader of Boston medicine early in the century. After graduating from Harvard College in 1866 and Harvard Medical School in 1870, he spent two years in Europe studying with such masters as Virchow, Theodor Meynert, Hughlings Jackson, and Jean Martin Charcot. Specializing in neurology, Putnam helped to establish the new field in the United States and eventually became Harvard's first professor of diseases of the nervous system. He conducted experiments on the localization of brain function and studied diseases of the spinal cord, brain tumors, and other problems of organic neurology. Having absorbed the somatic orthodoxy of his mentors, Putnam in 1876 severely condemned a colleague's paper on "mental therapeutics," a method he found unscientific, deceitful, and ineffective. Putnam's anger resulted as much from his fear that the sufferings of nervous patients would be dismissed as unreal as it did from intellectual conviction.

Two decades later Putnam endorsed psychotherapy; probably no American did more to make it respectable. Convinced by his clinical experience that the scientific method had its limitations, by the mid-nineties he welcomed the new theories of subconscious mental states and the therapies derived from them. He was one of the first reputable physicians to practice hypnotism, but what he called the "Grand Pasha" approach did not appeal to him. He preferred techniques that would *"help the patient exert his own reasoning and will,"* free the patient from his "humiliating" dependence on the physician, and enable him to cure himself in the future.[10] Putnam thought of himself as a teacher of his patients and insisted that he was their pupil as well. He ultimately found in psychoanalysis the most democratic, effective, and scientific of all the new therapies. Although Putnam resisted determinism in psychoanalysis as in philosophy, Freud's explanatory model appealed to the desire for scientific certainty that had been apparent in his youth. It also permitted him to integrate the moral and scientific interests that somatic orthodoxy had forced him to keep quite separate.

Richard Cabot, less touched by the orthodoxies of somatic medicine, was equally concerned with extending the responsibilities of the profession beyond the healing of physical illness.[11] No one did more to suggest what the physician's new role might be, or to implement it. Cabot was born in 1868 into a strongly Unitarian family in which idealism and community service were equally blended. His father was the friend and biographer of Ralph Waldo Emerson; his mother, a dedicated member of the Brookline School Committee for a quarter of a century. After graduating from Harvard College *summa cum laude,* Cabot entered Harvard Medical School because he believed medicine offered those of his generation a greater opportunity to serve humanity than did the ministry, his initial choice. Cabot's commitment to service was evident from the start. At the age of twenty-five, he hesitated on receiving the flattering offer to become the first bacteriologist at MGH because "I feel all my bent in the other half of medicine, the *practitioner's* part, the looking after bodies with souls in them, rather than bodies without." [12] Still, in the next few years, the intensely ambitious Cabot established himself as a specialist in blood diseases, a master diagnostician and clinical teacher. Cabot, a prodigious worker who was quick to grasp essentials, published books on blood diseases and serum diagnosis, several textbooks on differential diagnosis, and articles on an impressive range of illnesses. Paul Dudley White called Cabot's paper on "The Four Common Types of Heart Disease," which classified cardiac diseases on the basis of etiology rather than structural defects, a "landmark in medical history" and the "greatest contribution to cardiology of our generation." The achievement was all the more remarkable because Cabot did not consider himself a cardiologist.[13]

Cabot was also a dynamic and innovative teacher. He introduced systematic case teaching to medical students and the use of autopsies in the famous clinico-pathological conferences for MGH house officers and visitors. He saw these conferences as a means of overcoming the separation between clinicians and pathologists, and subjected his own diagnoses as well as those of colleagues to the rigors of post-mortem analysis.

As his reputation grew, Cabot gave considerable thought to how physicians might be more helpful to their patients. "The business of medicine," he asserted, "is to get people out of difficulties through the application of science and of dexterity, manual and psychical." Eschewing the therapeutic nihilism of many of his colleagues, Cabot argued for an "aggressive" therapeutics. By this he meant neither excessive reliance on drugs nor insistence on the doctor's authority, which he considered an unfortunate consequence of medical education: "We get to think that we are little tin gods—surrounded as we are by a clientele in whose minds our word is authoritative." Although proud of the physician's expert skills—accurate diagnosis was a passion—Cabot was equally cheered by what he considered a democratic trend in modern medicine whereby doctor and patient united in pursuit of health. Skeptical about the efficacy of most medicines, Cabot urged the physician to be a friend to the patient, doing everything possible to shore up the body's natural tendency to self-healing. He considered the patient a teacher as well as a recipient of aid. The physician must not only listen carefully to what a patient says, but learn to overcome the prejudices he or she brings to the clinical encounter. More than once Cabot told how he had learned to see Abraham Cohen as an individual rather than as a generic Jew. "The pity of it is that we see only what we have seen before. But the man, himself, is just precisely that which I have never seen before. So he is for me invisible: to him, as he sees himself, I am usually blind."[14]

Cabot also became an ardent champion of professional honesty. This meant not only dispensing with placebos (their use was then a common practice), but telling the patient only the truth (although not necessarily all the truth or all at once). As a young practitioner, he had been urged to lie for the "patient's own good." Once caught in an ambiguous situation by a patient, Cabot concluded that lies benefited the physician more than the patient. He began "the hazardous experiment of telling the truth," and to his surprise found it "innocuous"; even the most fragile patients admirably rose to the occasion.[15]

In short, Cabot was an iconoclastic physician who frequently outraged his colleagues. Skeptical of the skill of most practitioners, he championed lay participation in the therapeutic process. He also charged physicians with serious failings: dispensing useless if not harmful drugs, deception, and discouraging patients from seeking accurate diagnosis in hospitals. Cabot was also an early advocate of medical insurance, an innovation opposed by organized medicine. He was so outspoken that the Massachusetts Medical Society considered expelling him for advertising the profession's faults to the public.

His appointment to the outpatient department at MGH in 1898 gave Cabot a vehicle for implementing his medical philosophy. Hospitals like MGH had recently transformed themselves from charitable enterprises that served the poor into institutions where middle- and upper-class patients came for surgery and diagnostic tests, expecting to recover. The outpatient department remained "the tag end" of the hospital, a receptacle for patients who were poor and often foreign-born, cases of "chronic malnutrition, hygienic bankruptcy and mental torment." Between eight hundred and a thousand patients came each day, but aside from the interesting cases that were brought to the attention of medical students or those referred to the wards, they received little assistance. There was nothing that resembled a plan of treatment. A physician might hand a diabetic patient a sheet of dietary instructions without inquiring whether the patient understood them or had the funds to follow them.[16]

To the outpatient department Cabot brought his skill in diagnosis, commitment to the whole person, and passion for action. He hoped not only to bring the department up to the standard of the rest of the hospital, but to make outpatient work as much a part of public or preventive medicine as the new diagnostic laboratories. Above all, he wanted to end the impersonality of the clinical encounter, in which the physician attended only to the patient's immediate physical problem but knew nothing about the poverty and emotional stress that often interfered with recovery. Cabot insisted that each patient had a right to scientific diagnosis and effective treatment, both impossible under the hurried conditions in which a physician saw fifty or sixty patients in a morning, without the assistance of a nurse or even a secretary.

Cabot estimated that about 40 percent of those who visited the outpatient department suffered from functional complaints, which he defined as those which could be "ameliorated chiefly by a change in the patient's habits and by the correction of hygienic faults." The most important of these were the psychoneuroses, dyspepsia, constipation, and headache. Even tuberculosis and the diseases of infancy classified as organic could be ameliorated by similar techniques. Cabot estimated that the "quick cure" cases—those which could be treated by simple medical means—constituted less than half the total.[17]

In October 1905, Cabot raised funds privately to employ a social service worker to "make treatment more effective." Restricting themselves to patients referred by physicians, the social worker and a staff of volunteers saw 684 people during the first year, and more than twice that number in the second. The idea of hospital social service was not new—William Osler at Johns Hopkins and others had sent workers to patients' homes in the 1890s—but the "corner" at MGH became not only the first full-fledged department, but a model for others; by 1913, over one hundred hospitals and dispensaries had them.[18]

The primacy of MGH was only partly due to Cabot's inspirational leadership and genius for publicity. It also owed much to the foresight and organizational talents of Ida M. Cannon, a trained nurse who became head social service worker in 1908. Relations with the hospital administration were not at first entirely cordial, and Cabot was inclined to look for allies among social reformers outside the hospital. But Cannon insisted—and her policy prevailed—on making social service an integral part of the hospital. She initiated a supervisory committee, which drew in physicians from many parts of the hospital. By 1914, the superintendent acknowledged the need for social service work in the wards, and in 1919 the hospital finally made the department part of its regular program. Cannon also established the department as a training center for prospective social workers and later for medical students as well.[19]

Under the leadership of Cabot, Cannon, and Putnam, the department became a creative force in the hospital. Cabot variously defined social work as *"the study of character under adversity,"* "the attempt to interpret to patients the meaning of their illness," and the integrating force in the hospital. The emphasis was always on improving treatment, preventing future illness, and attending to the patient's varied needs. Staff members attempted to live up to Cabot's dictum that what every patient needed was a friend. For example, a social worker arranged for a woman who could not support herself during the winter because she suffered from Raynaud's disease, a painful affliction of the hands, to move to Florida where she could live and work in comfort throughout the year. Eleven members of one family had been attending the outpatient department for three years, mainly for scabies. All still had the affliction when a social worker first encountered them. After she supervised the treatment for one week, the condition disappeared and had not returned two and a half years later. Cabot helped at least one long-time invalid regain her confidence by giving her dictation and paying her for the work.[20]

Cabot believed that nothing restored a person to health so quickly as finding a useful purpose in life. Acting on this conviction, he encouraged former patients to work in the department, on a paid or voluntary basis, where they could help others worse off than themselves. The most dramatic instance was a seamstress who had lost both her legs and whose plan to train people to become self-supporting evolved into a Bureau for the Handicapped. Cabot befriended his co-workers and wrote them inspirational letters in difficult times. In many ways he sought to minimize the distinction between the sick and the well, between doctor (or social worker) and patient. Indeed, he claimed that he had learned to appreciate social work by having his wife practice it on him.[21]

Much of the department's work followed the specialized lines of the hospital's clinics. Social workers cooperated closely with the orthopedic, pediatric, and neurological departments, among others. Putnam, who was in charge of neurology, delegated the patients with organic diseases to his assistants and concentrated on what was variously called neuropsychological or psychiatric work. He employed as his first social worker a woman who had been hospitalized for mental illness. He also found funds to hire a psychologist interested in psychoanalysis and thus made available a rich man's therapy to the urban poor attending his clinic.[22]

MGH may have been unusual in having such gifted leaders as Cabot and Putnam, but the innovations there were very much a part of what can be called "Progressive" medicine. Nothing more aptly illustrates the environmental approach to illness than the social service department's pioneering work in industrial diseases. Working closely with David Edsall, chief of medicine, the department engaged in what may have been the first systematic work in industrial medicine in any U.S. hospital. Physicians knew little about lead poisoning and did not collect the social information that might contribute to a diagnosis. Only after a social worker stationed herself at the entrance of the outpatient department and asked the occupation of everyone who entered did it become possible to establish an accurate diagnosis of industrial diseases. The hospital subsequently changed its case-record forms to include the occupation of every male patient. It also established an Industrial Clinic which, in addition to diagnosis and treatment, sent circulars to factories in the community to inform workers of the early symptoms of industrial diseases.[23]

A few pioneers tried to integrate the new perspectives into the medical curriculum. No one was more innovative than Charles P. Emerson, who as early as 1902 had his students at Johns Hopkins work closely with the Charity Organization Society of Baltimore. Every medical student was assigned one or two poor families, whom they came to know over a period of weeks, months, or possibly years. The object was not to study disease—some of the families had no discernible illness—but to learn "how the poor man lives, works and thinks; what his problems are; what burdens he must bear." When Emerson became dean of the Indiana University Medical School in 1911, he introduced a compulsory course in medical sociology, in which students visited factories as well as public welfare and philanthropic agencies. He also organized a permanent department of environmental medicine, chaired by a sociologist.[24]

Changes of this sort remained the exception, but they highlight the importance physicians of the era attached to the environmental causes of disease. They frequently cooperated with lay men and women to secure legislation that would guarantee at least minimal standards of health and welfare. These included minimum wages and maximum hours, safety provisions in mines and factories, housing reforms, and the prohibition of child labor. Cabot even endorsed a proposal for health insurance on the grounds that it would diminish anxiety among the sick poor and thus alleviate many illnesses caused or aggravated by mental strain.

Such measures aimed mainly at preventing disease. But just as social reformers like Jane Addams believed that "increasing the positive value of life" should replace prevention as their primary concern, physicians often went beyond the attainment of "minimal" standards of health to consider what might be desirable or even ideal.[25] It is possible that this concern for the ideal, with its implication that the sources of health were principally within the individual, contributed to the neglect in later years of the minimal standards that still have not been attained by all Americans. But physicians in the Progressive era assumed that these would be achieved and went on to consider the attributes of health itself.

2

Interest in defining health was new. In the late nineteenth century, physicians believed that health was the absence of illness, rather than a quality in its own right.[26] One physician illustrated the point with a popular metaphor: "Health is like the silent existence of those happy nations that have no history. But disease represents the commotion, the storm and stress, the drama and convulsions into which the disturbed history of our race has usually been thrown." [27] Disease, in other words, was the norm; health, a welcome respite that could not be counted on.

Clinicians, whose work is with the sick, have sometimes viewed health as the opposite as well as the absence of illness. In the late nineteenth century, physicians assumed that since the mentally ill lacked control over their emotions, were self-absorbed, and suffered from delusions or hallucinations, it followed that the person who was emotionally temperate, but not unduly introspective or egotistical, must be healthy. Thus, one physician claimed: "Perfect inhibition is the sign of perfect mental health." Another recommended cultivation of emotional impassivity on the ground that "healthy and justly proportioned indifference is essential to healthy equilibrium." [28]

The thrust of this advice on preserving health was clearly toward self-restriction—of emotional attachment, aspiration, imagination, creativity, even individuality. Physicians were offering a formula for reducing anxiety that transcended their own clinical experiences and revealed more about their own values, and particularly their fears, than about the nature of health. In the late nineteenth century, physicians believed not only that each individual possessed a limited amount of nervous energy but that contemporary U.S. life placed inordinate demands on that supply. To this generation, the metaphors of the overloaded electrical circuit and the overdrawn bank account illustrated what happened to those profligate with scarce resources. Physicians viewed the individual as a passive being—the "tinder waiting for the spark"—with few options other than the prudent husbanding of resources for the inevitable dangers ahead. Health, finally, was the "successful adaptation to the conditions of existence." And in the era of Herbert Spencer, adaptation meant the *"continuous adjustment of internal relations to external relations"*; the organism must mold itself to a fixed environment rather than shaping that environment to its own ends.[29]

The restrictive outlook suggested by this "minimal" conception of health—freedom from incapacitating symptoms and the ability to withstand stress—characterized other aspects of U.S. culture as well. The Gilded Age did not call forth the heroic virtues in politics or economics any more than in matters of health. Liberals of the era favored what Grover Cleveland called "safe, careful, and deliberate reform." Saving and scarcity were still the watchwords of an economy geared to production rather than consumption. Workers and farmers struggled to make ends meet; and the two major depressions that delimit the period provided ample warning of the dangers of extending oneself too far. The high mortality and morbidity rates, particularly among infants, served as constant reminders to all classes of the precariousness of health and of life itself.

Against this background, Putnam's description in 1895 of the healthy person is arresting:

In health there is a certain degree of co-ordination and mutual support between all the vast activities of the mind, binding them to the consciousness on the one hand and to the vital functions of the body on the other.... The healthy man feels himself a consistent character, and can predict what he will do, not only as regards those new exigencies which require logical thought, but also as regards those which depend upon the promptings of all the deeper-lying and subconscious processes with which his mind is stocked. His reactions to the various problems which present themselves are as prompt as the conditions of the case permit, and the attention of his consciousness is at liberty to devote itself, unembarrassed, to the interest of each new question as it arises.[30]

Putnam's emphasis on internal dynamics, vital engagement, control—perhaps most of all his confidence—all point toward the more expansive cultural, political, and economic life that flowered in the first two decades of the new century.

American sensibilities changed dramatically within a single generation. Although difficult to explain, the signs of change were everywhere apparent. Some time during the 1890s, U.S. culture entered a more dynamic phase. The rages for competitive college sports (particularly football), for the outdoors, and for ragtime and martial tunes were among the more evident manifestations of the new consciousness. Women were exhorted to greater vitality, men to be more virile. A new magazine, *Physical Culture*, took as its motto "Weakness Is a Crime." Jingoism also flourished, with more serious consequences; the United States entered a war with Spain and landed an overseas empire.[31]

The new century brought prosperity to many—per capita gross national product almost quadrupled between 1889 and 1920—and a consumer orientation in business. Simon N. Patten, professor of political economy at the University of Pennsylvania, found in this transition from a "pain or deficit economy" to a "pleasure or surplus economy" a heartening "new basis of civilization." Patten believed that the unprecedented abundance, which made "equitable distribution of a surplus" rather than meeting deficits the central problem of economic life, would provide a basis for the intellectual as well as material liberation of those who had hitherto lived in poverty and ignorance.[32]

Politics also took an expansive turn, at the state and local level in the 1890s, and, with the presidency of Theodore Roosevelt, nationally as well. Men and women of the comfortable classes, particularly those who went to live in urban slums, strove to make industrial society more humane. They not only worked to correct the worst abuses (through remedial housing and factory legislation) but pioneered as well in public health nursing, school hygiene, and the playground movement in the hope of improving the general well-being of the urban poor. State and local politicians also began to regulate corrupt or dangerous business practices that had previously gone unchecked. Despite the meager results of these reforms at the national level, the idea that the environment could be controlled for human welfare—that the public need no longer tolerate adulterated food and drugs, unnecessary death due to poor sanitation, and other indignities— was of central importance to men and women of the Progressive generation. "Mastery," in the terms popularized by the young Walter Lippmann, was to replace the "drift" that had previously characterized American life.[33]

To this generation, no one exemplified the heroic virtues more completely than Theodore Roosevelt, big-game hunter, Rough Rider, and wielder of the Big Stick in foreign policy. In a famous address on "The Strenuous Life" in 1899, Roosevelt captured the new spirit of risk-taking: "It is a base untruth to say that happy is the nation that has no history. Thrice happy is the nation that has a glorious history. Far better it is to dare mighty things, to win glorious triumphs, even though checkered by failure, than to take rank with those poor spirits who neither enjoy much nor suffer much, because they live in the gray twilight that knows not victory nor defeat." [34]

William James was to philosophy what Roosevelt was to politics: His work not only embodied the new sensibility but helped to generate it in others. Although James opposed Roosevelt's unrestrained jingoism, his "Moral Equivalent of War" was a plea for finding peacetime equivalents for the exhilaration hitherto attained only in war. James's emphasis on the heroic virtues was partly a means of overcoming his own recurrent struggles with depression and neurasthenia, but his message struck a responsive chord in his countrymen. As a young man, James had pulled himself out of his worst depression by a conscious decision to believe in free will. For the rest of his life, he rejected determinism and stood for spontaneity, free choice, and a pluralistic universe. James early attacked Spencer's static view of the evolutionary process, his emphasis on the passivity of human intelligence, and his neglect of the noncognitive elements of human behavior. In *The Principles of Psychology,* published in 1890, James made much of the directing powers of intelligence. Even unruly subconscious mental states, which might lead to illness, could be controlled and channeled to higher ends.

James took up the theme of health in two popular essays. In "The Gospel of Relaxation," written in the mid-nineties, James agreed with the observation of a British psychiatrist that Americans " 'lived like an army with all its reserves engaged for action' "; his solution was a "toning down of . . . moral tensions." In James's view, "we must change ourselves from a race that admires jerk and snap for their own sakes, and looks down upon low voices and quiet ways as dull, to one that, on the contrary, has calm for its ideal, and for their own sakes loves harmony, dignity, and ease." As late as 1901, James wrote a friend: "Happiness, I have lately discovered, is no positive feeling, but a negative condition of freedom from a number of restrictive sensations of which our organism usually seems to be the seat. When they are wiped out, the clearness and cleanness of the contrast is happiness. That is why anaesthetics make us so happy." [35]

In "The Energies of Men," published in 1907, James pulled out all the stops. Far from prescribing anaesthetics, James argued that too many Americans were but "half awake." By this he meant that they did not live at the maximum rate of energy of which they sometimes proved capable, or even at their optimal level. Deploring the wasted potential of those "cut off from their rightful resources," James concluded: "In rough terms, we may say that a man who energizes below his normal maximum fails by just so much to profit by his chance at life; and that a nation filled with such men is inferior to a nation run at higher pressure. The problem is, then, how can men be trained up to their most useful pitch of energy." [36]

Lamenting the lack of "a topography of the limits of human powers," James tried to provide the contours for such a map. He considered the will "the normal opener of deeper and deeper levels of energy"; the difficulty was to use it. The best individuals, he thought, were often stimulated by *"excitements, ideas and efforts."* A man who moved from country to city, after his initial bewilderment, adapted to the new rhythms and permanently expanded his "efficiency-equilibrium." James attributed many of the most heroic acts to the classic emotional stimuli: "love, anger, crowd-contagion or despair." Ascetic discipline, such as Yoga, worked for some, sprees and excesses for others. James considered religion a particularly powerful spur, a theme he had developed earlier in *The Varieties of Religious Experience.*

So activist was his tone that James later felt it necessary to deny the charge that he had promoted a "gospel of overstrain." Indeed, the qualities James admired were precisely those considered inimical to health a generation earlier, probably by James as well as by clinicians. The fundamental premise was the same: that emotions, risk-taking, and excess stimulated energy. But what one generation feared, the next welcomed. In the more abundant world of the twentieth century, physicians were less concerned with the exhaustion of limited energy than with finding outlets for superabundant, and potentially dangerous, supplies. In the opinion of Cabot, himself a victim of ulcers: "The only possible preservation of our healthy activities against such a self-corrosive process as goes on to produce ulcer in the stomach is in setting one's energies—those restless, ceaseless energies—to work instead of allowing them to be turned in upon oneself." [37] It was a commonplace among physicians that fanatics were rarely invalids.

Far from assuming that health was the absence of illness, or its opposite, physicians began to equate it with various states of well-being. William Alanson White, superintendent of Saint Elizabeths Hospital and a pioneer psychoanalyst, claimed: "The business of life is to find the fullest and completest expression of one's personality. 'More life and fuller', as the poet says, is the formula." [38] More life and fuller to this generation variously meant happiness, vitality, or efficiency. Above all, the new behavioral mode was active rather than passive. *"Health is whole-hearted action,"* the president of the Playground and Recreation Association of America asserted. "If you cannot run a mile, run a hundred yards, or ten, or three—but run while you are about it. . . . Eternal moderation means health in moderation, life in moderation." [39]

Cabot went furthest in suggesting what wholeheartedness might mean. In a popular book, *What Men Live By*, he identified four sustaining human activities—work, play, love, and worship—each of which must be intensely pursued. Work was his "favorite prescription"; on the mantelpiece in his consulting room he had placed the framed motto "Employment Is Nature's Physician." He believed that women constituted such a large proportion of nervous patients because they had been denied meaningful work. [40] It is easy to interpret this invocation to work as simply a reincarnation of the Protestant ethic; but its standing as a health preserver was actually new. In the Gilded Age, physicians had warned against what they considered a national tendency to overwork and had prescribed a "rest cure" for those who succumbed to "wear and tear." In endorsing work and even a "work cure," physicians of Cabot's generation revealed their altered priorities. They were probably more consistent as well; the physicians who had issued the direst warnings against overwork in the Gilded Age had often ignored their own advice, sometimes to their personal peril. [41]

This generation was also the first to endorse play. Cabot correctly observed that, to his ancestors, the contemporary seriousness about play would have seemed "as blasphemous as a gospel of laxity." Physicians in the Gilded Age had actually recommended outdoor exercise or nature study for children's health rather than enjoyment. They had also preferred gymnastics to the more strenuous intercollegiate sports and feared that even roller skating, if indulged in at great speed, might prove too exhilarating. Although intensely serious about play, Cabot recommended it, not because it was good for one or even because it promoted rest or health, but because it made possible fuller use of human capacities. Cabot predictably preferred the "active" forms of play, with their promise of ecstasy, to such "passive" indulgences as gambling, gossip, swinging, and listening to lectures.[42]

In view of this emphasis on activity and control, it is not surprising that adaptation—although probably the single most frequent synonym for health—was no longer invariably considered the highest good. If it still seemed obvious that the mentally disturbed were "people who, for one reason or another, were not well adapted to their environment," the converse—that only the well-adapted were healthy—no longer seemed self-evident. As Putnam pointed out, contemporary physiologists did not equate disease with maladaptation. Rather, they believed that disease (or such symptoms as fever and fatigue) often represented the organism's efforts to right itself, to master the forces threatening it.[43]

But Putnam insisted that physicians go beyond normal physiology as well as pathology when considering what their patients were capable of and how to help them:

There has been a tendency among physicians to study the health and disease of the individual too much from the standpoint of his nervous mechanism. . . . In my opinion, we ought to reverse the process and study the individual as a conscious, self-active, creative force and ought, especially in talking with laymen, to throw the emphasis upon motive and obligation and social environment in the widest sense as influences making for health on the one hand or for disease on the other.[44]

Putnam hoped to make room for such considerations in psychoanalysis. As he wrote Freud: "I do not believe that we can study repressions adequately without having in our own minds an adequate idea of what there is in life over and above that which is repressed. . . . Friendship and love do not seem to me explicable on the basis of the conflicts of instincts." Like other U.S. analysts, Putnam considered sublimation an elevating, if painful, method of self-improvement, and analysis a means of creating more moral people. Always pessimistic about human nature, Freud dissented:

The unworthiness of human beings, including the analysts, always has impressed me deeply, but why should analyzed men and women in fact be better? Analysis makes for integration but does not of itself make for goodness. I do not believe, as do Socrates and Putnam, that all vices originate in a sort of obscurity and ignorance. I feel that one puts too great a burden on analysis when one asks that it realize each of one's dearest ideals.[45]

Against Freud's insistence on psychological determinism, Putnam held out the "creative power" of man's consciousness. He was "perfectly willing to admit that freedom characterizes only a millionth part of any act or thought. But this millionth part is, I believe, our most precious possession." [46] For Putnam, the sources of health existed mainly within the individual; it was the physician's task to liberate them. Influenced by James's ideas on purposive intelligence, Bergson's concept of *élan vital,* and the psychoanalytic view of the unconscious, Putnam included among the attributes of health: mental unity (by which he meant both conscious purpose and control of internal forces), creativity, spontaneity, and adaptability. The most complete health was that which allowed the greatest "spontaneity." If self-expression sometimes led the individual to defy conformity, it did not imply license; Putnam carefully distinguished genuine independence from egotistic individualism. He also viewed health "not as a 'place' or a 'condition,' but rather as a 'direction'.... For everyone, even for the 'well,' there are always new worlds to conquer, new adaptations to establish." [47]

For physicians like Putnam, health had a religious significance. Putnam was quite explicit about this. In his correspondence with Freud and elsewhere, he urged that the "narrow conception" of medicine, with its emphasis on physics and chemistry as the source of all knowledge, be transcended to make room for essentially religious values. Not only did religion provide many with the integrating principle considered essential for health; for some, health and religion were virtually the same. In Cabot's view:

"'Mental health' means ideal character—no less. . . . The healthiest mind is the most productive, sympathetic, self-forgetting, creative mind"; the object of the mental hygiene movement "was also that of the founder of Christianity."[48]

But if health in the Progressive era was an ideal of perfection, it was a relative ideal. Putnam believed that "one man's health is very different in quality and quantity from another man's health." Adolf Meyer, the most influential psychiatrist of the early twentieth century, acknowledged that there were *many standards of normality.* Indeed, physicians no longer assumed they knew what "normality" meant. When Cabot wanted a definition of the word *normal,* he asked a philosopher "how it is and should be used." He suggested two definitions, *"the average under certain conditions"* and *"what ought to be,"* and was inclined to dismiss a third, normal as *"an equilibrium."* He added: "That matter is getting hot! Here a reverent and marvellously industrious chemist [is] deciding that there's *no such thing* as normal urine—so that he has to write it 'normal' on the title page of his booklet." [49]

If neither health nor normality had a precise definition, health was no longer viewed as the opposite of illness. Putnam's experiences as friend and physician to members of Boston's upper class had taught him how difficult it was to distinguish the sick from the well, a view reinforced by psychoanalysis. Putnam's good friend William James was a case in point. James struggled for years with what he and his physicians called "nervous prostration," and in later years with a heart condition as well. Yet James left a remarkable intellectual legacy and at his best was a man of great buoyancy, an inspiration to his friends.[50] Putnam also observed that the historian Francis Parkman "was never able to sleep . . . and could only work a few minutes at a time, yet . . . accomplished such a vast amount of first-class historical research, and was of such splendid will and courage. Surely he represents a kind of person whom it would be a mockery to speak of as mentally weak in any usually accepted sense."[51]

Putnam, despite his perfectionism, was less inclined to label patients or to criticize their behavior than were physicians of an earlier era: "It is no longer enough to characterize a man as 'self-centered,' 'irresolute,' 'dominated by envy, suspicion, jealousy' or, on the other hand, as a person of 'fine' or 'strong' character, as if we had the right to assume that we had thereby added something material to our knowledge of him, in a scientific sense." [52] In a similar vein, William Alanson White, appalled by the prejudicial work of those who sought to establish a hereditary basis for mental illness, suggested that a patient's healthy as well as diseased ancestors be listed in the pedigree charts.[53]

Putnam believed that physicians must not impose their own values, but must help patients develop their own. But other physicians, less humble and more certain that they had the truth, sometimes claimed that their professional knowledge entitled them to impose their values, not only on their patients, but on society at large. Some physicians supported eugenic legislation to segregate or sterilize the insane or retarded—"the menace of the feeble-minded" was at its height in the Progressive era—or to restrict immigration of less favored nationalities. Such activities reflect the darker side of the expanding domain of medicine.[54]

If Putnam and his colleagues differed in the confidence with which they felt they could proselytize for a particular view of health, and in their attitudes toward patients, these differences presaged some of the fundamental tensions within the medical profession a half-century later. Indeed, little in the contemporary debate about human values and social responsibility is new. Putnam and Cabot advocated a balance between art and science in patient care, and called upon both physicians and patients to learn (or rediscover) skills of understanding and a sensitivity to the social and psychological determinants of well-being, including those arising out of the therapeutic situation itself. Against this view stood those doctors who would rely almost exclusively on a burgeoning technology, laboratory science, and the authority of the physician-expert as sole healer of the most varied ills. Cabot saw himself as an apostle of the future, but in many respects he was fighting a rear-guard action against the forces that came to dominate medicine in the twentieth century. In this context, it is perhaps significant that in later years Cabot was better known as a professor of social ethics than as a teacher of medicine.

Many of the essays in this volume point to the ways in which the cohesive image of medicine as art and science on which Putnam and Cabot relied has become blurred. They also constitute an attempt to recover and clarify that image. It would appear that medical history is more cyclical than linear, and that new forms of "progressive" medicine will involve not only scientific break-throughs and innovations, but also profound efforts at renewal and rededication.

NOTES

I wish to thank Diana Long Hall, Charles Rosenberg, Judith P. Swazey and members of the dialogue group for suggestions concerning this essay, and Catherine Lord for research assistance. Quotations from the Richard C. Cabot Papers, Harvard University Archives, are made with the permission of the Trustees, Clause IV, under the will of Richard C. Cabot. Quotations from the Personal Correspondence of William Alanson White, 1906–1937, Record Group 418, Records of Saint Elizabeths Hospital, National Archives, are made with the permission of Saint Elizabeths Hospital. Research for this paper was supported in part by a fellowship (MH-18,877) from the National Institute of Mental Health, U.S. Public Health Service.

1. *Report on National Vitality: Its Wastes and Conservation,* Bulletin 30 of the Committee of One Hundred (Washington: U.S. Government Printing Office, 1909), p. 14 and passim.

2. *Man Adapting* (New Haven: Yale University Press, 1965), p. 364.

3. For suggestive data on mortality, see Frederick L. Hoffman, "American Mortality Progress During the Last Half Century," in *A Half Century of Public Health,* ed. Mazÿck P. Ravenel (New York: American Public Health Association, 1921), pp. 94–117. See also other articles in Ravenel's volume and George Rosen, *A History of Public Health* (New York: MD Publications, 1958).

4. See especially Richard Harrison Shryock, *National Tuberculosis Association, 1904–1954: A Study of the Voluntary Health Movement in the United States* (New York: National Tuberculosis Association, 1957).

5. See John C. Burnham, "Medical Specialists and Movements Toward Social Control in the Progressive Era: Three Examples," in *Building the Organizational Society,* ed. Jerry Israel (New York: Free Press, 1972), pp. 19–30, 249–51.

6. Quoted in C-E. A. Winslow, *The Life of Hermann M. Biggs: Physician and Statesman of the Public Health* (Philadelphia: Lea and Febiger, 1929), pp. 230–31.

7. *Papers and Addresses III* (Baltimore: Johns Hopkins Press, 1920), p. 159.

8. On the psychotherapy movement, see Nathan G. Hale, Jr., *Freud and the Americans: The Beginnings of Psychoanalysis in the United States, 1876–1917* (New York: Oxford University Press, 1971), pp. 116–50; John Chynoweth Burnham, *Psychoanalysis and American Medicine, 1894–1918: Medicine, Science, and Culture* (New York: International Universities Press, 1967); and, for a contemporary account, E. W. Taylor, "The Attitude of the Medical Profession Toward the Psychotherapeutic Movement," *Boston Medical and Surgical Journal,* 157 (December 26, 1907):843–50.

9. An excellent guide to Putnam's life and work is Nathan G. Hale, Jr., ed., *James Jackson Putnam and Psychoanalysis: Letters Between Putnam and Sigmund Freud, Ernest Jones, William James, Sandor Ferenczi, and Morton Prince, 1877–1917* (Cambridge: Harvard University Press, 1971), especially the introductory essay. Putnam's papers are located at the Francis A. Countway Library of Medicine, Boston.

10. James Jackson Putnam, "Not the Disease Only, but Also the Man," *Boston Medical and Surgical Journal,* 141 (July 20, 1899): 53–57, (July 27, 1899):77–81; and idem, "Remarks on the Psychical Treatment of Neurasthenia," ibid., 132 (May 23, 1895):505–11.

11. There is no adequate study of Cabot, but see Neva R. Deardorff, "Richard Clarke Cabot," *Dictionary of American Biography,* Supp. 2, pp. 83–85; Paul Dudley White, "Richard Clarke Cabot, 1868–1939," *New England Journal of Medicine,* 220 (June 22, 1939): 1049–52; and Thomas Franklin Williams, "Cabot, Peabody, and the Care of the Patient," *Bulletin of the History of Medicine,* 24 (September–October 1950): 462–81.

12. Letter to Ella Lyman [Cabot], postmarked June 27, 1893, Box 14, Richard Clarke Cabot Papers, Harvard University Archives.

13. White, "Richard Clarke Cabot," p. 1051.

14. "Ethical Forces in the Practice of Medicine, an Address Delivered Before Students of Harvard College at the Harvard Union, on April 13, 1905," reprint, p. 1; "The Renaissance of Therapeutics" (1906), reprint; "The Doctor and the Community," *American Medicine,* 8 (October 22, 1904), reprint, p. 1; "Foregrounds and Backgrounds in Work for the Sick: An Address Delivered at the 43rd Annual Meeting of the New England Hospital for Women and Children, 1908," reprint, p. 5. All reprints of articles by Cabot cited here and elsewhere are from the Rare Book Room of the Francis A. Countway Library of Medicine.

15. "The Use of Truth and Falsehood in Medicine: An Experimental Study," *American Medicine,* 5 (February 28, 1903), reprint; "The Doctor and the Community," pp. 5–6.

16. See Richard C. Cabot, "Suggestions for the Reorganization of Hospital Out-Patient Departments, with Special Reference to the Improvement of

Treatment," *Maryland Medical Journal* (March 1907), reprint; idem, "Why Should Hospitals Neglect the Care of Chronic Curable Disease in Out-Patients?" *The St. Paul Medical Journal,* (March 1908), reprint; Ida M. Cannon, "Forty Years of Social Service," talk to students, October 15, 1945, in Archives of the Social Service Department, Massachusetts General Hospital (hereafter cited as SSD-MGH).

17. "Suggestions for Reorganization," p. 6.

18. For the early history of the department, see the annual reports of the Massachusetts General Hospital; M. Antoinette Cannon, "History of the Social Service Department: The First Ten Years—1905–1915," paper prepared for the fiftieth anniversary of the department, in SSD-MGH. See also Roy Lubove, *The Professional Altruist: The Emergence of Social Case Work as a Career, 1880–1930* (New York: Atheneum, 1969), pp. 23–35.

19. See Harriet M. Bartlett, "Ida M. Cannon: Pioneer in Medical Social Work," *Social Service Review,* 49 (June 1975):208–29; M. Antoinette Cannon, "History of the Social Service Department"; and Ida M. Cannon, *On the Social Frontier of Medicine: Pioneering in Medical Social Service* (Cambridge: Harvard University Press, 1952), pp. 63–154.

20. Richard C. Cabot, *Social Service and the Art of Healing* (New York: Moffat, Yard and Co., 1909), p. 55; idem, "Four Hopes for the Future of Hospital Social Work," *Hospital Social Service,* 24 (1931), reprint, p. 67; idem, "Suggestions for Reorganization"; and Ida M. Cannon, *Social Work in Hospitals: A Contribution to Progressive Medicine* (New York: Russell Sage Foundation, 1917), p. 104.

21. M. Antoinette Cannon, "History of the Social Service Department," pp. 17–18; Cabot, *Social Service and the Art of Healing,* p. 90. See also correspondence in the Cabot Papers, Harvard University Archives.

22. Annual reports of the Social Service Department of MGH; M. Antoinette Cannon, "History of the Social Service Department," pp. 15–17.

23. Ibid., p. 18.

24. Lloyd C. Taylor, Jr., *The Medical Profession and Social Reform, 1885–1945* (New York: St. Martin's Press, 1974), pp. 11–12, 43–45.

25. Jane Addams, "Charity and Social Justice: The President's Address," *Proceedings, National Conference of Charities and Correction,* 37 (1910):2–3.

26. For a fuller discussion of definitions of health in the late nineteenth century, see Barbara Sicherman, "The Paradox of Prudence: Mental Health in the Gilded Age," *Journal of American History,* 62 (March 1976):890–912.

27. Women's Medical Association of New York City, *Mary Putnam Jacobi: A Pathfinder in Medicine* (New York, 1925), p. xxiii.

28. Charles K. Mills, *Toner Lectures, Lecture IX: Mental Over-work and Premature Disease among Public and Professional Men* (Washington, 1885), p. 21; Mary Putnam Jacobi, "Some Considerations on the Moral, and on the Non-Asylum Treatment of Insanity," *Journal of Social Science,* 15, pt. 2 (February 1882):86.

29. Henry Putnam Stearns, *Insanity: Its Causes and Prevention* (New York,

1883), p. 47; Henry Maudsley, *The Pathology of Mind* (New York, 1880), p. 85; Samuel Osgood, "Health and the Higher Culture," American Public Health Association, *Public Health Papers and Reports*, 2 (1874–1875):202.

30. "Remarks on the Psychical Treatment of Neurasthenia," p. 506.

31. The examples are drawn from a suggestive article by John Higham, "The Reorientation of American Culture in the 1890's," in *The Origins of Modern Consciousness*, ed. John Weiss (Detroit: Wayne State University Press, 1965), pp. 25–48.

32. Simon N. Patten, *The New Basis of Civilization*, ed. Daniel M. Fox (Cambridge: Belknap Press of Harvard University Press, 1968); originally published in 1907.

33. For a summary of Progressive achievements in politics, see George E. Mowry, *The Era of Theodore Roosevelt and the Birth of Modern America, 1900–1912* (New York: Harper and Row, 1962); and in public health, Rosen, *History of Public Health*.

34. *The Strenuous Life: Essays and Addresses* (New York: Century Co., 1905), p. 4.

35. William James, "The Gospel of Relaxation," *Talks to Teachers on Psychology and to Students on Some of Life's Ideals* (New York: Dover Press, 1962), pp. 99–112, originally published in 1899; Henry James, ed., *The Letters of William James* (Boston: Atlantic Monthly Press, 1920), II, 158.

36. *The Energies of Men* (New York: Moffat, Yard and Co., 1917), pp. 11, 16, and passim.

37. "Work Cure—I," *Psychotherapy*, 3, no. 1 (1909):24.

38. Letter to James Hay, Jr., February 3, 1913, National Archives.

39. Joseph Lee, "The Unknown Basis of Mental Hygiene," *Proceedings, National Conference of Charities and Correction*, 42 (1915):236–40.

40. *What Men Live By* (Boston: Houghton Mifflin, 1914); "Work Cure—II," *Psychotherapy*, 3, no. 1 (1909):20–27.

41. Sicherman, "Paradox of Prudence," passim.

42. *What Men Live By*, pp. 89, 103, 136–40, and passim.

43. Richard C. Cabot, "The Analysis and Modification of Environment," *Psychotherapy*, 3, no. 3 (1909):5–10; James Jackson Putnam, "The Value of the Physiological Principle in the Study of Neurology," *Boston Medical and Surgical Journal*, 151 (December 15, 1904):641–47.

44. Letter to W. B. Parker, July 30, 1908, in the Putnam Papers, Countway Medical Library.

45. Putnam to Freud, May 19, 1915, in Hale, *James Jackson Putnam and Psychoanalysis*, p. 185; Freud to Putnam, June 7, 1915, ibid., p. 188.

46. Putnam to Freud, August 13, 1915, ibid., p. 192.

47. Putnam's views on health are most fully developed in his correspondence with Freud and in a series of four essays, "The Psychology of Health," published in *Psychotherapy*, 1, no. 2 (1908):24–32; no. 3 (1909):5–13; no. 4 (1909): 37–49;

and 2, no. 1 (1909):35–44. The quotation is from "The Psychology of Health—I," 1, no. 2, p. 30.

48. Quoted in Barbara Sicherman, *The Quest for Mental Health in America, 1880–1917* (New York: Arno Press, 1979).

49. Putnam, "The Value of the Physiological Principle in the Study of Neurology," p. 642; Meyer, "Mental and Moral Health in a Constructive School Program," in *The Collected Papers of Adolf Meyer,* ed. Eunice E. Winters (Baltimore: Johns Hopkins Press, 1952), IV, 366; Richard C. Cabot to Frances Rousmaniere (Mrs. Arthur S. Dewing), April 3, 1905, Box 16, Cabot Papers, Harvard University Archives.

50. James Jackson Putnam, "William James," *Atlantic Monthly,* 106 (December 1910):835–48, and the correspondence betwen Putnam and James and between Putnam and Frances R. Morse in the Putnam Papers.

51. Quoted in Hale, *Freud and the Americans,* p. 81.

52. "The Relation of Character Formation to Psychotherapy," in *Psychotherapeutics: A Symposium* (Boston: Richard G. Badger, 1910), p. 187.

53. Letter to Smith Ely Jelliffe, June 4, 1910, National Archives.

54. See, for example, Mark H. Haller, *Eugenics: Hereditarian Attitudes in American Thought* (New Brunswick: Rutgers University Press, 1963).

CHAPTER 6

Attitudes in Medical Ethics

Ernest Wallwork

The desire by health professionals to do the right thing needs informed exploration of the conceptual foundations of moral judgment, especially in a society with many disparate value systems. Ernest Wallwork describes some philosophical bases on which health professionals may develop reasoned moral concern for their profession and their patients. He uses ethics and the social sciences to build a perspective from which health care providers can approach specific problems of medical practice, such as advocacy, concern for social purposes, and humane treatment.

The basis of normative moral principles is, for Wallwork "recognition respect," which "involves acknowledgment of, and esteem for, the intrinsic integrity of another person as well as the fundamental interests that are constitutive of the other's self." Respect for persons, both attitudinally and conceptually, is the basis for normative moral principles, especially the key items of freedom and the welfare of others. In the latter half of his essay, Wallwork incorporates into the theoretical structure he has built observations about specific moral problems of health care delivery.

I intend to consider the following two questions: What fundamental attitudes underlie moral decision-making? How are these attitudes related to several central normative issues in ordinary medical practice—for example, the doctor-patient contract, truth-telling, informed consent in medical experimentation, and the social-policy question of adequate distribution of health care services? By highlighting the crucial significance of attitudinal sensitivities in moral judgment and relating them to the major principles governing particular cases, I intend to sketch a broad perspective on ethical judgments about medical care. My principal goal is to clarify, argue for, and systematically order some of the central moral evaluations that frequently arise (at least in discussions in which I have participated) in medical schools, hospitals, and conferences on medical ethics. The normative claims I shall be discussing are not new. They are commonly cited whenever physicians, nurses, educators, and administrators debate the ethics of medical care. What I intend to do is to relate these normative claims in a framework that is congruent with recent developments in philosophical ethics as well as with what we know about morality from the several social sciences, especially psychoanalysis as revised by ego psychology, cognitive developmental theory, and social research on role relationships.

1

The most important attitudes for moral judgment are those relating to persons. These attitudes are basic to the moral life, in the first place, because they have a profound and pervasive *casual* influence on the adoption of more specific principles of action, like truth-telling and promise-keeping. That is, one's basic attitude toward others tends to motivate the adoption of certain normative principles and the elimination of others. As I shall later observe, there is also a *logical* connection between attitudes and normative principles such that the attitude of respect for persons enters into the justification of our most basic, general normative principles.

Appreciation of the causal influence of attitudes on moral judgment and behavior is widespread in the medical profession, and thus scarcely controversial. It is generally recognized that doctors, nurses, and orderlies are motivated to make moral decisions by differing degrees of respect for the dignity and well-being of patients, their families, and medical colleagues. Partly for this reason, medical personnel often focus conversations about ethical issues on attitudes toward patients, their families, and other staff, as well as patient attitudes toward them. The unexpressed assumption in these discussions is that attitudes have an important causal influence, on both the kinds of moral decisions that are made and the quality of the resulting interpersonal relationships. A nurse who truly respects the dignity of patients is generally expected to avoid the extremes of both authoritarianism and oversolicitous interventions. Similarly, a "sympathetic" patient tends to exhibit not only "empathy" toward other patients and the medical staff, in the sense of "feeling with them," but also *active* "concern for others," as exhibited in acts of kindness, however small, and words of encouragement and gratitude.

Recognition of the crucial impact of attitudinal sensitivities on moral judgment and behavior is especially prominent in criticisms of contemporary health care. The distancing, technocratic orientation of some professionals, and the institutional practices that foster impersonal relationships, generate frequent criticism, precisely because the exclusive technocrat, by treating persons as things, lacks the respect for others that undergirds morality. To be sure, technocratically oriented professionals usually evidence respect for patients in treating specific health needs, and this is certainly a crucial moral aspect of most medical assistance. But a predominantly scientific or managerial orientation distances the professional from actively caring for the full range of patient interests that are affected by most medical interventions.

Ample evidence for the pervasive influence of attitudes on moral judgments is readily forthcoming from several very different traditions in the behavioral sciences. A central insight of psychoanalytic theory and practice, for example, is that ego attitudes toward others decisively affect normative judgments, a point Erik Erikson has most persistently mined in his developmental theory centering on varieties of interpersonal mutuality and their importance for moral judgment and action. "Cognitive consistency" research further reinforces clinical findings by demonstrating that individuals do not merely subscribe to random collections of attitudes and beliefs but rather maintain internally consistent beliefs and attitudes that dynamically affect behavior (Bem, 1970). Similarly, the cognitive developmental studies of moral judgment conducted by Jean Piaget and, more recently,

Lawrence Kohlberg show that responses to moral dilemmas form structured cognitive systems centering around, in Piaget's case, respect for authorities or peers and, in Kohlberg's research, evaluative attitudes toward human life (Piaget, 1965; Kohlberg, 1969, 1971). Sociological research on role expectations similarly demonstrates that institutional rules and roles foster the establishment of attitudinal patterns. An abundant literature in medical sociology shows, for instance, that socialization processes in medical schools and hospitals, as well as the norms of reference groups (such as professional associations, senior colleagues, and peers), foster the establishment of relatively coherent attitudinal and behavioral patterns toward physician-patient relationships, doctor-nurse-orderly interactions, and other role relationships.

The inescapable conclusion deriving from these various sources is that psychosocial attitudes, because they include modes of willing as well as thinking and feeling, motivate the adoption of some normative principles to the exclusion of others (Downie and Telfer, 1970, p. 17). An attitude, Gordon Allport rightly observed, is "a mental and neural *state of readiness,* organized through experience, exerting a directive or dynamic influence upon the individual's response to all objects and situations with which it is related" (cited in Merton, 1957, p. 253). This description, when applied to attitudes toward other persons, suggests a volitional "set" appropriate to the adoption of moral principles incorporating the positive or negative evaluations of persons. In short, attitudes toward others are more pervasive in their influence on the quality of the moral life than narrower principles of action.

So far, I have indicated that attitudes toward persons are causally influential in the moral life. There is, however, an important distinction between a psychosocial theory of causation and the meaning and justification of a moral judgment. From the fact that attitudes are causally important in making a moral judgment, it by no means follows that attitudes are essential to the definition of morality. Attitudes may well indicate something about the psychological make-up of human beings, who alone are capable of making moral judgments. But a psychological condition is quite different from, and should not be confused with, a moral judgment. Humans cannot make moral judgments without brains, but no one has suggested that the necessary condition of having a brain is part of the meaning and justification of a moral judgment. If we wish to recognize the importance of attitudes for the justification of moral judgments, we must take a different tack, although one suggested by the fact that attitudes are mental states that are more closely related to what a person means than are physiological events in the brain.

Attitudes have not received much sustained attention from contemporary ethicists, largely because of the unsatisfactory way in which they were handled within the now widely discredited emotivist theory of ethical meaning. In the writings of C. L. Stevenson, who best represented emotivism several decades ago, attitudes were identified with feelings, and moral judgments were held merely to express and evoke attitudes of approval or disapproval (Stevenson, 1944, 1963). Thus, moral disapproval of someone's behavior was identified with the disgust or revulsion that the speaker felt on witnessing it. All moral judgments were summarily reduced to utterances taking the form, "I approve (or disapprove) of *x*; do so as well." But clearly this was a mistaken approach to the meaning of moral judgments. A typical moral utterance like "You ought to do *x*" is not, explicitly at least, an expression of the speaker's attitudes. It is, rather, a prescription telling someone to make *x* the case (Hare, 1952, 1963). Furthermore, moral judgments are rational in a way in which mere expressions of emotional taste, delight, and disgust are not. The absence of a reason undermines a moral judgment, but it does not invalidate an expression of taste. The statement "You ought to do *x*" requires rational defense when "why" questions are asked. But it is sufficient to respond to the question "Why do you like *y*?" with "I just do." Emotivists tried unsuccessfully to account for the rational character of moral discourse by claiming that it is simply a way of persuading others to accept one's own emotional set. If this were the case, however, irrational methods would be as appropriate as rational deliberation in the defense of an ethical stance, since they are often very persuasive indeed.

These criticisms of emotivism may be accepted without abandoning the attitudinal foundations of ethics. In the first place, it may be granted that moral judgments seldom explicitly express attitudes. When I say "You ought to do *x*," I am clearly prescribing behavior to you, not expressing my attitudes. Nonetheless, attitudes may lie in the background, though often unexpressed. In technical jargon, attitudes may be present below the surface of the "speech act." And indeed, moral judgments do imply the presence of certain attitudes. One cannot without oddity claim that something is good or ought to be done and, in the same breath, indicate that one does not approve of it. Imagine how odd it would be if someone uttered the sentence "*x* is good," but we could not recognize anything at all in her or his behavioral stance that implied the slightest trace of approval. Would we not say that such a person did not understand what she or he was saying? An attitude of approval is part of what it means sincerely to express a positive evaluation of some action or state of affairs.

Not only is it characteristic of moral judgments to imply the presence of attitudes, but also the specific "primitive" or fundamental attitude of respect for some persons is always present in the background of a moral utterance. In other words, morality is characterized not only by its formal prescriptive or commendatory character (Hare, 1952, 1963), but also by its content—namely, the positive evaluation of at least some persons. This claim is supported, we shall see, by the way in which most basic moral principles imply such respect in one way or another. If "respect" in this context refers to valuing or esteeming the intrinsic integrity of a person, the fundamental needs or interests that are constitutive of the self are clearly valued along with the granting of such respect. This explains why we defend an ethical position by bringing forward the fundamental needs and interests of the persons affected by the action.

Although respect for persons is an attitude, it is not immune to rational deliberation, as some emotivists have supposed. In fact, attitudes in general are not cut off, in Humean fashion, from thought and cognition. Because they lean more toward beliefs than mere tastes and preferences, attitudes can be "taken up" and "given up," supported and attacked by reasons. The greater ease with which attitudes can be altered in this manner distinguishes them from deep-seated emotions, which can be changed only exceptionally. In contrast with the latter, attitudes are relational mental states connecting feelings to beliefs about objects (or persons). To discuss an attitude is to refer not merely to a subjective state, but to the relationship in which a person stands to some object. A polar reference is involved both to the experiencing subject and to the object experienced. The outward reference of attitudes explains why we tend to resist their reduction to mere subjective states of admiration or approval. Normally we insist that there is something about an object that evokes our admiration. When I say a patient is worthy of respect as a person, I do not merely mean that I do in fact subjectively feel esteem for the patient. My meaning is that the person in question is a fitting or worthy object of esteem. And I expect that others will share this attitude as well. Because attitudes are susceptible to reasoning, the universalizability criterion—that similar cases are to be treated similarly—assists in the extension of attitudes of respect for *some* persons to all persons equally.

The idea that respect for persons is the fundamental moral attitude is scarcely new in ethical theory, having received early formulation in the Golden Rule and its analogues in non-Western religions. Since the Enlightenment, the idea that every human being deserves respect qua human person has enjoyed a central place in such diverse philosophical works as Kant's *Groundwork of the Metaphysic of Morals,* John Stuart Mill's *On Liberty,* and Emile Durkheim's "Individualism and the Intellectuals" (Wallwork, 1972). Recent moralists who have defended the centrality of respect for persons include John Rawls, Bernard Williams, R. S. Peters, R. S. Downie, and Elizabeth Telfer in philosophical ethics, together with theologians like Paul Ramsey and Gene Outka. Respect for persons is also central to Erikson's (1969) ethic of generative care. In *Gandhi's Truth,* Erikson defines care in terms of equal regard for the essence of every other human being, a point of congruence between the implicit ethic of psychoanalysis and Gandhi's reinterpretation of the ancient Hindu concept of *ahimsa* (Wallwork, 1973). From the very different orientation of cognitive developmental theory, Lawrence Kohlberg (1971, 1973) argues that moral judgment proceeds from the first positive evaluation of other persons to a final, fully ethical stage in which all persons are equally respected.

My own position is that these diverse metaethical theories are right, because the attitude of respect for persons is constitutive of the moral point of view. To take up the perspective of morality is to assume the attitude of "recognition respect," as distinguished from "appraisal respect" (Darwall, 1977). Recognition respect involves acknowledgment of, and esteem for, the intrinsic integrity of another person as well as the fundamental interests that are constitutive of the other's self. To treat another with recognition respect is to acknowledge his or her claims as deserving of consideration or regard in all one's moral evaluations. This is very different from "appraisal respect," which involves a comparative evaluation of the excellences of actions or character traits resulting from voluntary choices. Whereas recognition respect is assumed upon entering the moral point of view, appraisal respect for another is acquired within that perspective. To be granted recognition respect, one need only possess the generic characteristics of human beings, whereas appraisal respect praises the excellences of the voluntary choices of those qualifying for recognition respect.

Although an extensive discussion would be necessary to justify fully the thesis that recognition respect is constitutive of morality, it is sufficient for present purposes to observe that such respect is implied by our most fundamental, general normative principles. These basic principles are generally thought to include nonmaleficence, truthfulness, promise-keeping, gratitude, reparation, beneficance, liberty, and distributive justice (cf. Ross, 1930, p. 21). These principles are basic in the sense that if someone delivers what purports to be a moral judgment, he or she usually uses these principles or, when pushed to state a more general principle covering lower-level rules, invokes at least one or more of the principles from this range.

The sense in which these principles *imply* respect for persons is roughly as follows. To say that a moral utterance implies recognition respect is to say that in performing it I give it to be understood, in the background presuppositions and sincerity conditions of the speech act, that I have such respect (Searle, 1969). Thus, noninjury of others, which is widely considered the most stringent of moral obligations, implies respect for the physical and psychological integrity of others. Truthfulness implies respect for persons as rational creatures capable of shaping their lives in accordance with reason. Promise-keeping implies respect for both the reasonable expectations raised in the promisee and the voluntary action of the promisor, who has restricted the range of his or her future behavior by freely accepting an obligation. Gratitude is an expression of appreciation for a freely given, usually unmerited, beneficence and implies respect for the kindly acts of a self-determining agent. Reparation, resting on acknowledgment of a previous wrongful and avoidable act of the agent, implies respect for the one who has been harmed or injured. Beneficence presupposes voluntary acts directed at intrinsically desirable states of affairs (for example, knowledge, pleasure, a sense of identity, and virtue) that are close to the center of a well-constituted self. Liberty is respect for others as self-determining moral agents, who have a right to noninterference except for very good reasons. And distributive justice respects the needs, the merits or deserts, and the social contributions of other self-governing agents.

These several principles are not to be interpreted as binding, legalistic rules. They are "abstract" rather than "actual" obligations; that is, they are *prima facie* right as abstract generalizations apart from concrete situations. They only engender a moral obligation when they are actually present in a specific context or situation. They are thus compatible with the particularistic focus of "situation ethics." Whether or not an "actual" moral obligation

exists depends upon the presence of one or more of these principles in human relationships as well as upon their relative weight.
When we are in a situation in which several of these claims are
incumbent upon us, we have to form a considered opinion that in
this circumstance one is more weighty than another. Then we are
actually bound morally.

The fact that the foregoing principles imply respect for persons
suggests that such respect enters into their justification. When
pushed to explain why one of these principles is right, we normally say something about the various ways in which we respect others—for example, by honoring their fundamental interests in freedom, well-being, health, truth, mutual aid, and noninterference.

Despite the importance of these implications for the coherence
of normative theory, all they really show is that respect for at least
some persons is presupposed in taking up the moral point of view.
But this limited result is what one would expect from an investigation of the most general characteristics of morality. Such a characterization must be broad enough to include all those codes we
recognize as moral, even if we disagree with their normative contents. For example, we recognize morality in children, although
their respect for others does not extend beyond parents and
peers. Elitist and nationalistic moralities are similarly restricted in
scope.

However, this account contains the means whereby these limited forms of respect are naturally extended to all human beings.
If I say "I respect you," it is on account of some quality such that I
would respect anyone who was similar in that regard. Insofar as
the qualities that lead me to grant recognition respect to a near
one are shared by all other human beings, universal respect for
persons qua persons is justified. Through this application of the
universalizability criterion, one reaches the normative perspective
shared by Kant, Mill, Durkheim, Rawls, Williams, Erikson, and
Kohlberg: that persons are of unconditional value, that each and
every person is valuable qua human existent, not because he or
she is such-and-such a person with idiosyncratic qualities and

accomplishments (Outka, 1972, p. 12). A fundamental equality is thereby recognized to exist among persons that prevents one from being more highly valued than another. From this perspective, differential treatment is still possible, but only on relevant grounds. Thus, respect for persons means that the claims and interests of everyone are equal in value to your own and your near one's unless there are relevant reasons for regarding these claims as unequal and hence deserving of differential treatment.

Two prominent normative claims are given with recognition respect. First, the fundamental needs and interests that are constitutive of every self's identity give rise to welfare rights. Because these basic needs must be met in order to do anything else, whether poorly or well, considerations of merit are inappropriate to distribution of primary welfare goods. Minimally, all persons require relief from acute physical pain as well as a package of subsistence goods that includes psychological as well as biological necessities, such as a certain minimal degree of affection, psychosocial identity, and sense of self-worth. Inasmuch as all human beings require these goods equally prior to differential degrees of effort, one person's claims are as good as another's. "Thus, to take a perfectly clear case, no matter how A and B might differ in taste and style of life, they would both crave relief from acute physical pain. In that case we would put the same value on giving this to either of them, regardless of the fact that A might be a talented, brilliantly successful person, B 'a mere nobody' " (Vlastos, 1962, p. 51). The natural equality of persons vis-à-vis basic needs calls for equal consideration, with each person's well-being given the same weight as another's.

A second normative claim acknowledged with recognition respect is individual liberty, or the unique freedom of persons to choose among alternative courses of action in accordance with rational purposes and decisions. Thus, every person's freedom of choice is as unique and inalienable as his or her existence itself. My freedom cannot be transferred to another and remain mine. To be sure, others can and often do make decisions for me, but only on the basis of their own capacities for free decision-making, not mine. Freedom, like basic welfare, is thus equally shared, at least among normal adults. Hence, we rightly believe "that choosing for oneself what one will do, believe, approve, say, see, read, worship, has its own intrinsic value, the same for all persons, and quite independently of the value of the things they happen to choose" (Vlastos, 1962, p. 51). Of course we distinguish among the uses people make of their freedom of choice, but, first of all, we value their exercise of that freedom, regardless of the outcome. And we value it equally for all. In brief, one person's freedom is as valuable as any other's.

Normally, respect covers both the welfare needs and liberty of others. But where freedom of choice is not yet fully developed, as in the case of children, there is an obligation to meet welfare needs, while responding to them in such a way as to maximize current capacities for choice and the chances for reasonably free decisions later in life. Since there is a close connection between how we treat children and what they become, respect means treating them as capable of choices from a very early age. This also entails acknowledging their responsibility for the consequences of the decisions made. Where freedom of choice has been severely reduced, as with the senile and many seriously ill patients, the capacities for choice that are retained should be respected and, in the case of the elderly, enhanced as far as possible—a task that current treatment programs for the elderly have only begun to tackle. Where individuals have lost consciousness, as with comatose patients, we continue medical care of basic welfare needs on the presumption that, if they were conscious, this is what they would value; but we respect them primarily for the potentialities they may regain when recovered.

My argument, then, is that respect for persons is morally basic in the double sense that a weak form is partly constitutive of morality and enters into the justification of our most important general moral principles. Insofar as recognition respect is directed toward the psychosomatic integrity of persons, the universalizability criterion of rational choice implies that all persons deserve equal regard for those basic needs and interests, including freedom of choice, that are constitutive of the self. This egalitarian attitude is not incompatible, it should be noted, with recognizing the moral claims deriving from special relationships, such as those created by previous acts of one's own (promise-keeping, reparations) and previous acts of others (gratitude). The grounds of these obligations are such that one would be equally bound to any other person with whom one had these ties. It is also compatible with acknowledging special merits or deserts, again assuming that one would respect similar achievements by anyone. But someone with the attitude of equal regard will tend to appeal to the generic characteristics of all persons before acknowledging the idiosyncratic achievements that distinguish persons from one another. One reason for this is that merit can be justified as a basis of distribution "only if every individual has an equal chance of achieving all the merit he is capable of (and it cannot simply be assumed that they have had this chance)" (Frankena, 1975, p. 254). If competing individuals have not had an equal chance to achieve all the merit of which they are capable, then merit is not a fair basis for distributing the benefits of cooperation among them:

If this is so, then, before merit can reasonably be adopted as a ground of distribution, there must first be a prior *equal* distribution of the conditions for achieving merit, at least so far as this is within the power of human society. This is where such things as equality of opportunity, equality before the law, and equality of access to the means of education come into the picture. In other words, recognition of merit as a criterion of distribution is reasonable only against the background of a recognition of the principle of equality, the primary basis of distribution is not merit but equality, substantive or procedural. (Frankena, p. 254)

The consequences of this position for selected issues in the ethics of health care will now be explored.

2

The first section of this essay has argued for the underlying attitude of respect for persons in the moral life. We will now consider how this attitude is related to normative principles that arise in routine medical care. This second section is limited to principles integral to the general practice of medicine, largely because the attitudinal sensitivities and insensitivities embodied in the principles governing everyday practice establish the normative ethos of the profession. It is within the normative context of ordinary practice that special ethical dilemmas involving exceptions and uses of new technologies arise. Spectacular, headline-generating medical problems also require careful ethical scrutiny, but the spirit with which medical personnel approach these issues is largely conditioned by the principles governing ordinary practice. The normative ethos of a demanding profession like medicine is especially important because the urgent pressure of constant decision-making often means that practitioners have little time for the reflection necessary for complex ethical justifications.

From the standpoint of an ethic focusing on respect for persons, every person has an equal claim to those minimal standards of subsistence and health care without which it is impossible to use or develop capacities necessary to live the life of a human person. Thus, relief from physical pain, to take one example, is a particularly urgent moral claim precisely because without such relief there is precious little that one can effectively do or become. The value of medical care, whatever else it may achieve in terms of optimal human functioning, begins with the desirability of relieving pain, sustaining life, and restoring health. A physician's moral responsibility to relieve suffering and to restore health is increased beyond that of the ordinary citizen by proximity to, and knowledge about, health needs as well as by specialized professional competence and commitment to acting helpfully. Here, as in other human relationships, moral responsibility increases with proximity, knowledge, capability, and commitment (Simon, Powers, and Gunnemann, 1972, pp. 22–25).

When the seriously injured or ill cannot clearly communicate their choices regarding medical assistance, the presumption should be that they desire the health values shared by humankind. But insofar as patients are capable of rational choice, respect for the other as a self-determining agent prevents trespass upon their bodies without voluntary consent. Acknowledgment by one who performs medical procedures of the principle of reasonably free and informed consent reflects the underlying attitude of respect for the personhood of the patient on whom the procedures are performed. Other aspects of medical care—for example, tests and surgery—may treat individuals as passive participants, but human beings are more than patients—they are persons whose consent to actions involving their bodies initially constitutes the doctor-patient relationship as a human encounter. Reasonably informed consent not only establishes the doctor-patient relationship, but continues to legitimate it. The consent requirement implied or explicitly granted in the original contact legitimates the relationship *only* to the extent that the continuing relationship is "not incompatible with the demands of an ongoing partnership sustained by an actual or implied *present* consent and terminable by any present or future dissent from it" (Ramsey, 1970, p. 6). As far as possible, the patient should be fully engaged as a conscious and willing partner in medical procedures, because this is basic to what it means to treat a human being as a person rather than as a manipulable object.

These initial points about the nature of the physician-patient relationship are all fairly widely understood by medical practitioners, and most of them are embodied in law. Yet it is also common knowledge that patients are often treated in ways that disregard their dignity as persons, both in the initial encounter and subsequently. Indeed, many contemporary medical practices undermine the very respect for persons that justifies medical care itself. The numerous factors weakening respect for persons extend from the bases for selecting medical students, through the socialization procedures of medical schools, to the everyday practices of the profession. The selection of students, for instance, tends to gather into the field those who are more object- than person-oriented. Admissions are based on quantitative, scientific skills rather than interpersonal sensitivities and abilities. Medical school education focuses on tissues, symptoms, diagnoses, pharmaceutical remedies, and surgery—all of which support I-It rather than I-You or I-Thou relationships. Paradigm experiences, like the corpse dissection, distance medical students from empathetic identifications. Hospital jargon, like SPOS (subhuman piece of shit) and "to dork" (meaning "to die"), serves the same depersonalizing function as "gook" during the Vietnam war. Patients spared these derogatory designations are too often tacitly assumed to be ignorant, incompetent, passive, and weak rather than self-determining moral agents. Trained to interrogate, inspect, test, and prescribe, young physicians too frequently adopt authoritarian, technocratic forms of interaction, so that telling the patient the truth becomes a question rather than a recognized obligation. Since income is based on the number of office visits, extensive time involvements tend to be avoided in favor of quick diagnoses and unilateral prescriptions. Too frequently, talking with patients comes to be perceived as boring in comparison with the interest of symptoms, diagnoses, and prescriptions. Symptoms, not people, become fascinating—so much so that some physicians gradually become bored with the day-to-day maintenance required of general practitioners.

For this litany of dehumanizing processes, there are a variety of reasonable explanations. Technological competence is obviously crucial for adequate patient care. A degree of distancing and even numbing is probably a prerequisite for psychic balance in the face of acute physical suffering and death. The powerful desires of patients unquestionably contribute to the physician's often exaggerated sense of self-confidence, although the desirability of physicians reinforcing exaggerated expectations in the face of malpractice suits might well be questioned on grounds of professional self-interest alone. Certainly, seriously ill patients are helpless, weak, and often ignorant of medical technology, and all too readily regress to infantile patterns in relation to authority figures, especially in "total institutions" (Goffman, 1961). Shared social-role expectations about the traditional, unilateral diagnosis and the importance of the professional's time tend to support abrupt relationships. Yet the lay critic cannot help but be disturbed by the scarcity of educational policies and professional procedures that effectively "lean against" these developments, understandable as they may be. Where in this training and practice, one asks, does "reverence for the patient come in—not just politeness or civility—but reverence?" (Pruyser, this volume).

One place where reverence ought to be shown is in diagnosis. As Paul Pruyser persuasively argues, depersonalization and degradation would be considerably diminished if diagnosis were to become bilateral through inclusion of the patient as a full partner in egalitarian diagnostic processes. Pruyser correctly believes that widespread institutionalization of physicians as "counselors at medicine" would help counter elitist, authoritarian, technocratic, and managerial orientations.

Another point where respect for persons needs institutionalized reinforcement is in truth-telling. From the research surveys I have read, it appears that most physicians consider truth-telling in cases involving serious or fatal illnesses as an issue for the physician to decide on the basis of whether it will cause the patient harm. Apparently few physicians consider the patient's right to know the truth as primary, and the danger of harm resulting from truthful communication as an exception to the general rule of truth-telling. Yet patients have a right, as free and rational agents, to know the truth necessary for responsible decision-making. To respect another is to recognize in all one's dealings with the other that he or she is a rational creature capable of shaping his or her life in accordance with reasons, and that to veil, misconstrue or distort the truth is to fail to treat the other as fully human. The common practice of veiling the truth presupposes an authority over another's life which is often not justified, because only a patient is sufficiently informed about his or her life situation and sufficiently concerned about various personal interests to decide how best to act in the light of the truth. As Joseph Fletcher (1960) observed, "without their freedom to choose and their right to know the truth, patients are only puppets. And there is no moral quality in a Punch and Judy show; at least there is none in Punch or Judy! It was not because we are only automatons or pawns in the flux of nature ('red in tooth and claw') that Hamlet marvelled, 'What a piece of work man is!' " (p. 33).

The use of patients in experimental research also requires institutional safeguards against disregard of patient rights. With the proliferation of research alongside health care, especially involving indigent patients in large research hospitals, respect for the dignity of potential experimental subjects and donors is subject to continuing assault. What is often ignored in a technological age in which professional prestige rests on experimentation is the fact that any human being is more than a patient or experimental subject; he or she is a personal subject—every bit as much a person as the physician-investigator (Ramsey, 1970, p. 5). When we fail, in an experimental situation, to treat another human being as a person, we are in effect erasing the distinction between how we acceptably respond to human beings and how we acceptably respond to animals or inanimate objects. "Our responses to the human being are determined, not by his choices, but ours in disregard of or with indifference to his" (Morris, 1970, p. 124). When we "look upon" an experimental subject as something less than a person or not a person, we consider the other as incapable of rational choice. As a consequence of not treating the other as a person, we feel justified in interfering with the "person in such a way that what is done, even if the person is involved in the doing, is done not by the person but by the user of the person" (Morris, p. 125).

However, potential research subjects are persons, equal in dignity to medical personnel. Correlatively, the rights of researchers are limited by the equal rights of patient-subjects. And this means that only by their reasonably informed, voluntary consent may persons properly become participants in experimental projects (Wallwork, 1975).

Of course, problems continually arise regarding what it means to be fully informed. The Nuremberg Articles provide one clear set of guidelines. An "enlightened decision" by potential research subjects, the articles declare, "requires that before the acceptance of an affirmative decision by the experimental subject there should be made known to him the nature, duration, and purpose of the experiment; the methods and means by which it is to be conducted; all inconveniences and hazards reasonably to be expected; and the effects upon his health or person which may possibly come from his participation in the experiment." Obviously, phrases like "all inconveniences," "hazards," and "effects" upon health are capable of various interpretations, but they place a heavy burden of moral responsibility on medical investigators to inform patient-subjects adequately about realistic expectations regarding discomforts, risks, and probable consequences. This does not mean, as some caricatures of informed consent suggest, that one must frighten patients out of their wits by listing all procedural details as well as the most remote consequences. But it does mean that potential research subjects have a pressing moral claim to be adequately informed of the relevant inconveniences, hazards, and probable effects. Given the well-known tendency of experimenters to understate these matters in order to entice research subjects, careful institutional safeguards are required.

Other problems surround the much discussed issue of "free consent." This is especially the case where the incentives offered for research participation or the confusion of experimentation with therapy casts doubt upon the freedom of choice involved. It is imperative, for consent to be freely given, that patients "be able to exercise free power of choice, without the intervention of any element of force, fraud, deceit, duress, overreaching, or other ulterior form of constraint or coercion" (Articles of the Nuremberg Tribunal). Again, the line separating coercion from adequate rewards for participation may be difficult to draw in practice, but the fuzziness of this line does not legitimate heavy psychological pressure, deceit, fraud, or force. Safeguards are necessary to counter laissez-faire attitudes toward unrestricted research and to assure reasonable freedom of choice.

The issue of informed consent among potential experimental subjects raises the closely related, but broader, issue of *intervention* by physicians in the lives of others, where such intervention is

initially perceived as deleterious by those affected but where the
physician believes that intervention is right. For example, the
question sometimes arises whether morally offensive decisions by
parents regarding the treatment of their children obligate the
physician to intervene. The problems facing the intervener, as
Charles Powers points out in an unpublished paper, are several.
In the first place, we normally have much less information about
the effects of intervening in someone else's normal life pattern
than we have about actions among our intimates. Second, there is
a presumption against intervention, given respect for the self-
determining decisions of others. Third, we are seldom in a position to compensate or remedy whatever harm might result from
the intervention; that is, the intervener usually withdraws after
stepping into another's affairs, leaving the scene in the hands of
the original parties. Thus, the physician-intervener, in breaking
into the life of a family, may not be fully aware of the complexities
involved, and he or she does not become a part of the family in
the postintervention adjustment. For these reasons, a strong justification for intervention is required, but this does not mean that
respect for persons may not justify intervention despite its being
initially perceived as deleterious. It is in fact especially necessary
to insist on the importance of intervention in certain circumstances in order to counter the widespread tendency in a pluralistic society "not to get involved" even though there are overriding
ethical reasons for doing so.

A strong case for intervention is usually present when third
parties are being harmed. A case in point would be one in which
parents refused medical treatment for their child. The justification here is the presumption that the child would choose, if he or
she were able to make a decision, to have the care indispensable
for the continuation of existence. As Powers points out, there are
a number of interventionist strategies an attending physician who
disagreed with the parental decision could take to protect the life
of the child. The physician-intervener, for example, could seek to
persuade the parents in private consultation, or wider staff support could be sought in an effort to persuade the parents. These

weaker interventions failing, the physician could seek a court order to provide treatment, either by direct order or by removing the parents as "representative agents" of the child. As a final step, the physician could unilaterally treat the child without parental or court consent. Each of these strategies calls for a stronger justification. But, in each case, justification would rest on the overriding moral claims of the third party for protection of her or his fundamental interests. The strength of these claims when survival is at stake leads to a closing of the respectful distance normally separating one person from the decision-making of another.

Because physicians are confronted more frequently than most people by complex moral issues of this sort in which a variety of considerations, including several plausible strategies, are involved, opportunities are needed for hard-headed ethical debates both during medical training and in subsequent practice. The experiments with "ethics rounds" and ethics committees that are being tried in some hospitals provide one opportunity of this sort. But these fledgling efforts suffer badly from weak legitimation and institutional support, even at otherwise innovative hospitals.

The final issue I wish to discuss has to do with the justice of the entire health care system within which physicians and other medical personnel operate. Is the current distribution of health services just or fair? Since this is a question of social justice, the answer revolves around which among the following standard criteria of distribution is relevant:

1. To each according to his or her merit or desert
2. To each according to his or her societal contribution
3. To each according to his or her contribution in satisfying whatever is freely desired by others in the open marketplace of supply and demand
4. To each according to his or her needs

As Gene Outka (1974) has shown in a careful analysis of these principles, the first two are inappropriate justifications for the receipt of medical care (p. 189). Merit is especially irrational as a basis for distribution in most cases, because health crises tend to fall "without discrimination on the (according-to-merit) just and unjust, i.e., the virtuous and the wicked, the industrious and the slothful alike" (p. 191). To be sure, some health needs apparently arise from voluntary acts of patients (for example, obesity, alcoholism, automobile accidents, and drug addiction). But it is impossible to apply criteria of merit within even these few categories, given the complex factors, including unconscious neurotic motivations, affecting individual cases. In any case, ill health is by and large completely unrelated to moral merit or demerit of any sort. Not only is it caused by morally arbitrary factors, but ill health generates prior claims to those of merit by virtue of its damage to the integrity of persons. Acknowledgment of the value of health is given with minimal recognition respect for persons, in contrast with appraisal respect for merit or for what those granted initial moral respect do with their capacities.

The second distributive criterion, "societal contribution," is as difficult to assess as moral merit, since it requires an overall evaluation of the qualitatively different contributions a person makes in all spheres of life—religious, economic, aesthetic, political, and interpersonal. As Paul Ramsey (1970) observes, "we have no way of knowing how really and truly to estimate a man's societal worth or his worth to others or to himself in unfocused social situations in the ordinary lives of men in their communities" (p. 256). But even if we could make these calculations, societal contribution would be an inappropriate criterion for distribution of health care, primarily because an exclusive emphasis on contribution counters recognition respect for persons by supposing that individuals are to be valued, not for what they are, but as mere means to social benefits. This obviously goes against our considered judgment that persons deserve medical treatment even when their social contributions are marginal or declining, as is true of the chronically disabled or the aged.

The third criterion, "to each according to his contribution in satisfying whatever is freely desired by others in the open marketplace of supply and demand," is the primary justification of the current fee-for-service approach within market economies. Justification of this system of private medical consumers and producers involves an appeal in three values—liberty, fairness, and efficiency. First, a decentralized market economy contributes to individual *liberty* in that both potential consumers and medical personnel freely choose their jobs as well as the items they will consume or sell. Such a conception accepts the choices persons make as reasonably rational expressions of what makes them better off. Second, rewards are said to be *fair* in the light of a mixed set of criteria, including ability, desert, effort, and social contribution. Finally, the incentives of differential incomes enhance *efficiency* and, hence, the total goods available for want-satisfaction by a population.

It is not my present purpose to contest these claims for a decentralized market economy outside medicine, except to note the obvious fact that widespread restrictions on the pure market model are now widely recognized as legitimate. Restrictions are especially thought to be necessary when the interests of some bargainers are likely to be deleteriously affected by their inherently unequal bargaining power or when the freedom of a large number of consumers is adversely affected by the power of a few producers.

Clearly the advantages of personal liberty, fair opportunities for advancement, and the incentives provided by differential incomes can be retained without tying health care to a fee-for-service structure. At least society does not have to tie either medical fees or access to medical services to the competitive market to secure these values. One reason for not doing so is the inappropriateness of the competitive market model in considering fair allocations in contemporary medicine. On the supply side, most medical services are made possible not by the inventiveness or isolable contribution of independent physician-entrepreneurs but by a complex, interdependent system in which the attending physician's role is relatively minor. "Modern physicians depend on the achievements of medical technology and the entire scientific base underlying it, all of which is made possible by a host of persons whose salaries are often notably less. Moreover, the amount of taxpayer support for medical research and education is too enormous to make any such unqualified case for provider-autonomy plausible" (Outka, 1974, p. 196). Yet many physicians charge for their time as if they were the sole producers of the benefits dispensed.

Another set of arguments for abandoning the fee-for-service system derives from the physician's excessive power in relation-ship to consumers. I am thinking here not only of monopolistic practices, like the American Medical Association's past efforts to curtail the supply of physicians and local examples of fee-fixing, but more generally of the consumer's unequal bargaining power. Not only is the consumer's knowledge limited in comparison to that of the physician, but the latter often makes the decisions about diagnostic services, visits, hospitalization, and so forth. Normally "the consumer knows very little about the medical serv-ices he is buying—probably less than about any other service he purchases" (Schultze, Fried, Rivlin, and Teeters, 1972, p. 214). Consumers also seldom have much choice over whether or not to purchase health services, given the overriding importance of health care, in contrast to consumer choices among nonessentials such as a new television or dishwasher.

Although the preceding arguments against the physician-supply side of the current fee-for-service system are admittedly controversial, the most important reason for abandoning this sys-tem lies on the demand, or ability-to-pay, side. The chief problem is the lack of a meaningful relationship between the rationale for differential incomes and that for health services. Income dif-ferentials are justified by their incentive effect. But is better medi-cal care (in the likelihood of need) an appropriate incentive for the healthiest and best-endowed members of society? It seems highly unlikely that many of the most productive members of society are significantly motivated by the reward of improved access to better medical care. Yet a system that ties the quality of medical care to the ability to pay is really meting out health services in accordance with success in the competitive marketplace, in complete disregard of the real reasons why people seek medical help.

The only criterion that is relevant for health care is need. Moral merit, social contribution, and success in the marketplace are irrelevant when compared to this criterion, at least insofar as basic health care is concerned. The connection between need and medical treatment is, in Bernard Williams's words, "a necessary truth" (1976, p. 240). Because this need takes priority over most other interests of a person, being tied to the essential integrity of the self, it enjoys the sort of priority given with recognition respect for persons as such. Health care stands alongside food and shelter as one of the essential conditions of minimally decent human existence.

Since all persons need health, a policy that considers need as the ground of care treats everyone equally. But, inasmuch as specific health needs vary, equal concern for the health of everyone also requires differential treatment. In other words, it is just to treat people unequally according to need, because the goal is the equal health of everyone, given age, debilitation, and so forth. Since health needs vary randomly in a kind of natural lottery, it seems only fair to establish an insurance program that spreads the costs through progressive taxation.

A national health insurance program would undoubtedly be costly. This is one reason why we have collectively decided to muddle through with an uncertain system that meets the needs of many, but by no means all, impoverished persons. For the needy, health care is available where they can find it. Often, proof of dire need extracts a toll of shame in lieu of cash. Middle-class families faced with financial ruin often lack even the resources available to the poor. A national health insurance program, despite its costs, would certainly seem warranted by these and other well-documented injustices of the current system. And the overriding importance of health for the achievement and enjoyment of all other goods would seem to place such a program high on the list of national priorities.

Not all these normative consequences follow directly from respect for persons. My claim is only that, when such respect is recognized at the heart of morality, good reasons support welfare guarantees. However one balances the pros and cons of national health insurance, respect for persons brings coherence to our dominant ethical concerns about doctor-nurse-orderly-patient relationships. Because "respect" is an attitude, medical educators and administrators should pay special heed to the kinds of attitudes fostered by the implicit curricula of medical schools and hospitals. In the formation of attitudes, everyday socialization is a far more potent force than anything that is likely to happen in occasional ethics discussion groups. Nevertheless, medical students and workers certainly should have frequent opportunities to reflect critically upon the moral assumptions that sustain and guide their professional life. Anything less denies medical personnel the very respect that they ought to display toward others.

REFERENCES

Bem, Daryl J. *Beliefs, Attitudes, and Human Affairs*. Belmont, Calif.: Brooks/Cole Publishing Co., 1970.

Darwall, Stephen L. "Two Kinds of Respect." *Ethics*, 88 (October 1977):36–49.

Downie, R. S., and Telfer, Elizabeth. *Respect for Persons*. New York: Schocken Books, 1970.

Erikson, Erik. *Gandhi's Truth*. New York: W. W. Norton and Co., 1969.

Fletcher, Joseph. *Morals and Medicine*. Boston: Beacon Press, 1960.

Frankena, William K. "Some Beliefs About Justice." In *Philosophy of Law*, ed. Joel Feinberg and Hyman Gross, pp. 250–58. Calif.: Dickenson Publishing Company, 1975.

Goffman, Erving. *Asylums*. Garden City, N.Y.: Doubleday, 1961.

Hare, R. M. *The Language of Morals*. Oxford: Clarendon Press, 1952.

Hare, R. M. *Freedom and Reason*. New York: Oxford University Press, 1963.

Kohlberg, Lawrence. "Stage and Sequence: The Cognitive-Developmental Approach to Socialization." In *Handbook of Socialization Theory and Research*, ed. D. Goslin. New York: Rand McNally, 1969.

Kohlberg, Lawrence. "From Is to Ought: How to Commit the Naturalistic Fallacy and Get Away with It in the Study of Moral Development." In *Cognitive Development and Epistemology*, ed. T. Mischel. New York: Academic Press, 1971.

Kohlberg, Lawrence. "The Claim to Moral Adequacy of a Highest Stage of Moral Judgment." *The Journal of Philosophy,* 70 (October 1973):630–46.

Merton, Robert. *Social Theory and Social Structure.* Glencoe, Ill.: Free Press, 1957.

Morris, Herbert. "Persons and Punishment." In *Human Rights,* ed. A. I. Melden, pp. 111–34. Belmont, Calif.: Wadsworth Publishing Co., 1970.

Outka, Gene. *Agape.* New Haven: Yale University Press, 1972.

Outka, Gene. "Social Justice and Equal Access to Health Care." In *Love and Society,* ed. James T. Johnson and David H. Smith, pp. 187–207. Missoula, Mont.: American Academy of Religion and Scholars Press, 1974.

Piaget, Jean. *The Moral Judgment of the Child.* New York: Free Press, 1965.

Powers, Charles W. "Understanding and Justifying Intervention." Unpublished manuscript.

Ramsey, Paul. *The Patient as Person.* New Haven: Yale University Press, 1970.

Ross, David. *The Right and the Good.* Oxford: Clarendon Press, 1930.

Schultze, Charles L.; Fried, Edward R.; Rivlin, Alice M.; and Teeters, Nancy H. *Setting National Priorities: The 1973 Budget.* Washington, D.C.: Brookings Institution, 1972.

Searle, John R. *Speech Acts.* London: Cambridge University Press, 1969.

Simon, John; Powers, Charles W.; and Gunnemann, Jon. *The Ethical Investor.* New Haven: Yale University Press, 1972.

Stevenson, Charles L. *Ethics and Language.* New Haven: Yale University Press, 1944.

Stevenson, Charles L. *Facts and Values.* New Haven: Yale University Press, 1963.

Vlastos, Gregory. "Justice and Equality." In *Social Justice,* ed. Richard Brandt. Englewood Cliffs, N.J.: Prentice-Hall, 1962.

Wallwork, Ernest. *Durkheim: Morality and Milieu.* Cambridge: Harvard University Press, 1972.

Wallwork, Ernest. "Erik H. Erikson: Psychosocial Resources for Faith." In *Critical Issues in Modern Religion,* Roger Johnson, Ernest Wallwork *et al,* pp. 322–61. Englewood Cliffs, N.J.: Prentice-Hall, 1973.

Wallwork, Ernest. "Ethical Issues in Research Involving Human Subjects" and "In Defense of Substantive Rights." In *Human Rights and Psychological Research,* ed. Eugene Kennedy, pp. 69–81, 103–25. New York: Thomas Crowell, 1975.

Williams, Bernard. *Problems of the Self.* New York: Cambridge University Press, 1976.

CHAPTER 7

Toward the Optimal Human: Images of the Future and Genetic Engineering

Thomas K. McElhinney

Medical practice has been altered by a new knowledge of genetic mechanisms which has provided a key to understanding organic development as well as the nature of some diseases. In addition to the once dramatic changes that have already become routine in diagnosis and care, current research should add significant new interventions. Indeed, the importance of drugs, for the last half-century a major factor in medicine's ability to deal with human ailments, may soon be surpassed by interventions in genetic structure (although drugs may be among the agents used to effect change).

Thomas K. McElhinney argues that individuals bring to the task of genetic intervention certain concepts of what optimal human functioning is. These concepts are identified as ideals for the human, or images of possible evolution, which are important because people seem to favor or disfavor specific interventions according to the future they deem most desirable. Thus, health professionals may better understand disagreements about specific genetic manipulations if they recognize the differences in beliefs about the optimal human.

The problems associated with various forms of genetic intervention, sometimes grouped under the rubric *genetic engineering*,[1] are related to conceptualizations of the human, to the degree to which humanity is considered adaptable, and to the desirability of attempting to direct the future biological evolution of the human. In this essay, competing views of human nature and of the desirability of attempting planned change are examined as presuppositions that are associated with ethical arguments about specific genetic interventions. A claim is made that differing views of optimal human functioning are related to evidence advanced for or against specific genetic interventions. When these competing views remain unrecognized, major disagreements among medical specialists responsible for implementing the techniques remain unresolved. Discussion of these views, however, can lead to better understanding of, if not reconciliation about, the issues in genetic interventions.

An increasing ability to alleviate distress and to cure or control illness has been made possible through new technologies. As more has been discovered about mechanisms that determine the structure and functioning of the body, methods of intervening have become more sophisticated and health professionals ever more reliant upon complicated equipment. Information about genetics, largely arising from work done in the past few decades, has provided new methodologies and the promise of further interventions that may be used to adjust an individual's genetic constitution or to attempt a more ambitious planned biological alteration of the species.

The understanding of genetic mechanisms and the new powers of intervention have made it possible to select genetic types upon which therapies might be practiced routinely. The U.S. government battles to "cure cancer," and it has sponsored programs to identify the carriers of Tay-Sachs and sickle-cell anemia. A controversy rages about the safety of research on recombinant DNA. Such campaigns indicate that massive attempts at engineering human genetic factors to achieve social goals are at least possible. Attempts to eliminate genes that produce negative effects could be extended by enlarging the concept of what a negative gene is, and attempts to control negative traits could easily become efforts to produce positive features. In the special case of genetics, knowledge is *not* power; but increased knowledge can provide the base for powerful and widespread interventions—for good or for ill.

Although many of the planned interventions seem remote from the practice of medicine, some of the information learned about human genetics has already been introduced into medical procedures, for example, in genetic counseling and screening. In addition, research money is being channeled into projects related to the control of aging, to *in vitro* fertilization, and to the causes of mental retardation. More distant prospects, such as algeny (genetic surgery) and organ regeneration, are possible therapies.[2] These current and future methods raise the questions of both what is possible and what is desirable. Much that may be hoped for may never be realized, and perhaps some things that may be feasible should not be done.

Just as medical ethics involves many problems common to other areas of applied ethics (such as respect for persons, truth-telling, and promise-keeping), so also do these problems arise in genetic engineering. It is virtually impossible to speak responsibly of genetic engineering without encountering the problem of the degree to which humans ought to be restrained—morally if not legally—from doing all that they become capable of doing; similarly, it is necessary to remember that genetic engineering techniques must be considered in view of principles such as "Do no harm." Thus, every proposal for genetic engineering calls for reassessment of some traditional and enduring ethical concerns. It is not my purpose to review again these issues, which have been discussed in many places.[3] Instead, I intend to direct attention to the possibilities of human change that influence the weight given to considerations of ethical issues; for the potential devices of genetic engineering not only pose some old debates in new guises, but add the ethically significant factor of planning human genetic change, of attempting to control the type of humans we wish to be. We have visions and dreams of what humanity can become, and these visions are related to the way we will act. Mortimer Adler has said, "The image that we hold of man cannot fail to affect attitudes that influence our behavior in the world of action, and beliefs that determine our commitments in the world of thought."[4] I shall show some of the conflicting images of the human that are present in writings about the ethical problems of genetic engineering. Because these images are related to our actions, it becomes difficult to ascertain the proper ethical course among several competing images. Since the interventions have already begun and may be expected to increase, it is highly important that competing hopes for the human future be examined.

The problem of the images of the human is important because humanity has a dynamic nature that is constantly subject to the pressures of biological and cultural evolution. The awareness of our changing nature and the ability to accomplish increasingly refined manipulations of genetic characteristics not only destroy our innocence of the fact that political, social, and medical decisions will determine what our nature will be and can become, but also raise hopes and fears about the changes that may be made. With a loss of innocence about our evolutionary biological nature, we are now aware that *not* introducing techniques is also a decision about the human future. As Robert Sinsheimer has so well outlined the situation:

For the first time in all time a living creature understands its origin and can undertake to design its future.

This is a fundamentally new concept. Even in the ancient myths man was constrained by his essence. He could not rise above his nature to chart his destiny. This day we can envision that chance and choice.[5]

The views considered in this study are responses to the challenge that theories of evolution evoke. They are reactions to the knowledge that evolution has introduced, based upon wagers about human nature and destiny. They are, above all, images from which people make choices about work in genetics and medicine, work they believe is ethically justifiable.

Before considering the images of the human that are in conflict, I shall briefly review movements that are related to the current debate about the ethical problems of genetic engineering. These are the sources from which some of the conflicting images arise. They are also the locus of reports that confuse the arguments, because of the sensationalism and passion raised by some issues.

Movements and Themes in the Debate About the Genetic Future

The idea of planning for a certain type of humanity has antecedents in ancient Greek writings. Herodotus, for example, may have recorded the first positive eugenic program (as a plan to promote an improved breed of man) when he described the origin of the Sauromatae. He reported that the Sauromatae were the result of the union of shipwrecked Amazon women and Scythian men. The Scythians met the Amazons and were defeated in an attempt to subdue them. After the defeat, the Scythians sent over some of their most handsome men to try to win by charm what they had been unable to gain by force. "All this they did," says Herodotus, "on account of their strong desire to obtain children from so notable a race." [6]

Plato proposed a planned eugenic program based on the breeding of animals. He advocated marriages for the good of the state and felt that any plan would need to include "falsehood and deceit" on the part of the rulers. Mates would be chosen by lot, but in a lottery that was fixed by the rulers. Most people were to have marriage without procreation (because of their undesirable traits), and the newborn children were to be screened, with the good ones going to a nursery and the others "put away." [7] Aristotle also recommended exposing defectives, exposing infants in the case of overpopulation, and abortion before sensation.[8] These ideas of the Greeks were ignored until the rise of the eugenic movement in the nineteenth century.

Meanwhile, the Judaeo-Christian heritage became the dominant religious tradition in the Mediterranean basin and later in the Western world. The major view of the Christian theologicans, which in turn influenced Western philosophical thought and early scientific argument, centered on individual salvation and final judgment. The main emphasis in Christian proselytizing was the "good news" of salvation in which the individual who accepted Jesus became, as Paul claimed, "a new creature" (2 Corinthians 5:17). The redeemed Christian put away the "old man" to become a "new man." A second vital interpretation of the future was associated with apocalyptic visions of a new heaven and a new earth (Revelation, chapter 22). Thus, both individually and corporately, the West believed in the possibility of change through spiritual renewal.

The concept of an evolving humanity, popularized by Darwin and others in the latter half of the nineteenth century, soon wedded the ideas of Plato and others to the hopes expressed in Christianity. A Eugenic Movement with the goal of species improvement through genetic manipulation was founded by Francis Galton, Darwin's cousin. The strong influence of the Eugenicists in the first three decades of the twentieth century was demonstrated through legislation passed in the United States to prevent immigration (unchecked immigration was seen as a genetic threat to the Anglo-Saxon stock), and through other laws that were enacted to provide for involuntary eugenic sterilization of "undesirables." [9] The excesses practiced by the Nazis in the name of eugenics harmed the eugenicist cause and forced a reconsideration of their proposals in order to provide answers for critics who argued that even the most innocuous measures were the edge of a wedge leading to abuse.

Many eugenicists were also utopians, but utopian thought has its own place in Western literature. Utopian hope developed from Judaeo-Christian origins and was a meld of ideas of the goodness of humans and the development of the idea of progress.[10] The primary emphasis was on social change that would provide better conditions for individual development, and the rise of a "Kingdom of God on earth." The American and French revolutions may be seen as part of this general desire to make changes and provide a new basis for social interaction to improve the human condition. By the mid-twentieth century the possibility of constructive change was being questioned, and several antiutopias had been written.[11] Yet even the antiutopians were captured by ideas of progress; and thus they often spoke only to those selected forms of technological development which they feared. Utopian literature and its antiutopian backlash and eugenic programming of the period from 1870 to about 1950 provide parts of the background for the current discussion of desirable futures.

We can identify a third group of writers who are involved in the discussion leading to the problem of the relation of genetic intervention and the future of humanity. These are the futurists, who are generally recognized as a special breed of technician. From the Rand forecasts to magazines dedicated to the future, through conferences and in books, contemporary humans are learning to think about their future and to try to take action to make desirable changes. Humanity is being presented with possible futures (technically, scenarios of futuribles) from which it is expected to choose. While much of this material concentrates on social, economic, or military forecasts, some attention has been given to attempts that might be made to use technology arising from genetic discoveries.

Futurists, eugenicists (ancient and modern), and utopians have contributed to thoughts about the future of humanity and planning for social, economic, political, and personal goals—including the manipulation of biological nature. Popular attention has been called to the question of possible futures in two other ways: through science-fiction writing and through the sensationalism of many reports in the news media. The movie *2001* and a number of articles in leading popular journals and newspapers have made many people aware of potential interventions, without separating immediate interventions from those which are not now possible and may never be realized.

The thought of changing human nature is not new, however. Although a more static view of the human was dominant in Western Europe until recent centuries, eugenic and utopian movements with their hope of improvement have been present in most periods of human history.

In the time following the Second World War, many advances were made in the understanding of genetics. In the same period, the atomic age and then the computer age led to considerations of the perils as well as the promises of technology. Professional journals, which formerly gave scant notice to value questions, began to publish articles on political, social, and moral questions. *Bioethics, biomedical ethics,* and other terms came to be used for studies that gave new meanings to traditional medical and scientific ethical work. A group of articles and books, mostly written after 1959 (the centennial of Darwin's *Origin of Species*), explored the possible consequences of genetic interventions. The authors came from several scientific disciplines including genetics, biochemistry, physics, and medicine; the ethicists involved were primarily theologically trained.[12]

Several of these authors argued for specific images of the human and chastised opponents for seeking different futures. However, a systematic appreciation of the conflicting images is conspicuously absent in this literature.[13] Since, as Adler claimed, our image of what the human is, is closely related to the actions we take, it becomes important to understand conflicting images of the future if we are to appreciate fully the choices that are being made. In the next section, the interpretations of the future that these writers use are described and contrasted and two specific genetic techniques are examined.

Interpretations of the Future and Specific Techniques

The possibilities of genetic intervention and manipulation raise both hopes and fears. The requisite knowledge is available for attempts to impose our fancies, wills, and longings on human biological evolution, and this knowledge itself is part of our cultural evolution. What shall we do with this new understanding of the human? What is the most desirable course of action? I shall show that three irreconcilable views about the future can be identified. Each represents a set of value assumptions about the optimal conditions that humanity can achieve, given that humanity has lost its innocence about evolutionary process and at the same time has gained knowledge about the mechanisms of genetics. They are labeled "desired futures" because those who hold each view want the scientific and medical communities to direct their energies toward means that will give the best chance to accomplish their hoped-for future. But first, two positions that deny these claims must be considered. Both of these are called "pseudo-futures" because they ignore the reality of the human situation;

the first rejects evolution; the second, technological intervention. The five views are summarized in the following chart.

Possible Views of the Future

Pseudo-Futures	Claims
1. Denial of evolution	All humans are descended from an original couple whose nature was created directly by God. This nature has remained constant.
2. Denial of intervention	Humanity should reject all genetic understanding and refrain from intervention. Knowledge has reached its limits.

Desired Futures	
1. Preservation as a goal	Present humanity is to be protected, with any engineering restricted to care of existing individuals. Some social restrictions may be permissible to prevent deterioration.
2. Intervention as a goal	Present humanity is an open system upon which it is possible to develop improvements without creating a new species.
3. Transformation as a goal	Present humanity is the repository of developments in evolution which can be improved by the introduction of new biological forms.

Pseudo-Futures

1. Denial of evolution. The pseudo-future that rejects evolution posits a static view of the human derived from a particular religious perspective. Its proponents are entangled in a limited view of divine revelation that fosters a separation between knowledge achieved through nature and knowledge believed to be from God. The biologist Theodosius Dobzhansky said this about those who hold such views:

Those who choose to believe that God created every biological species separately in the state we observe them but made them in a way calculated to lead us to the conclusion that they are products of evolutionary development are obviously not open to argument. All that can be said is that their belief is an implicit blasphemy, for it imputes to God appalling deviousness.[14]

Contrary to this static view, which Dobzhansky so ably criticizes, humans must be seen as a part of general evolution with an existence that is but a moment in time. Evolutionary consciousness means that, in the continuum of time, we understand a time when human beings were not, this period of time when they are, and a future when they will no longer be. Of course, it is the future that is puzzling to humans as they exist at this particular moment— and perhaps all the more puzzling to those who now understand that they are themselves a part of evolution.

   2. Denial of intervention. The second pseudo-future, that humanity should forsake any genetic interventions, is a form of Luddism that not only ignores the potential good which may be developed, but also negates several useful methods including screening for PKU and other defects, genetic counseling, voluntary eugenic sterilization (self-elected sterilization of a carrier of certain genetic defects), and artificial insemination by donor (to avoid eugenic problems where both husband and wife are carriers of a particular recessive gene). Although these techniques pose ethical problems and all can be abused, it is difficult to believe that it would be desirable to cease applying the very limited means of help that are now available.

   We have lost our innocence about our evolutionary development, and neither a rejection of evolutionary theory nor a move to forgo our present capacity for assisting in the alleviation of genetic distress seems intellectually valid or morally correct.

Desired Futures

Three futures are possible when evolution is accepted and knowledge is not denied. These futures are held by those who are attempting to create a frame of reference that will maximize the hopes and minimize the fears that are raised by the forces possible in genetic interventions. Health professionals are now, and probably will continue to be, the chief agents responsible for the use of genetic techniques on individuals and populations. Through understanding which futures they hold to be desirable, health professionals will better be able to recognize their feelings about the uses and abuses of various methods. They also will find that questions which reveal the images held by patients and other colleagues will clarify the source of some misunderstandings and disagreements about specific interventions.

1. Preservation as a goal. The first view of the desirable future is one in which the preservation of present human biological nature is a foremost consideration. The biologist Leon R. Kass summarizes this position:

The new technologies for human engineering may well be the "transition to a wholly new path of evolution." They may therefore, mark the end of *human life* as we and all other humans have known it. It is possible that the non-human life that may take our place will be in some sense superior—though I personally think it most unlikely, and certainly not demonstrable. In either case, we are ourselves human beings, therefore it is proper for us to have a proprietary interest in our survival, and in our survival as *human beings*. This is a difficult enough task without having to confront the prospect of a utopian, constant remaking of our biological nature with all powerful means but with no end in view.[15]

The point about ends is well taken. If one thinks about directing genetic change, the question of a desirable goal becomes obvious.

To assert an "optimum" is to assume a knowledge of what is

best. Kass uses picturesque language, and it is worthwhile to offer another of his statements:

We are witnessing the erosion, perhaps the final erosion, of the idea of man as something splendid or divine, and its replacement with a view that sees man no less than nature, as simply more raw material for manipulation and homogenization. Hence, our particular moral crisis. We are in turbulent seas without a landmark precisely because we adhere more and more to a view of nature and of man which both gives us enormous power and, at the same time, denies all possibility of standards to guide its use. Though well-equipped, we know not who we are nor where we are going. We are left to the accidents of our hasty, biased and ephemeral judgments.

Let us not fail to note a painful irony: our conquest of nature has made us slaves of blind chance. We triumph over nature's unpredictabilities only to subject ourselves to the still greater unpredictability of our capricious wills and our fickle opinions. That we have a method is no proof against our madness. Thus, engineering the engineer as well as the engine, we race our train we know not where.[16]

It is possible to concur with Kass on the primacy of a knowledge of goals without accepting the premise that the only legitimate future is one in which humans work for self-perpetuation. Values other than the existence of this species (for example, consciousness) may be introduced. As more knowledge of evolution is gained, new meanings may be found for human development and new goals determined. Kass prematurely closes off the future. Furthermore, if humanity is itself a part of evolution, a course designed to preserve rather than modify may lead to atrophy and occasion a premature species extinction.

Basically, Kass and others are willing to use some genetic interventions in therapeutic ways. Thus, the theologian Paul Ramsey states:

Remove the messianic faith that has been added to scientific capabilities, and there remains ample room for significant interventions that are not only morally justifiable but *morally required* of men who have come to possess these capabilities. It has always been the tradition of our Western religions that in *procreation* of the transmission of human life (block that manufacturing metaphor, "reproduction"!) men and women stand at the point where they should assume responsibility for future generations of mankind by assuming responsibility for their children. This would cut across a number of presently cherished social practices.[17]

Ramsey claims that the capability to intervene is thus a power that humans should use. But what limits, if any, must be placed on such help? A number of factors, including risks and costs, also enter into the decision to use or not to use a specific therapy.

Each intervention has its genetic consequences. If it is the moral duty of humans to intervene to alleviate genetic distress, then humans are affecting their biological evolutionary future. Indeed, many dire warnings have been presented about the cost in an increasing genetic load of therapies for retinoblastoma, diabetes, and other interventions. The biologist Bentley Glass draws this portrait of a future human: "Will the Man of Tomorrow need to spend a large part of his day getting ready to face the world, putting on his spectacles, and adjusting his hearing aid, inserting his teeth, adding his false hair, taking insulin shots in one arm and allergy shots in the other, and topping it off with a tranquilizer before venturing to step into his car?"[18] Glass does not believe this situation need occur, but he is willing to attempt a more positive directing of the human genetic future than either Ramsey or Kass. No interventions will mean change, limited interventions for individual help will mean change; why then should humans not try to guide change in beneficial ways?

This first future assumes that humans can never understand their own nature and its place in evolutionary process well enough to "engineer the engineer." It is enough to attempt to help individuals. Yet, so opponents of this future argue, these interventions appear to increase the prophylactic interventions without reducing the number of affected individuals—and perhaps even dramatically increase the number who will need therapeutic intervention in the future.

2. Intervention as a goal. A second future seeks to improve human performance while trying to determine and preserve those qualities which are essential to humanity. The optimal condition is thus one in which individuals are not only treated to relieve problems caused by genetic distress but also assisted toward fuller development. Human nature is understood as dynamic, not fixed, and no preference is given to maintaining present biological limitations if and where improvements may be introduced. Not only are humans understood to have an open nature, but change is assured. James F. Crow, for example, describes the alternatives:

We must remember that natural selection has been cruel, blundering, inefficient, and lacking in foresight. It has no criterion of excellence except the capacity to leave descendants. (Not necessarily a particular species.) It is indifferent as to whether living is a rich and beautiful experience or one of total misery. . . .

Selection under individual human control, on the other hand, could be greatly different. Its means are birth selection, not death selection. . . . It can have foresight. It can have criteria of health, intelligence, or happiness—not just survival and fertility. And it can make use of the various scientific and technological advances (sperm storage, egg transplant, and other more distant prospects) as they are discovered.

We must remember that the decision is not as to whether man should influence his own evolution. He is already doing this by his revolutionary changes in the environment, by medical advances, by the intervention of contraceptives. The issue is not whether he is influencing his evolution, but in what direction.[19]

Although the direction may not be known, and although the criteria are not well defined (for example, what is *health?*), the assumption is that human control is preferable to that of nature (which is essentially described as control without consciousness).

In this second future it is recognized not only that humanity has developed from more primitive forms but also that further improvements must be justified. In this view, genetic interventions might be used to accomplish social change. An imperfect world seems capable of change, yet the limits of our present knowledge to understand which changes might be most suitable and beneficial restrict the means to be employed. The future, like a sword, is two-edged. Humans must be wary if they are to maintain their humanity.

But what of the opportunities for change? On what basis should it be assumed that present humanity is biologically normative? The genetic constitution of humanity is constantly shifting (minor alterations with each birth and death), so that no one normative point may be identified. Why, then, should the present be the maximum condition? It may be possible to introduce conditions that will benefit humanity. It may be that some biological state in the past was superior. Why is it not possible that the splendid idea is humanity, not as it now exists, but in what it may become?

3. *Transformation as a goal.* A third future that determines how some feel toward genetic interventions has a more distant perspective. The goal is altered from considering a *changing human* in a changing world to a *transitional creature* in a transitional world, from an enriched human to a posthuman creature.

Although this view, which seems closely related to science fiction or popular television shows, might be quickly dismissed as frivolous because the dreams so outstrip our present ability to manipulate genes, it is yet difficult to ignore the hope expressed in this future. The writers favoring it do not pretend to know what goals ought to be sought. They are, in fact, generally certain that humanity is not now ready to make such grand plans. What is important is that the possibilities suggested by this image of the future guide some people into making dramatic decisions about present activities. Bentley Glass, a biologist, draws this picture:

We must, then, seek a change within man himself. As he acquires more fully the power to control his own genotype and to direct the course of his own evolution, he must produce a Man who can transcend his present nature. The Erect Ape-Man had little vision of the power that his 20th-century descendant would wield in really so short a span of evolutionary time. For the Erect Ape-Man a club was the acme of power. Even so, if man can avoid the ultimate follies which our present powers have bestowed upon us, and can survive a few centuries more, we today can little perceive what he may be. Perhaps the Golden Age of no progress will be but a passing phase and history may resume. We can only hope.[20]

The interventionist's wish to mitigate or subvert the forces of natural selection through humanly directed methods is carried further by Glass, who substitutes human direction, not only to alleviate the apparent waste and cruelty of natural selection, but also to replace a product of evolution—man—by a new species, a transformed man. Glass and others of similar views believe this goal is desirable, but they are well aware of the follies that may prevent humans from making the wisest choices and that might bring on genetic disaster.

The future evolution of the human might, by chance, be salutary; the transformers argue that humans themselves will some day possess the knowledge necessary to increase the odds that a beneficial change will occur. It is very important to grasp the distinction between using methods appropriate to present ability and knowledge and the belief that sufficient research, adequate preparation and safeguards, and the proper social and political climate will, in some distant but attainable future, provide an opportunity for a "fairer species" to arise.[21] If the transformer view were merely a utopian hope, a vision of "nowhere," then this position would be of little use to people wrestling with the ethical problems of genetic engineering. However, as the image defines the actions, so does this view become a distinct position from which judgments about specific techniques can be made. This connection of images and proposals for action will be considered shortly.

The transformers and, to some degree, the interventionists make an argument about the use of genetic interventions that differs from the proposals of Plato. Plato saw genetic intervention as a tool to be employed by the state to produce the kinds of people who would best serve it. Modern writers view with ambivalence the relation of species good to social utility. On the one hand, the danger may lie in failing to protect society by a laissez-faire attitude toward threats that would damage the human gene pool.[22] On the other hand, the present social, political, and moral climate is generally viewed as unfavorable to long-range planning. Part of the problem is a lack of sufficient knowledge about biological nature, but the level of cultural evolution is also judged inadequate. Basically, the present is generally classified by these writers as a time of breakthrough toward a new age. Humanity is judged to be on a developmental plane, one that may have lasted for ten thousand years or more, but one that may be transcended—or degraded—by the choices that are made. Unfortunately for their hopes, the transformers generally do not believe that society has yet evolved to the condition necessary to cope with the biological development of the species.[23]

Thus, three divergent images of the future may be found among those who are considering genetic interventions. Each future is deemed desirable by its proponents and conflicts with the others. A few of these conflicts are:

1. We are no longer innocent and therefore recognize that every decision affects our genetic future, but we do not know how to evaluate the present (the state of the gene pool) nor do we know how other factors (political, economic) produce changes. We do not even know whether one action cancels another to produce a quasi equilibrium. Yet we are aware that we are subject to change.

2. The problem of ever understanding what we are doing is raised. Can humanity interpret evolution sufficiently to make beneficial alterations? How much wisdom is needed?

3. What agencies will be required to control genetic intervention? If techniques are developed, can they be restrained?

4. To what extent is the irreversibility of biological mutations to be considered? How can humans effect changes that will not be impossible to remedy if they prove to be biological cul-de-sacs?

The tragedy of the Karen Ann Quinlan case illustrates how little concurrence there is about what is essential to human life. The data provided by the measurements of scientists and the studies of anthropologists and historians, the writings of philosophers and poets, and the records of religion still leave an inchoate image of the human qualities that are to be valued.

Almost all the writers who hold these different futures agree that humans do not now possess the wisdom to chart their own future; they disagree over the possibility of attaining such knowledge. They further agree for the most part that the political and social conditions that would guard against abuse of genetic interventions do not now exist. But those who see the possibility of improving the human species and those who would move toward transforming the human are more concerned that the present genetically linked ills of humans be addressed through scientific development and social control than those who favor more restrictive use of genetics.

Each of these futures is a wager about what humanity is and can become, a value statement about human nature that is only partially dependent upon evidence, an interpretation of data that are common to all three groups. Even with the limited capabilities that are presently available, some differences arising from the variant hopes and fears may be seen in the normative judgments that are given about specific techniques. Two examples of attitudes toward specific techniques that are now possible illustrate different value commitments toward the desirable future.

Eugenic Sterilization

The discovery of the genetic basis of heredity has enabled humanity to understand many of the causes of birth defects and, in turn, to develop means of providing treatment (if not cures) for some individuals. Unfortunately, the ability to sustain many lives once lost to genetic disease creates a problem, as these "saved" individuals often go on to produce children, many of whom will also be affected by the disease or, at least, will have the gene to pass on to their descendants. Retinoblastoma (a cancerous condition of the eyes), for example, was once invariably fatal in childhood. Surgical removal of the affected eye now generally permits the individual to retain sight in the other eye and to live an otherwise normal life. Since this is a dominant condition (needing only one gene in a pair to cause the disease), about half the children of a person who has suffered from retinoblastoma will also have the condition.

An increased genetic load, and the economic, personal, and social costs that arise from the use of new medical procedures which lessen the mortality rate of certain genetic defects, have produced questions about control of human reproduction. In one sense this is an entirely new human problem. It has been common and accepted to place some restrictions on marriage relationships (such as incest laws and caste laws); however, it has been generally conceded that married couples have a right, if not a duty, to have children. Now, with the knowledge that certain people have a potential for producing children who will suffer debilitating diseases because of their genes (and not, for instance, as God's judgment), and because medicine is permitting more people with certain genetic infirmities to survive to reproductive age, the *right to reproduce* is being questioned. Furthermore, an understanding that certain people will have problems only if they marry someone with the same recessive gene (both partners must have this gene for it to be operative) also raises the question of the right of these people to reproduce or even to marry.

Several *possible* solutions are available to combat the problem of the effect of deleterious genes. For example, algeny (surgery on the genes to correct or replace defective genes or gene action) would provide a cure by introducing genetic changes in the somatic (body) cells of an individual. Algeny could also be used to prevent future problems in the affected person's progeny by changing germ (reproductive) cells. Most scientists feel that algeny, unfortunately, will not be available in the immediate future. A less subtle method of control, now commonly used, is fetal diagnosis followed by therapeutic abortion where indicated. Yet another method of attacking the problem of genetic defects is to identify all carriers and to restrict marriages between individuals who have a similar deleterious gene. This method would work only for recessive genes.

A more significant step which is now possible would be to limit the ability to reproduce. This method, called eugenic sterilization (sterilization for genetic purposes, as opposed to sterilization to limit family size), was widely used in the United States in the earlier part of this century.[24] The ethical principle involved is that individuals have no *right* to reproduce. This is a movement away from more traditional doctrine. This principle is acceptable within all three views of the future that have been presented. However, in each future a different attitude toward the enforcement of sterilization may be seen.

In the maintenance perspective, Paul Ramsey speaks of a preventive eugenics that will necessitate the development of an "ethics of genetic duty," built on the freedom of parenthood, which is "a freedom to good parentage, and not a license to produce seriously defective individuals to bear their own burdens." [25] Ramsey advises a wider use of premarital counseling with genetic tests included, and the possible use of the marriage-licensing power of the state to enforce genetic duty. Finally, Ramsey says that couples who are aware of the possibility that they might produce a child with a grave genetic defect may use contraception or even sterilization.[26] Ramsey is quite clear that the state *might* intervene by refusing to license a marriage, which would, in effect, mean (for Ramsey) that the bond between conjugal love and procreation could not lawfully be established; however, once a couple is married, the only control that is possible comes from their voluntary action (continence, contraception, or sterilization) made as a response to moral duty.

In the second future, stronger methods of suasion could find legitimation. The theologian Charles Curran, for example, agrees with Ramsey as the situation is *now*, but Curran holds open the possibility that a different historical situation might call for more community control.[27] Theodosius Dobzhansky has taken different views of the need for sterilization, ranging from a positive feeling that it can be justified to a belief that it will be inefficient for eugenic purposes.[28] Those who hold the preservationist and interventionist views agree that reproduction is not a right and that voluntary sterilization is morally justifiable, but the interventionist is more open to situations that might call for compulsory sterilization measures.

The transformers emphasize the social cost of the genetically handicapped, which means not only that individuals have no right to reproduce, but that there is no right to be born (or, conversely, that there is a right to be born sound).[29] In addition, society has a right to prevent people from reproducing. The biologist Robert T. Francouer poses the problem this way: "Does society have a right to protect itself against the irresponsibility of an individual who seeks to benefit from modern medicine and with its aid escape the scythe of natural selection, but is unwilling to accept the obvious responsibilities which accompany this gift?" [30] Francouer's answer to his own question is yes, society does have a right to protect itself. The major problem Francouer and others face is the determination of which traits require what degree of force; that is, is there a difference between the treatment of someone with retinoblastoma and someone with allergies? between diabetes and Tay-Sachs? If these are treated differently, where is the dividing line?

In summary, a common solution, eugenic sterilization as a valid moral means of controlling birth defects, finds favorable response in all three futures. The preservationist seeks voluntary means (although the possibility of preventing marriages between carriers is discussed). The interventionist foresees situations that call for compulsory measures, but prefers more "tender-hearted" means. The transformer, placing an emphasis on social needs, is prepared to justify mandated sterilization. The three positions show some agreement that the technique may be used, but little correspondence about the legitimate degree of enforcement. Which of these positions may the health professional adopt? What are the obligations of society to control the health profession in the application of any given measure? Which image will dominate?

Eugenic sterilization and the other techniques for combating birth defects that were mentioned earlier are designed to reduce the suffering of the afflicted and their families, the personal and social economic burdens these defects create, and the load placed on medical facilities and personnel in the care of genetically defective people. Some writers have proposed further eugenic interventions that would go beyond the attempt to eliminate genetic defects and seek, in addition, to "improve" the quality of the genetic stock. For example, algeny (genetic surgery) could be used not only to correct or replace defective genes, but also to introduce designed changes; cloning (asexual reproduction) could be used to replicate the genetic qualities of people judged to be of special worth; and the artificial synthesis of genes could be used to introduce new abilities within humans. None of these techniques is now available for use with humans. Although they provide material for science fiction and other popularizations, the benefits of many of these methods, *within* the standards of present medical practice, are enormous.

Eugenic Insemination

Another method of introducing positive change, eugenic insemination, is based on the generally accepted technique of artificial insemination by donor, and therefore could be used at this time. Artificial insemination is a medical procedure used to aid infertile couples. It is generally estimated that ten to twenty thousand AI children are born in the United States each year. When a husband's sperm count is low, several ejaculations are kept and mixed to increase the number of viable sperm, and then these sperm are implanted in the wife at the most fertile moment of her cycle. When the husband is incapable of producing sperm, the sperm of a donor may be used.

The late Hermann J. Muller for several decades argued for the use of eugenic insemination and for a transformer view of the future. He believed that eugenic insemination presented no moral difficulties because it relies on an existing technique. He also advocated eugenic insemination because he felt the gene pool was being polluted by environmental hazards (radiation) and advances in medicine. Finally, Muller was convinced that mankind would find the use of eugenic insemination a step toward new and finer levels of existence. It must be carefully noted that Muller believed in ideals, and not the development of an Ideal Man; felt that the procedure *must* be voluntary; and suggested that the procedure would only gradually win acceptance as more people had "better" children through artificial insemination.[31] Muller's main assumption was that many of the characteristics that are most admired have a genetic origin and, therefore, the use of eugenic insemination would in the long run provide more people of higher types through the simple distribution of more of the desirable genes. If improvement was noted, the practice would be more popular, and a cumulative effect would occur.

Challenges to Muller's position include the basic argument that normal people produce geniuses and geniuses often have normal children; in other words, not enough is known about heredity to establish the correlations that Muller makes. Does this effectively counter the long-run view?

Robert Francouer similarly sees problems in the technical questions about the efficacy of Muller's proposals, but Francouer believes that Muller is raising some significant points, including the egoism involved in insisting that children carry one's own genetic heritage, and the possible advantage of having the involved couple, rather than the attending physician, make the choice of a donor.[32] Bentley Glass carries Muller's proposals for eugenic improvement further. Glass suggests that prenatal adoption (embryo selection) might be preferable to artificial insemination, because it would provide more opportunity to ensure a sound genetic constitution and also the choice of sex. Glass summarizes the benefits: "In the future age of man it will become possible for every person to procreate with assurance that the child, either one's own or one prenatally adopted, has a sound heritage, capable of fully utilizing the opportunities provided by society for optimal development." [33] The key words in this quotation are "provided by society" and "optimal development," for Glass is assuming that society has an obligation to provide such intervention. Glass is aware that what Muller presents, as well as his own plan of prenatal adoption, share the as yet unresolved problem of identifying good genotypes.[34]

Paul Ramsey, who is among those who would limit genetic interventions to care (the preserving future), gives several reasons for rejecting eugenic insemination on the basis of questionable science that is involved in proposals for the method.[35] The broader ethical questions, which for Ramsey are decisive even for the common use of artificial insemination, center in the conflict that he identifies as the clash between an "ethics of science" (represented by Muller) and an "ethics of genetic duty" in the Judaeo-Christian sense (by which Ramsey means the bond or union between conjugal love and procreation).[36] Ramsey summarizes his concern for eugenic insemination, as well as for other plans for alteration of the human, in the following: "In general, grand designs of positive or progressive eugenics should be opposed in the name of the right and the good, in the name of the more urgent and practical applications of genetics in medicine— and because of our lack of wisdom to create, by favoring selected phenotypes, an evidently stronger and more adaptable species than nature has achieved in man pluralistically." [37] Ramsey fails to see that Muller and others argue for eugenic insemination specifically because it is a method that is presently available, one that as "artificial insemination by donor" is now a practical application of genetics in medicine and would not introduce an alternative to urgent needs in medicine. The "right and the good" to which Ramsey refers are primarily the "union of sex and procreation," but this notion is not necessarily valid for those who do not accept the Judaeo-Christian premises upon which Ramsey constructs the argument, or for theologians and others in the Judaeo-Christian tradition who do not see artificial insemination as a threat to conjugal love. Ramsey's major point is thus his view of natural selection as opposed to artificial means directed by the limited wisdom of humans—an image not shared by other writers who have different views of the human.

Eugenic insemination is also generally unacceptable to those who would use methods for limited improvements. Charles Curran, for example, rejects Muller's proposals for many of the same reasons that Ramsey uses. Curran, however, couples his objections—which are based on the limitations of human judgment, the potential loss of certain human values, and the danger of utopian schemes[38]—with an openness to the possibility that a different historical situation might legitimate new methods. Curran says: "One can envision a possibility in which greater values might be at stake and call for some type of altering the way in which Christian marriage now tries to preserve these important values. For example, if the dire predictions of Muller were universally accepted and mankind did face a genetic apocalypse in the near future, then the entire situation might be changed." [39] Curran's opposition to Muller is thus, in part, based on what Curran believes the present is like and the future should be. Unlike Ramsey, Curran is open to the new moral directives that may arise in a changing historical context. Curran's image of the human is flexible and, therefore, for him, means that what today may be considered invalid can, in the future, become morally acceptable.

Theodosius Dobzhansky also opposes Muller's schemes. Dobzhansky rejects the Ramsey assertion that Muller's schemes are "unnatural," because Dobzhansky is more concerned with the end Muller has in view, reasoning that humans cannot now know what "will be best for mankind centuries or millennia hence." Dobzhansky argues, in agreement with Ramsey, that the problem is technical, that humans cannot know the ends to be sought; unlike Ramsey, but in agreement with Curran, Dobzhansky also opens the possibility that at some time, with proper preparation, mankind might learn the requisite information. [40]

Thus, for interventionist writers such as Dobzhansky and Curran, eugenic insemination is rejected as a means for use *at this time*. This rejection is not absolute. With a regard for changing circumstances, Curran believes that a different historical setting might validate these means, whereas Dobzhansky is open to the possibility that more knowledge might lead to a different conclusion about the practice; however, neither Curran nor Dobzhansky appears to be enthusiastic about the proposed intervention.

Although some of the disagreement about eugenic insemination focuses on factual information (the efficacy of the method and the available wisdom to select traits), different images of the human future are also involved in the arguments. The transformers are trying to alter the species, but the two other groups would not approve such methods. However, these two groups differ over the question of whether the prohibition is absolute (the preservers) or a matter of the present state of human knowledge (the interventionists). The images of the desirable future thus in part define the acceptability of the techniques of eugenic insemination.

Conclusion

Conflicting images of the optimal human destiny are present in debates about genetic engineering. Desirable ends or goals are not prescinded solely from facts and data but also from deeply rooted beliefs about the nature and purpose of human existence. It is not clear that any specific intervention is justified on the basis of improving or transforming the human, nor yet again that it is more desirable not to intervene. Are humans to be limited to their present development, with its losses and pain as well as its glories? Or is it reasonable to use an increased knowledge of methods of intervention to plan and facilitate change? Human problems—including suffering caused by environmental factors that stimulate faulty gene responses, external accident, the distress of bearing a child with a hereditary disease, or the anguish of not being able to conceive—must be balanced against the impact and moral weight of the means that will be employed to solve them. The good of individuals must be protected at the same time that the well-being of the species is assured. New knowledge about the hereditability of certain genetic diseases has caused a revaluing of parenthood; more information about the mechanisms of genetics will doubtless cause a rethinking of many traditional norms and values. Because we have no final answers to these conflicts now, and no clear picture of human evolution is yet available, questions about the techniques of genetic engineering are unresolved.

At present a lack of knowledge means that humans must act while their basic suppositions are in serious conflict and their information is incomplete. Human knowledge of evolution is rudimentary for those questions raised by the capacity to perform interventions. What one person calls an action of importance to the species is to another an unconscionable invasion of individual freedom. Where one writer proposes genetic intervention as a way to relieve suffering for an infertile couple, another speaks of unnatural means of procreation. The dilemma exists: Humans know enough about the origin of the human species to recognize that piecemeal interventions will affect the future of the race; but they do not know enough about the place of humanity in evolution to know what either intervening or not intervening will mean. The introduction of new techniques may be deleterious, or it may be the alternative to a degradation of the species. In any case, people are suffering and interventions are used.

Because of the power of our images to dominate our actions, the acquisition of more knowledge about evolution, the creation of social and political settings that could inhibit abuses, and the development of agreement about some enduring ethical questions (such as distributive justice) will perhaps not provide guidance about the proper goals of genetic intervention. The deep-seated nature of the basic beliefs held by individuals is often unrecognized. Discovering the underlying conflicts and exposing them to dispassionate reasoning, even among those who most strongly espouse logic and the scientific method, will not assure that agreement will be reached about the human future.

Geneticists and others have introduced a variety of techniques for use by health professionals. When these professionals are unaware of the conflict between their own basic images of the human and those of other health professionals or their patients, they will experience frustration as they attempt to pursue their own projects. The abortion controversy has shown the persistence of competing images and the difficulty of using scientific methods to determine the nature of human existence. After much debate and significant legislative review, the status of the fetus remains morally unclear, and a division exists between pro- and anti-abortionists.

The expectations embodied in institutions and the impact of government may not only redirect the course of medical practice but also cause serious divisions among health professionals. Researchers or practitioners will find apparently unreasonable obstacles and apparently unrealistic expectations from others who do not share their hopes or recognize their fears. These conflicts will appear not only in the laboratory, when a city council or the federal government starts to enact legislation, but also in questions about decisions that need to be made about the results of an amniocentesis test, in advice to be given to people seeking genetic counseling, or in the structure of genetic screening programs.

In his presidential address to the American Society of Human Genetics,[41] Barton Childs reported on the state of genetics in medical education and practice. He indicates that a general knowledge of medical genetics has increased among physicians, yet the use of the information in medical schools and practice still falls far short of its potential. In order to use genetics fully, Childs suggests, it is necessary to adopt a view of disease as an abstraction, with the reality being "the inability of one person's homeostasis, conditioned by his genotype and a lifetime of special experiences, to maintain equilibrium." [42] With this view of disease and an awareness of the social character of genetic conditions, students in the health professions can, according to Childs, be exposed to the rudiments of genetics, apply genetic principles to the study of human variation, and note the relation of genetics to medical practice.[43] Of special importance is the need to further the learning of the mechanics of genetics by emphasis on genetics in the clinical exposure of students.

Educators will, I believe, also need to attend to the different conceptions of the human that they and their students hold. They will need to see the role of the conflict in images among practicing health professionals and to attend to the different preconceptions of the human that students hold. Without a specific guide to determine the most desirable image, the educator will need to explore with students the conflicting values in these images and the relation of arguments about the use of specific techniques to the images of the human, which affect judgments of sanctioned application. Legal and moral constraints, as well as arguments related to particular practices, will be more clearly grasped if the problem of identifying the optimal human is understood as derived from both available information and basic beliefs.

A humanity aware of its origins and, at least dimly, of the genetic factors involved in the development of the species, has begun to consider the interventions that might be desirable. But competing images about the basic human exist, and these images determine both the actions that are considered desirable and those judged to be morally proper. Addressing the conflicting hopes and fears of the future is necessary if the tangled legal, social, and human considerations are to be unraveled. Health professionals and geneticists who are seriously attempting to use genetic techniques must address the issue of the desirable future and, with philosophers, theologians, lawyers, and other professionals, as well as legislators and the general public, look to the competing hopes and fears. To avoid the discussion may mean not only continued frustration for the health professions, but also the introduction of unnecessary restraints. Finally, it may affect the ultimate destiny of humanity.

Which future should be supported? Humans know present humanity with its evident weaknesses as well as its many strengths; they also know, however dimly most believe it, that the species *Homo sapiens* is doomed; and therefore they dream. The dangers of intervening are clear: abuse of power, the development of genetic "haves and have nots," the limitation of genetic variety, the censuring of tolerance for the genetically handicapped or the "different," the loss of liberty, too hasty action, and the ruin of the "flower of evolution" through misguided good intentions. Yet people are suffering; and more knowledge of genetics will undoubtedly bring powerful means for intervening, both for individual welfare and for species good. With restraint and caution in the immediate future, and until the evidence is firmly on the side of arguments that the meaning of interventions is understood, why should humans not believe that their own interventions can lead to finer forms of evolutionary development? The primacy of human life as it is now formed may be agreed upon without holding that the present system is not itself subject to change as more about the "genius" of human life in evolution becomes known.

Thus, with respect for the limitations of present human wisdom, I would support the position of the transformer, emphasizing the promises more than the threats of the new technologies, and accepting the possibility of some vigorous intervention in the present.

Individuals need protection from the constraints of their society. When these constraints are unreasonable or selective because of the whims or caprices of others, including well-intentioned politicians, physicians, and prelates, the individual needs the intervention of his society. But it is difficult to argue that individuals enjoy *any* rights that may never be compromised by their obligations to society. Even a "right to life" may be qualified by a duty to undertake a hazardous assignment, as in obedience to military commands. A transformer position senses not only that individuals have duties because of their specific genetic constitution but also that moral suasion and even legal restrictions are permissible against those who would knowingly neglect their genetic responsibilities.[44] Such a doctrine lies on the thin edge of a multitude of possible abuses, and the inequity of present societies and the general incompleteness of genetic knowledge mitigate against enforced measures. Nevertheless, if genetic restraints are located even within the limiting conditions of the present, they may be morally preferable to unchecked and irresponsible genetic parenting.

I argue here not that the reader accept my image of the optimal future, but rather that the different futures be recognized, with both their powers and their limits. While I believe that an increased knowledge of the place of the human in evolution will provide stronger evidence for the transformer view of the desirable future, I also believe that the strength of the competing images will, for some time, remain an important factor in arguments about genetic engineering. Belief, not knowledge, dominates; and beliefs about the nature and destiny of man are firmly rooted and not easily changed.

NOTES

1. Several terms have been suggested for techniques involving genetics. In adopting *genetic engineering* to cover the many modes of intervention I am following the usage in a report to the Congress: U.S. Congress, House, Committee on Science and Astronautics, Subcommittee on Science, Research, and Development, *Genetic Engineering: Evolution of a Technological Issue,* prepared by the Science Policy Research Division, Congressional Research Service, Library of Congress, Serial W, 92d Cong., 2d sess., 1972, p. 3.

2. David M. Rorvik's largely discredited claim that a cloned child is now alive (*In His Image: The Cloning of a Man* [Philadelphia: Lippincott, 1978]) shows not only how subjects considered to be distant prospects may become immediate concerns, but also how important to medicine the subject of genetic interventions is. How many infertile couples will now approach their physicians for this solution to parenting?

3. See, for example, the continuing debate between Paul Ramsey and Joseph Fletcher in their several works, but especially in Ramsey, *Fabricated Man: The Ethics of Genetic Control* (New Haven: Yale University Press, 1970); and Fletcher, *The Ethics of Genetic Control: Ending Reproductive Roulette* (Garden City, N.Y.: Doubleday-Anchor, 1974).

4. *The Difference of Man and the Difference It Makes,* based on the Encyclopaedia Britannica Lectures delivered at the University of Chicago, 1966 (New York: Holt, Rinehart and Winston, 1967), p. 294. See also Wallwork's article in this volume, especially his discussion of attitudes.

5. "The Prospect for Designed Genetic Change," *American Scientist,* 57 (Spring 1969):134. Sinsheimer is correct that humans for the first time understand something of their origin, but in the past the knowledge of breeding practices did lead to some consideration of human genetic mating. See my comments on the early Greek thinkers.

6. *The History of Herodotus* 3.110–16.

7. *Republic* 5.459–62; *Timaeus* 19; *Statesman* 269–74; *Laws* 5 and 6. Plato did not intend for the plan to be voluntary nor did he uphold the right of the individual to procreate as having precedence over the right of control by the state.

8. *Politics* 7.16.

9. Two studies of the eugenic movement make these points. Mark H. Haller, *Eugenics: Hereditarian Attitudes in American Thought* (New Brunswick: Rutgers University Press, 1963); and the more recent work by Kenneth M. Ludmerer, *Genetics and American Society* (Baltimore: Johns Hopkins University Press, 1972). The impact of the eugenic movement on U.S. society in the first several decades of this century should be better known because of its influence upon many of the medical actions performed in that period.

10. The controversy over the relation of thinking by man and machine led to an excellent discussion of utopian proposals by Harold E. Hatt, *Cybernetics and the*

Image of Man: A Study of Freedom and Responsibility in Man and Machine (Nashville: Abingdon Press, 1968), chap. 7. See also Ernst Benz, *Evolution and Christian Hope: Man's Concept of the Future from the Early Fathers to Teilhard de Chardin,* trans. Heinz G. Frank (Garden City, N.Y.: Doubleday-Anchor, 1968).

11. Including Aldous Huxley's *Brave New World,* George Orwell's *1984,* and Anthony Burgess's *A Clockwork Orange.* These three important antiutopias have been made into motion pictures and have reached wide audiences. The effect these antiutopias have on popular opinion about genetic engineering cannot be measured, but is undoubtedly important.

12. Several Nobel Prize winners are listed among those from the scientific community, and the theologians include several of the most respected ethicists in the nation. Many have written popular articles which have appeared, among other places, in *Saturday Review, Harper's, Atlantic Monthly,* and *Esquire.* Their approaches, whether cautious or optimistic, are attempts to take seriously matters which easily become sensationalized by their subject matter. Even a careful and thoughtful writer such as Willard Gaylin had an article in the *New York Times* surrounded by pictures of cloned Hitlers. See "We Have the Awful Knowledge to Make Exact Copies of Human Beings," pt. I, March 5, 1972, pp. 12–13, 41, 43–44, 48–49.

13. Two writers who do make some distinctions among the possible futures are Victor Ferkiss in *Technological Man: The Myth and the Reality* (New York: George Braziller, 1969), and Paul Ramsey in *Fabricated Man.* Neither writer explores the categories or defines the positions as they are outlined in this essay.

14. *Mankind Evolving: The Evolution of the Human Species* (New Haven: Yale University Press, 1962), p. 6.

15. "Making Babies—The New Biology and the 'Old' Morality," *Public Interest,* 26 (Winter 1972):54.

16. "The New Biology: What Price Relieving Man's Estate?" *Science,* 174 (November 19, 1971):785–86.

17. *Fabricated Man,* p. 150, first emphasis added.

18. "The Effects of Changes in the Physical Environment on Genetic Change," in *Genetics and the Future of Man,* ed. John D. Roslansky (New York: Appleton-Century-Crofts, 1966), p. 45.

19. "Mechanisms and Trends in Human Evolution," in *Evolution and Man's Progress,* ed. Hudson Hoagland and Ralph W. Burhoe (New York: Columbia University Press, 1962), p. 20.

20. "Science: Endless Horizons or Golden Age," *Science,* 171 (January 8, 1971):29.

21. A phrase used by Robert L. Sinsheimer, "Prospects for Future Scientific Development: Ambush or Opportunity?" *Hastings Center Report,* 2 (September 1972):7.

22. The human gene pool is the aggregate genetic composition of the human race measured at a particular time. Much debate centers around the effects on

the gene pool of various genetic interventions and general environmental factors. Basically a case may be made that those who take the position that intervention should be limited to care of individuals do not see the gene pool being seriously affected, whereas those who seek to move toward transformation are very concerned about the addition of deleterious genes, of gene load, which they feel is now occurring. The interventionists are liable to say that humans cannot now know what is happening, but there may be room for concern.

23. Even the optimistic view of Robert Sinsheimer has become more cautious. In discussing controlled evolution he admits that his doubts about forecasting the future have increased; still he closes the article by saying: "As individuals men will always have to accept their genetic constraints, but as a species we can transcend our inheritance and mould it to our purpose—if we can trust ourselves with such powers. As geneticists we can continue to evolve possibilities and take the long view" ("Troubled Dawn for Genetic Engineering," in *Contemporary Issues in Bioethics,* ed. Tom L. Beauchamp and LeRoy Walters [Encino, Calif.: Dickenson Publishing Company, 1977], p. 612).

24. See above on the rise of eugenic laws. Forced sterilization is a rare occurrence today, and public outcry is quick to follow even the suggestion that such measures are contemplated. If a clear danger is shown to exist, then public opinion may again change. The role of propaganda and the threat that could be posed to minorities are obvious concerns.

25. *Fabricated Man,* pp. 57, 98.

26. Ibid., pp. 41, 118, 120.

27. Charles E. Curran, "Theology and Genetics: A Multi-Faceted Dialogue," *Journal of Ecumenical Studies,* 7 (Winter 1970):74–75.

28. Most often Dobzhansky was against enforced sterilization, but in one writing he does endorse it (*Mankind Evolving,* p. 333).

29. Glass, "Science: Endless Horizons," p. 28.

30. "Medical Progress and the Inalienable Right to Reproduce," *Relevant Scientist,* 2 (November 1972):8.

31. "Better Genes for Tomorrow," in *The Population Crisis and the Use of World Resources,* ed. Stuart Mudd (The Hague: Dr. W. Junk Publishers, 1964), pp. 314–58.

32. Robert T. Francouer, *Utopian Motherhood: New Trends in Human Reproduction* (Garden City, N.Y.: Doubleday, 1970), pp. 35–37.

33. "Science: Endless Horizons," p. 28.

34. Ibid.

35. In chap. 1 of *Fabricated Man,* Ramsey gives an account of his differences with Muller.

36. Ibid., p. 33.

37. Ibid., p. 99.

38. "Theology and Genetics," esp. pp. 80, 82, 86.

39. Ibid., p. 71.

40. "Changing Man," *Science,* 155 (January 27, 1967):411.

41. "Persistent Echoes of the Nature-Nurture Argument." *American Journal of Human Genetics,* 29 (January 1977):1–13.

42. Ibid., p. 6.

43. Ibid., p. 9.

44. Laws restricting many expressions of sexuality have been overthrown, for example, in the acceptance of homosexuality and other sexual activities once labeled "deviant." Could not someone argue that parent-child or sibling sexual love be recognized as legitimate human activities? Even if such relationships were to be tolerated, would they not have unwise genetic consequences that society might bar?

CHAPTER 8

Toward Measures of Equity in the Delivery of Health Care Services

Frank A. Sloan

Another area in which the ethic of respect for persons becomes important is the equity of health care services available to people of different economic classes. Frank Sloan examines several forms of equity, starting with ease of access to health services. Drawing on several types of national survey data in the United States, he shows that differences from area to area (for example, rural to urban) and from low to high income are not so great as one would expect. Yet he also demonstrates some of the problems in measuring the complex issues relating to satisfaction with quality of care. Travel time, waiting time, and appointment delay intervals yield exact data, but until recently there has been little emphasis on patient-oriented measures of quality, or of attitudes toward caretakers.

Sloan's research draws both types of data together. On the whole, physicians appear to be perceived as both caring and accessible. To enhance this perception would take large increments of recruitment and training that he suggests may have questionable merit, although the quality of training clearly has a bearing.

The place of economic research in medicine is important, not only for medical education priorities but also for national health policy and planning. Sloan examines some of these relationships, criticizing the relatively uninformed political assumptions about inequities in access, and raising some thorny questions about national health insurance (using comparative data from Canada's program). Like McElhinney, Sloan sees the need for a coordinated planning effort that includes concerned physicians, public-policy analysts, social scientists, and ethicists. His sense of the reforms needed, however, is certainly more modest than that of Lifton, Pruyser, or Stoeckle.

As was noted in a November 1973 conference on ethical issues in health and the delivery of health care services, "the value (or ideal, or societal goal) of equal access to comprehensive health services, irrespective of income or geographic location, has now virtually the status of a platitude. Political leaders on both left and right give it at least verbal endorsement." [1] Many arguments cited by proponents of government programs in health care services use concern with equity in the distribution of these services as their rationale. Some of these programs have had the objective of improving the health care consumer's ability to pay; others have concentrated on medical education and facilities.

Only rarely is political change the result of scholarly writing, either theoretical or empirical. In some cases, however, scholarly evidence has been used as an instrument for bringing about change. For this reason, it is not at all surprising that billions of dollars have been spent on public programs with the specific intent of achieving greater equity in the distribution of health care services; yet only recently have there been efforts by scholars and policy analysts to develop theoretical concepts of equity that are operational empirically, as they apply to health and the delivery of health care services. Without these concepts or measures, there is really no way to predict the effects of public programs with regard to equity, *ex ante,* or to gauge the results of these programs, *ex post.*

The focus of this essay is on equity in the distribution of health care services, not in the distribution of health status by income status or geographic location. Many health experts regard health as important but maintain at the same time that the impact of health care services is low, certainly in comparison with other potential sources of improvements in health, such as housing, recreation, nutrition, and education. However, as Rashi Fein cogently argues:

Persons have come to believe that medical care services and intervention by the physician make significant contributions to health. This view is not likely to change. . . . groups who today receive less than what they consider their fair share of services are hardly likely to be impressed by an argument that they translate: "Some people do get more of certain services, but after all the services don't—on the average—yield high benefits (relative to their costs). Therefore, though the rich may waste their money in purchasing the services, we shall not invest government funds to increase the availability of the services. The poor should not be

distressed—they are not being denied things of considerable value! . . ."
[Most consumers] will behave as if medical services do count for more
and public policy will respond to their concerns.[2]

The next section of this essay considers three alternative kinds
of equity measures pertinent to the delivery of health care services. It is followed by a presentation of recent empirical evidence
from the United States relating to these broad types of measures.
As will be apparent, alternative types of measures do not always
point in the same direction. In the following section, empirical
evidence from foreign countries, as well as from the United
States, is reviewed as a basis for evaluating the potential impacts of
national health insurance and of expenditures on medical education on the distribution of health care services. As seen in that
section, there has been a clear tendency for national health insurance to redistribute health care services in favor of people with
low incomes. Although the general intent of such programs has
been to raise health care services consumption levels of the less
affluent up to the levels of the rest of society, this has not been
achieved (even to the extent it has been desirable) because health
resources—manpower and capital—are reasonably fixed in the
short term. The final section summarizes conclusions from the
data and conceptual discussion.

Three Types of Equity Measures

One possible objective of programs to attain greater equity in
the use of health services involves equality in the use of services
in relation to need. A more modest objective is the use of services
in relation to need above some minimum threshold of health
services utilization.

According to one proponent of this type of measure:

Equitable distribution does not imply that everyone should receive the
same amount of health services. Instead, I propose that an "equitable
distribution" of health services is one in which illness (as defined by the
patient and his family or by health care professionals) is the major
determinant of the distribution. . . . Perceived need and evaluated need

are the major determinants of health services use in such a system, because of the well-established relationships between health and age, sex and marital status. On the other hand, social structure, health beliefs, family resources, and community resources should have less impact on utilization. Inequity is suggested, for example, if the distribution of services is determined by race, income or availability of facilities. Empirically, a distribution of services may be defined as more equitable, the stronger the association between utilization, perceived and evaluated need and demographic variables on the one hand, and the weaker the association between utilization and social structure, health benefits, family resources and community resources on the other hand.[3]

Although this type of measure has many attractive features, it also has problematic aspects. The most important of these involve the definition of need. Social science has established systematic variations in perceptions of need and the ways medical symptoms are presented according to measurable characteristics of the person and his or her environment. If, for example, one subculture tended to have, in sociological terminology, a higher acceptance of the "sick role" than another, holding such factors as income constant, this definition would in effect argue in favor of a redistribution toward the former subculture.[4] Moreover, illness may sometimes be used to legitimate absences from work and school; [5] attempts to achieve greater equity in the delivery of health services may effectively subsidize absenteeism as well and in this respect violate other ethical principles held by a large segment of the population. These points emphasize that no one measure, at least an operational one, is likely to be fully consistent with the ethical principles held by most members of society.

Proponents of public education do not typically argue for equality in the use of educational services, or for that matter, for utilization of educational services in relation to some external measure, such as native intelligence. Lower bounds on educational attainment are established by state statutes. Below these thresholds, which establish minimum quantities of schooling all children are to receive, there is concern about the nature of the child's educational experience—qualitative dimensions. Achievement of equality in use below statutory thresholds has by no means eliminated interest in distributional issues. Above them, there is greater emphasis on price, which includes various time costs borne by the student—such as those associated with travel to the educational facility and forgone earnings—as well as direct out-of-pocket payments for books and tuition. There is comparatively little concern about equality in use; in fact, substantial differentials in use, in the presence of a low price of education, are widely tolerated, or even advocated, by "liberals" in education.

An important implication for health care delivery is that equality in use, or equality in use relative to need, would not likely lead to a lack of public interest in distributional issues. One gets an indication of this from critics of the present Medicaid program. If Medicaid has raised the consumption of services by the poor in relative as well as absolute terms, it still has not eliminated complaints about impersonal care received by the poor, long waiting times, and so on.[6]

In my view, proponents of use-need measures of equity have sometimes been too harsh in their criticism of an alternative type of measure, namely those describing the process according to which people receive health care services. For example, David Salkever, in arguing the superiority of a use-need measure of equity, states that "a norm based on these [process] characteristics might specify that travel times to primary care sources should be equal across population groups. But substantial divergences from this specification are not necessarily inconsistent with complete or almost complete equality of use."[7]

Salkever's point is correct *if* one accepts the premise that equality of use or use relative to some measure of need is of primary importance, but it is by no means certain that this is so. Clearly, recent concern with "humaneness" in health care delivery is less with the efficacy of health services in improving health status or with a lack of uniformity in visits to physicians in relation to a measure of need. Rather, it is primarily a concern about the nature of services received. It is possible to justify such features of the current delivery system as long waiting times in clinics and physicians' offices, especially on the part of the poor, in terms of economic efficiency. Yet society may be willing in this, as in many other instances, to sacrifice economic efficiency in delivery of health care services in return for greater equity in the delivery of these services.[8]

As noted earlier, political decisions are generally made in response to various forms of constituent pressure rather than in response to scholarly studies. Evidence of widespread constituent dissatisfaction or concern about a particular issue is more likely to elicit a political response and ultimately affect legislation and influence administrative decisions than is a series of scholarly papers. In this regard, it may be useful to examine attitudinal measures relating to individuals' satisfaction with the medical care they now personally receive and measures relating to the same individuals' satisfaction with the care those outside their families receive.

The case for a redistribution in favor of the comparatively poor is somewhat stronger, all other factors being equal, if the more affluent are willing to pay for improved services for the poor; but this is clearly not a necessary condition for such a redistribution. Although there may be some question as to degree, most would agree that votes in the political marketplace are more equally distributed than are votes in the economic marketplace. And although measures of citizen satisfaction taken at a single point in time have some interest, measures obtained before and after the imposition of a major public program, such as national health insurance, may command even greater interest. In this way one can, at least in principle, obtain a measure of overall welfare gains (or losses) from the program and the distribution of such gains by income class or geographic location.

It is quite possible that substantial differences in the first two classes of measures may not be reflected in attitudinal measures, particularly those dealing with the respondent's own health experiences. For example, in assessing the courtesy of health professionals, there may be a tendency to compare experience in health care with experiences in other areas. From the vantage point of a low-income individual, the brusqueness of, for example, social service agency employees may be substantial in comparison to that of health professionals. Assessments of the quality of care rendered by health professionals may be somewhat marred by the respondent's apprehensions that the quality of care she or he is likely to receive in life-or-death situations may be less than adequate. Responses to questions relating to such process variables as time spent waiting for doctors and time traveling to doctors may reflect the fact that the person spends a great deal of time obtaining a number of goods and services, and there is really no reason to single out health care.

In this last case, for policy makers to single out health care is to place a higher value on one type of time expenditure than on others. Some would argue that this is not justified. For example, people living in rural areas may be gaining clean air and access to outdoor recreation at the cost of access to services most likely to be located in urban areas, including health care.[9]

The Recent U.S. Experience

With one exception, the tables presented in this section depict the relationships between specific measures of access to physicians' services and family income. Most of the tables also contain breakdowns by age. The age variable, probably better than any other *single* measure, accounts for differences in patient medical needs. Sorting on any one variable, of course, may be expected to leave a large portion in need unaccounted for.

All tables are based on two national data sources, Health Interview Surveys (HIS) conducted by the National Center for Health Statistics, and a comprehensive survey of health services utilization for 1970 conducted by the University of Chicago's Center for Health Administration Studies in 1971 (CHAS). The tables from the latter survey have been prepared from unpublished data. The emphasis in this empirical discussion is on physicians' services rather than health care services as a whole.

Utilization and Utilization-Need Measures

Table 1 shows estimates of the number of visits per person per year and the percentage of people with at least one physician visit in the past year, by family income and age. Considering all ages together, it is apparent that visits per capita decline with increases in income. The percentage seeing a physician at least once rises with family income, but only slightly. The disaggregations by respondent age reveal a distinctly positive relationship between use and family income for children; in the other age groups, this relationship is either negative or essentially invariant with respect to income. Thus, except for children, table 1 indicates that use is not presently dependent on an individual's financial resources.

It is well known, however, that people with low incomes have traditionally tended to have higher levels of morbidity than those

TABLE 1. Visits to Physicians by Family Income and Age, U.S., 1973

Age and Family Income	Number of Visits per Person per Year	Percentage with a Physician Visit in Past Year
All ages		
Under $5,000	5.7	73.8%
$5,000–9,999	4.8	72.9
$10,000–14,999	4.9	75.3
$15,000 and over	5.1	77.4
Ratio, highest to lowest income category	0.89	1.04
Under 17 years of age		
Under $5,000	3.9	67.2
$5,000–9,999	3.8	70.0
$10,000–14,999	4.3	74.9
$15,000 and over	4.6	78.1
Ratio, highest to lowest income category	1.18	1.16
Ages 17–44		
Under $5,000	5.9	78.9
$5,000–9,999	4.8	75.3
$10,000–14,999	5.1	76.5
$15,000 and over	5.1	77.2
Ratio, highest to lowest income category	0.86	0.98

TABLE 1—*Continued*

Age and Family Income	Number of Visits per Person per Year	Percentage with a Physician Visit in Past Year
Ages 45–64		
Under $5,000	6.5	71.3%
$5,000–9,999	5.6	70.5
$10,000–14,999	5.2	72.6
$15,000 and over	5.4	76.4
Ratio, highest to lowest income category	0.83	1.07
Age 65 and over		
Under $5,000	6.6	75.7
$5,000–9,999	6.5	77.0
$10,000–14,999	7.5	79.5
$15,000 and over	6.7	81.4
Ratio, highest to lowest income category	1.02	1.08

Source: Data from the 1973 Health Interview Survey conducted by the National Center for Health Statistics. Published in U.S. Department of Health, Education, and Welfare, *Health: United States 1975* (Washington, D.C.: U.S. Government Printing Office, 1976), DHEW pub. no. (HRA) 76-1232.

with high incomes. The use-need measures of equity of access take this factor into account. At present, there is conflicting empirical evidence on measures of this type.

Lu Ann Aday and Ronald Andersen have developed two need indexes for gauging access of various population groups.[10] One need measure is based on the individual's disability days. The other is a symptoms-response ratio based on reported symptoms, weighted according to illness severity (as judged by a panel of physicians). With measures of physician contact as the numerator and these need indexes as the denominator, differences are found according to whether the person is above or below the "poverty" line.

Lee and Alexandra Benham employ a more comprehensive measure of family income, one that identifies a broader range of income categories than simply poverty versus nonpoverty. The Benhams find that utilization of physicians' services by low-income people rose relative to utilization by other groups between 1963 and 1970 and that, by 1970, the impact of income on utilization was small. Moreover, when health-status measures are included in their regression equations, even the small impact of income disappears.[11] Salkever assesses the relationship between need and the probability of entering the health care system for treatment. He reports essentially no differences in use relative to need for adults, but children from higher-income families do have better access. Salkever's analysis is based on data from Canada, England, Finland, and Poland as well as the United States, and surprisingly, these conclusions seem to hold irrespective of the health system examined.[12]

Although empirical studies of utilization and utilization-need have not always yielded consistent results, there are several studies reporting negative findings—that is, access independent of family income. Using this class of measure alone, it is doubtful that those concerned with inequities in access would become very alarmed.

Process Measures

Process measures have often been defined as characteristics associated with the delivery of health care services that affect the rate at which these services are utilized.[13] An alternative to assessing utilization differences themselves is to assess differences in the preconditions for utilization. Once equity in the preconditions or utilization determinants is achieved, one may let the utilization differences fall as they may.

Access to health care services decreases as the cost per unit of services received increases. These costs should be measured not only in fees paid to providers, but also in travel and waiting-time costs, out-of-pocket transportation and child care costs, embarrassment and various types of anxieties associated with the receipt of medical care, and the like.

Table 2 reports mean total and out-of-pocket expenditure on physicians' services by income class. A larger proportion of the

TABLE 2. Mean Expenditures and Out-of-Pocket Payments for Physicians' Services per Person by Family Income, U.S., 1970

Family Income	Mean Expenditure	Percentage Paid Out-of-Pocket	Mean Out-of-Pocket Expenditure
Under $5,000	$72	42%	$30
$5,000–9,999	61	53	32
$10,000–14,999	56	59	33
$15,000 and over	62	58	36

Source: Derived from CHAS data reported in U.S. Department of Health, Education, and Welfare, *Expenditures for Personal Health Services: National Trends and Variations, 1953–1970* (Washington, D.C.: U.S. Government Printing Office, 1973), DHEW pub. no. (HRA) 74-3105.

Note: In performing the calculations, I have eliminated certain small miscellaneous expenditures not specifically identified in the HEW report.

poor's expenditure is covered by third parties or provided free by the physician, as is evident by examining the second column of table 2. The total expenditure includes all costs, irrespective of who pays—the private or public third party, the physician (by providing free service), or the patient. One may argue that "equity in access" implies that the poor should pay *even* a smaller proportion of expenditure out-of-pocket, but it is at least somewhat reassuring that the out-of-pocket proportion rises with family income. Tax burdens are not so equitably distributed.

Table 3 presents mean travel, waiting, and appointment delay times by family income and patient age derived from the CHAS survey. In all cases, the time estimates refer to "typical" situations with the patient's "usual" source of physicians' services. Responses from patients without usual sources are not included. Travel time is the time typically required to reach the patient's usual source of physicians' services (one way). Waiting time is the usual interval between the patient's arrival at the doctor's office or clinic and the time he or she is seen by the physician. The appointment delay is the period between the date the patient contacts the usual source and the date he or she is seen.

The CHAS survey requested interval responses to its time questions. Before calculating the means, I recoded each response at the mean of the interval; depending on the specific variable, re-

TABLE 3. Mean Travel, Waiting, and Appointment Delay Times by Family Income and Age, U.S., 1970

Age and Family Income	Travel Time (Minutes)	Waiting Time (Minutes)	Appointment Delay Time (Days)
All ages			
Under $5,000	25.0	77.9	2.85
$5,000–9,999	20.7	58.7	3.09
$10,000–14,999	17.5	45.8	3.73
$15,000 and over	17.1	36.5	3.67
Ratio, highest to lowest income category	0.68	0.47	1.29
Under 17 years of age			
Under $5,000	24.7	94.0	2.12
$5,000–9,999	20.2	63.2	3.24
$10,000–14,999	16.9	46.6	3.73
$15,000 and over	17.5	33.4	3.89
Ratio, highest to lowest income category	0.71	0.36	1.83
Ages 17–44			
Under $5,000	27.0	79.7	3.02
$5,000–9,999	20.9	60.1	2.89
$10,000–14,999	16.9	44.9	3.70
$15,000 and over	16.4	37.9	2.93
Ratio, highest to lowest income category	0.61	0.48	0.97
Ages 45–64			
Under $5,000	25.6	71.8	3.08
$5,000–9,999	21.8	55.6	2.82
$10,000–14,999	18.7	45.7	3.39
$15,000 and over	17.8	38.7	4.78
Ratio, highest to lowest income category	0.70	0.54	1.55

TABLE 3—*Continued*

Age and Family Income	Travel Time (Minutes)	Waiting Time (Minutes)	Appointment Delay Time (Days)
Age 65 and over			
Under $5,000	23.3	59.9	3.46
$5,000–9,999	20.0	41.3	3.73
$10,000–14,999	21.1	45.7	5.67
$15,000 and over	17.3	36.5	2.89
Ratio, highest to lowest income category	0.74	0.61	0.83

Source: Unpublished data from CHAS.
Note: Table includes all people in sample.

sponses in the highest, open-ended category were coded at or near the lower bound of the category. In some cases, the patient typically "walks in," with no appointment. I assumed the mean appointment delay in such instances to be 0.5 days.

The delay to an appointment does not exact a cost from the patient in the same ways that travel and waiting times do, since delay time can often be used for other purposes. But as Charles Phelps notes:

For patients whose ability to function is limited by their illness, and whose illness could be cured by immediate physician contact, the delay does indeed exact a price in the usual sense, the price being the value of the foregone productive time. For other patients, however, the delay simply postpones access to the physician. This may still reduce demand for care if many of the illnesses traced to this group are self-limiting in nature, so that illness goes away before the physician visit may be obtained. In either case, additional delay to appointment should reduce demand for care, just as any other form of a higher price for care should, and we can expect demand to fall for patients facing longer appointment delays.[14]

Table 3 shows marked differences in travel and waiting time by family income, irrespective of patient age. The contrast is particularly evident for waiting among children under seventeen years of age; children from families with incomes of $5,000 or less, and their parents or guardians, wait nearly three times as long as their counterparts in the highest income group.

The mean travel and waiting times may be expressed in monetary terms with estimates of the value of forgone productive time by age and income class. Without a doubt, the differentials shown in table 3 would narrow considerably if such calculations were made. In fact, in some instances, the relationship between time costs and family income could conceivably be positive.

Techniques have recently been developed by economists that allow one to derive estimates of the value of time of people not engaged in market work. Thus, failure to consider the value of forgone productive time as a result of traveling or waiting on the part of the nonemployed is not a valid objection to developing monetary equivalents for the time individuals spend in obtaining health care services. To the extent that society regards extensive waiting time in the offices of providers as demeaning, one may object to the implications of such calculations on distributional grounds.

Overall, table 3 shows appointment delays to rise with family income, but this pattern probably reflects variations in diagnostic mix by income. In another study using data from the District of Columbia, Bruce Steinwald and I controlled for patient diagnosis and found a weak negative relationship between appointment delays and income.[15]

In a recent article, I presented estimates of mean travel and office waiting times derived from the 1969 Health Interview Survey of the National Center for Health Statistics for the twenty-two largest Standard Metropolitan Statistical Areas (SMSAs), aggregates of smaller SMSAs for the four U.S. Census Areas, and aggregates of nonfarm and farm areas, again by U.S. Census Area.[16] All SMSA estimates are given for the central city and non–central city areas of the SMSA. A central city includes the largest city in the SMSA and, in some cases, additional comparatively large cities within the SMSA. The remainder of the SMSA, which is likely to be largely suburban, falls into the non–central city category. In total, travel and waiting time estimates are presented for 60 distinct locations.

Table 4 contains the locations with the five highest and lowest totals of time expended per visit. Total time is derived by multiplying the travel time by two (to reflect time spent on a round trip to a physician) and then adding the estimate for office waiting time. Time spent with physicians and staff, and time spent waiting once the patient has seen the physician, are not included. A weighting scheme has been used to adjust for systematic family income differences by location. Therefore, income is not a source of the time differences evident in table 4.

TABLE 4. Mean Travel and Waiting Times by Location, U.S., 1969

Location	Travel Time (Minutes)	Waiting Time (Minutes)	Total Time (Minutes)
Five highest total times			
Atlanta, central city	24.3	62.1	110.7
Chicago, central city	22.6	60.9	106.1
Farm, South	29.3	43.0	101.6
Houston, central city	24.9	51.0	100.8
St. Louis, central city	19.7	59.5	98.9
Five lowest total times			
Cleveland, non–central city	16.3	19.3	51.9
San Diego, central city	14.9	26.0	55.8
San Diego, non–central city	20.3	17.0	57.6
Boston, non–central city	17.2	24.0	58.4
Dallas, non–central city	15.7	27.6	59.0

Source: Abstracted from Frank A. Sloan, "Access to Medical Care and the Local Supply of Physicians," *Medical Care,* 15, no. 4 (April 1977):341-43.

Table 4 and the article on which the table is based indicate that, on the whole, total time is longest for people living in central cities of the largest SMSAs, not those living in smaller communities or, with the exception of the South, on farms. Although inner cores of central cities are frequently deficient in medical resources, the same cannot be said, as a rule, for the central city as a whole. In comparison to people who live in the central cities of the largest SMSAs, residents of non–central city areas of the same SMSAs frequently spend far less time in transit to the physician or waiting once they arrive. As will be discussed more fully, this finding has implications for the use of medical education programs as a means of achieving more equitable access by patient location.

Whether or not a person has a particular physician or clinic to whom he or she usually goes when sick or in need of medical advice is often considered a process measure. In important ways, the presence or absence of a usual source is a price variable, as are the time variables. A patient who has a usual source can spend less time searching for and obtaining appointments when physicians' services are desired. In fact, the patient without a usual source may have difficulty obtaining an appointment at all.[17] Moreover, the physician is likely to have better medical and personal information about the patient and is likely to arrive at a diagnosis and course of action in less time.

Table 5 gives the percentage of patients without usual sources of physicians' services by both family income and age. Substantial

TABLE 5. Choice of Usual Physician Provider by Age and Family Income, U.S., 1970

| Age and Family Income | No Usual Source | Usual Source | | |
		Clinic	Office-based GP	Office-based Specialist
All ages				
Under $5,000	20.0%	36.2%	31.5%	12.3%
$5,000–9,999	15.1	27.5	41.4	16.1
$10,000–14,999	12.3	20.8	42.3	23.9
$15,000 and over	8.8	13.9	45.1	32.1
Ratio, highest to lowest income category	0.44	0.38	1.43	2.61

TABLE 5—*Continued*

Age and Family Income	No Usual Source	Usual Source		
		Clinic	Office-based GP	Office-based Specialist
Under 17 years of age				
Under $5,000	19.1%	47.3%	26.0%	7.8%
$5,000–9,999	14.7	31.2	38.3	15.7
$10,000–14,999	8.1	23.0	41.6	27.2
$15,000 and over	3.1	17.1	41.8	38.1
Ratio, highest to lowest income category	0.16	0.36	1.61	4.88
Ages 17–44				
Under $5,000	23.3	40.1	26.3	10.3
$5,000–9,999	16.7	27.1	42.1	14.7
$10,000–14,999	16.1	19.1	43.7	21.0
$15,000 and over	12.7	12.5	46.2	28.5
Ratio, highest to lowest income category	0.55	0.31	1.76	2.77
Ages 45–64				
Under $5,000	20.9	28.3	36.7	14.0
$5,000–9,999	16.8	23.1	43.6	16.4
$10,000–14,999	12.6	20.8	43.3	23.3
$15,000 and over	10.1	12.7	45.7	31.4
Ratio, highest to lowest income category	0.48	0.45	1.25	2.24
Age 65 and over				
Under $5,000	17.7	21.8	41.2	19.3
$5,000–9,999	6.0	20.0	47.4	26.7
$10,000–14,999	13.3	19.2	43.4	24.1
$15,000 and over	7.3	11.6	52.2	29.0
Ratio, highest to lowest income category	0.41	0.53	1.27	1.50

Source: Unpublished data from CHAS.
Note: Rows may not add to 100% because of rounding.

differences in the percentages presented in this table are apparent by both income and age. As in some of the previous tables, children living in poor households appear to be at a particular disadvantage.

The type of provider of those reporting a usual source has implications for a study of the distribution of health care delivery. Although hospital outpatient departments and emergency rooms offer entry and clinical services for large numbers of patients, they have definite limitations in the provision of comprehensive family care services. Only rarely is there an attempt to assign a patient to a particular physician. For this reason, many of the primary advantages of having a usual source of medical services are lost.

On the whole, private office-based physicians serve much more satisfactorily as the usual sources of physicians' services. Whether an office-based general practitioner or a specialist is more appropriate depends on such factors as the presence of an important chronic condition and, in the case of pediatric services, age.[18]

Unfortunately, the meaning of the term *clinic* could have been more precise than it was in the CHAS survey. Individuals using a hospital outpatient clinic or an emergency room as their regular source are undoubtedly included under the heading "clinic," but members of large prepaid group-practice plans may be included as well. The latter are thought by many to be a very appropriate usual source. Prepaid practices still deliver a very small fraction of physicians' services in the United States. Thus, even though responses to the CHAS survey are probably not as clear as one would like, it does yield a reasonably reliable picture of the distribution of usual sources by family income class. If anything, the imprecise definition of clinic probably leads to an overstatement of the proportion of higher-income people using clinics.

According to table 5, there are substantial differences by income class in the proportion of people who have a clinic as a regular source. The differences narrow somewhat in the two higher age groups. Reliance on office-based specialists is likewise highly dependent on family income but, as anticipated, in the opposite direction.

Attitudinal Measures

The CHAS survey requested a substantial amount of attitudinal information relating to the care presumably received by the survey respondents and about preferences concerning the distribution of health care services. Many of the questions relating to the individual's own medical care correspond to the kinds of process measures specifically considered earlier; others involve assessments of the overall quality of care received.

Table 6 contains the percentages of respondents dissatisfied (combining those who were "unsatisfied" or "very unsatisfied" in

TABLE 6. Percentage of Respondents Unsatisfied with Aspects of Medical Care Received by Family Income, U.S., 1970

Aspect	Family Income			
	Under $5,000	$5,000–9,999	$10,000–14,999	$15,000 and Over
A. Overall quality of medical care received	8.8%	9.2%	10.8%	6.7%
B. Information given to you about what was wrong with you	16.1	17.2	16.8	11.9
C. Information given to you about what you should do at home to treat illness	10.8	10.6	9.8	8.5
D. Concern of doctors for your overall health rather than just for an isolated symptom or disease	12.6	18.5	17.0	13.5
E. Courtesy and consideration shown you by:				
1. Doctors	7.1	7.7	7.4	5.9
2. Nurses	9.9	11.2	8.2	8.3

TABLE 6—*Continued*

Aspect	Family Income			
	Under $5,000	$5,000– 9,999	$10,000– 14,999	$15,000 and Over
F. Follow-up care received after an initial treatment or operation	6.8%	8.3%	8.7%	4.1%
G. Waiting time in doctors' offices or clinics	40.9	40.1	37.3	34.6
H. Availability of medical care at night or on weekends	40.1	44.8	45.2	42.0
I. Ease and convenience of getting to a doctor from where you live	19.7	14.7	11.2	7.9
J. Out-of-pocket costs of medical care received	37.6	43.6	41.2	30.8

Source: Unpublished data from CHAS.
Note: Table includes answers of respondents only (not respondents speaking on behalf of other family members); excludes blank answers (always a small percentage).

response to the CHAS survey questions) with specific aspects of care-seeking. The patterns in the full distribution of responses ("very satisfied," "satisfied," "unsatisfied," and "very unsatisfied"), not shown here for reasons of space, have essentially the same implications as does table 6. With few exceptions, dissatisfaction with care personally received is reasonably invariant with respect to family income. The most notable exceptions are "information given to you about what was wrong with you" and "ease and convenience of getting to a doctor from where you live." Rates of dissatisfaction with the "overall quality of medical care received" are invariant with respect to income, as are those corresponding to "waiting time in doctor's office," which demonstrated a great deal of variation by income when reported in terms of minutes typically spent waiting.[19]

According to responses to the CHAS survey, there is very little dissatisfaction in the aggregate and across income groups with regard to quality of services, information received about what to do at home, levels of physician and nurse concern, and the physician's follow-up care subsequent to initial treatment or surgery. Waiting time, availability of physicians' services during off-hours, and out-of-pocket medical costs appear to be much more important sources of dissatisfaction, but in no aspect covered in table 6 is the majority of respondents dissatisfied.

Table 7 reports responses to two questions concerning political attitudes about medical care. Judging from answers to a question about whether or not "medical care is a right," it is evident that the vast majority, irrespective of income class, regard medical care to be a right. Responses to the second question, however, reveal substantial variation by income class in reactions to a possible method for actually achieving more equitable distribution in the delivery of health care services. Although minorities in the lower two income categories favor keeping the Medicare program as it is or "doing away with the program," 58 percent of respondents in the highest income group take these conservative positions. One may infer from the pattern of responses to the latter question that there is, on the whole, less enthusiasm among those who would in fact pay for the redistribution.

Effects of Government Programs

The types of public policies most likely to be relied upon to improve access to ambulatory care services involve extending insurance to cover all segments of the population, especially low-income groups, and increasing student places in medical schools.

Potential Effects of Universal Health Insurance Coverage

The United States is the last major industrialized country to contemplate enacting a national health insurance system. In one important sense, it is fortunate to be last, as the experiences of

TABLE 7. Political Attitudes About Medical Care, U.S., 1970

Question and Responses	Family Income			
	Under $5,000	$5,000– 9,999	$10,000– 14,999	$15,000 and Over
A. Do you agree or disagree with this statement? All people have a right to medical care whether they can pay for it or not.				
1. Strongly agree	49.2%	46.5%	38.7%	36.0%
2. Tend to agree	44.3	46.2	53.3	53.1
3. Tend to disagree	4.7	5.5	5.6	8.6
4. Strongly disagree	1.7	1.7	2.3	2.3
	99.9%[a]	99.9%[a]	99.9%[a]	100.0%
B. As you probably know, Medicare is the government-sponsored health insurance for people 65 and over. It is paid for mainly through Social Security taxes on workers and employers. By increasing the taxes that workers and employers have to pay, Medicare could cover other people in the population as well. Do you favor:				
1. Keeping it as it is	34.6%	39.6%	45.7%	49.9%
2. Extending it to cover all people under 65 who cannot afford their own health insurance	45.1	36.3	29.8	27.0

TABLE 7—*Continued*

	Family Income			
Question and Responses	Under $5,000	$5,000–9,999	$10,000–14,999	$15,000 and Over
3. Extending it to cover all people in the country	17.6%	19.7%	17.5%	15.2%
4. Doing away with the program.	2.7	4.3	6.9	7.9
	100.0%	99.9%ᵃ	99.9%ᵃ	100.0%

Source: Unpublished data from CHAS.
Note: Table includes answers of respondents only (not respondents speaking on behalf of other family members); excludes blank answers (always a small percentage).
a. Does not add to 100% because of rounding.

other countries can be used to forecast effects likely to occur in the United States. The closest country to the United States, in terms of both the population's demographic mix and the health care system before universal health insurance, is Canada. "Before" and "after" data, comparable to the data presented in the previous section, are available for one Canadian province, Quebec. Data were obtained during two eight-month periods immediately before and soon after Medicare, the Canadian universal plan, was introduced (1969–1970 and 1971–1972). These data permit one to gauge Canadian Medicare's short-term impacts on access to physicians' services.

Table 8 presents mean estimates on utilization, process, and attitudinal measures by family income for the "before" and "after" periods. The income categories have been made as close to the categories used in the tables in the previous section as the data published in the source article will allow. As in the United States, visits per capita were negatively related to family income before universal health insurance. Introduction of Medicare in Canada accentuated these differences; utilization by the affluent declined both absolutely *and* relatively. With one exception, all income

TABLE 8. Changes in Pertinent Access Measures

Family Income	Mean Visits per Person			Mean Travel Time (minutes)		
	Before	After	% Change	Before	After	% Change
Under $5,000	6.0	6.8	13.3	23.6	24.7	4.7
$5,000–8,999	4.7	4.7	0.0	20.6	20.9	1.5
$9,000–14,999	5.1	4.9	−3.9	20.9	20.2	−3.3
$15,000 and over	5.3	4.8	−9.4	17.9	18.9	5.6
Total	5.0	5.0	0.0	21.2	21.3	0.4
Ratio, highest to lowest income category	0.88	0.71	—	0.76	0.77	—

Source: Based on Philip Enterline, Vera Salter, Alison McDonald, and J. Cosbett McDonald, "The Distribution of Medical Services Before and After 'Free' Medical Care—The Quebec Experience," *New England Journal of Medicine,* 289,

groups experienced losses in terms of three process measures: travel, waiting, and appointment delay time. But the poor, while gaining relatively, experienced losses in absolute terms, as did those with higher incomes. Even though the vast majority rated the quality of care received very highly in the "before" period, there were slight declines in patient assessments of quality in the "after" period. Satisfaction among high-income people with care personally received fell the most, although not substantially. Responses to other satisfaction measures, not presented in table 8, are fully consistent with the measure presented in the table.

Estimates of "before" and "after" utilization rates are also available for Saskatchewan, England, Wales, and Finland. R. G. Beck presents estimates for Saskatchewan, Canada, of the percentage of people in each income class who report at least one contact with physicians in given years.[20] As in table 1, which represents the experience in a recent year in the United States, the percentage of people with at least one visit rose with family income, both before and after Medicare, but the differences by income in Saskatche-

After the Introduction of Universal Health Insurance: Quebec

Mean Waiting Time (minutes)			Mean Appointment Delay (days)			Percentage of People Who Considered Care Received at Last Visit Best Possible		
Before	After	%Change	Before	After	%Change	Before	After	%Change
45.9	48.2	5.0	6.3	9.0	42.9	90.6	90.1	−1.0
37.8	42.6	12.7	5.3	10.7	100.0	93.3	91.2	−2.3
30.8	37.5	21.8	6.3	11.1	76.2	93.7	91.4	−2.5
24.0	33.3	38.8	6.6	12.3	86.4	95.4	92.4	−3.1
36.0	40.1	11.1	6.0	11.0	83.3	92.8	91.4	−1.5
0.52	0.69	—	1.05	1.37		1.05	1.03	—

no. 22 (November 29, 1973):1174–78.

Note: Travel, waiting, and appointment times include only people with prior appointments. The CHAS tabulations, by contrast, include all responses.

wan were far more pronounced than those in table 1. Medicare in Saskatchewan has tended to narrow these differences, even though some still persist. Immediately before the introduction of the National Health Service (NHS) in the United Kingdom, both crude and need-adjusted physician utilization rates were higher for the poor. The NHS had the effect of widening differentials in utilization by income category.[21] Per capita visits were negatively related to income, and per capita visits adjusted for need were positively related to income immediately before implementation of a national sickness insurance program in Finland in 1964. Four years later, gains of the poor relative to the more affluent were seen in both the crude and need-adjusted visit rates.[22]

The potential impacts of increases in the physician-population ratio as a means of improving patient access to physicians' services have been evaluated in several articles. Since one of the primary methods for increasing physician-population ratios is by expanding medical school classes, results dealing with the effects of the ratios have important implications for medical education. Using regression analysis with data on individual physician practices from the American Medical Association, John Lorant and I found that a hypothetical (and substantial) increase in a county's physician-population ratio from 1 physician per 4,000 population to 15 per 4,000 population would reduce the county's mean waiting time in the physician's office by 4.9 minutes.[23] The 1:4,000 ratio is sometimes given by policy makers as the boundary between "shortage" and "nonshortage" areas. Compared to the mean waiting times shown in table 3 and 4, it is apparent that a reduction of this magnitude does not mean a great deal. With more detailed evidence of the type presented in table 4 and a set of simple correlations, and relying on U.S. National Center for Health Statistics Health Interview Survey data, my work largely supports the finding of the waiting time study.[24] The area physician-population ratios can explain no more than 6 percent of intercommunity variations in patient travel and office and clinic waiting time.

Although the CHAS survey requested information on a number of process measures, it did not use information on the length of time physicians and staff spend with patients per visit. It is very likely that courtesy and concern shown by physicians and staff, and pertinent health information shared with the patient, are associated with the length of time health personnel spend with patients.

With reference to a theoretical framework, John Lorant and I hypothesize that one factor responsible for variations in length of visit is the availability of physicians in a geographic area. Based on parameter estimates obtained by means of regression analysis, we calculate that an increase in the physician-population ratio of the same magnitude as the one considered earlier would raise mean visit lengths by about 4 minutes on the average.[25] The mean physician visit length in the United States, based on American Medical Association data, was 18.6 minutes in 1973. Physician availability clearly makes some difference, but as with travel and waiting time, manpower policies should not be viewed as a panacea.

Further Discussion, Conclusions, and Implications

In the 1970s, most U.S. citizens regard health care as a right. As evidence presented in this study indicates, the overwhelming majority, irrespective of financial circumstances, subscribe to this principle. Yet there is far less unanimity on specific methods to assure all citizens of this right in practice. It is probably in large part the lack of enthusiasm in the United States for what people in the upper half of the income distribution perceive as a redistribution against their own interests that accounts for the apparent delays in enacting universal health insurance in this country.

It is easy to speak of an equitable distribution of health services, but devising operational meanings of the term is by no means so easy. As we saw in the example of the two subcultures, one may readily devise a measure that is consistent with some ethical precepts but in conflict with others. Furthermore, plausible measures do not always move in the same direction empirically. Some may suggest that the current distribution is equitable, whereas others suggest quite the opposite. Substantial changes in health care delivery systems, such as those associated with the introduction of national health insurance, may cause what are thought by many to be improvements in the distribution of services; other measures, as we have seen, may show impacts that are less desirable or even undesirable.

Although there are some ambiguities with regard to patterns of utilization of physicians' services in the United States by income class, available evidence suggests less inequality with respect to the quantity of health care services than with some important qualitative, or process, aspects. The patient's time input in the consumption of health care services varies markedly by income class and location, even though the patterns are not always the same as conventional wisdom would have them. There are, moreover, substantial disparities by income in the proportions of people without a usual source of medical care. For people with a regular source, there are substantial income-related differences in the proportions of individuals using a clinic as opposed to a private office-based practice. Limitations of clinics as sources of primary care were briefly reviewed. To the extent that valid inferences about the United States can be made from the experiences of other countries, it would appear that universal health insurance might well achieve its quantitative objectives but perform unsatisfactorily with regard to some of the qualitative features.

On the whole, there is surprisingly little variation in dissatisfaction with medical care personally received by income category. There appears to be a high degree of satisfaction with overall quality, as well as courtesy and consideration of physician and staff toward patients. To the extent that there is dissatisfaction with care personally received, it seems to be concentrated on aspects relating to cost and convenience. There is little in the data presented in this study to suggest that inhumane or impersonal treatment by health professionals is currently a major concern to patients.

According to survey results presented in this study, patients rank nurses slightly lower than physicians in terms of courtesy and consideration. This does not mean that efforts medical schools may now make to teach awareness of the human being as a whole rather than as a collection of parts do not have merit. They do, however, tend to place such efforts in perspective. To the extent that it exists, inhumane treatment is by no means restricted to physicians, but is shared by other kinds of health professionals. Furthermore, and more important, this is only one dimension of access. If further equity in the delivery of health care services is to be achieved, efforts to broaden the viewpoints of health professionals must be coupled with approaches toward improving other dimensions of access.

Several statements in this essay may suggest that I am pessimistic about the efficacy of major public programs as vehicles for achieving a more equitable distribution of health care services. It would be more accurate to state that I seriously doubt that improvements across the board can readily be achieved. Although improvements may be evident using some criteria of equity, one must be prepared for much less satisfactory results on others. Ultimately, whether or not a program has indeed achieved greater equity will most certainly involve weighing a number of pluses and minuses.

NOTES

1. Eugene Outka, "Commentary," in *Ethics of Health Care,* ed. Lawrence R. Tancredi (Washington, D.C.: National Academy of Sciences, 1974), pp. 271–77.

2. "On Achieving Access and Equity in Health Care," in *Economic Aspects of Health Care,* ed. John McKinley (New York: PRODIST, 1973), pp. 24, 26.

3. Ronald Andersen, "Health Service Distribution and Equity," in *Equity in Health Services,* ed. Ronald Andersen, Joanna Kravits, and Odin Andersen (Cambridge, Mass.: Ballinger, 1975), p. 10.

4. A useful review of literature on cultural and social factors underlying illness and illness behavior is found in David Mechanic, *Public Expectations and Health Care: Essays on the Changing Organization of Health Services* (New York: Wiley-Interscience, 1972).

5. Stephen Cole and Robert LeJeune assess the use of illness as a means of coping with failure ("Illness and Legitimation of Failure," *American Sociological Review,* 37, no. 2 [June 1972]:347–56).

6. On trends in health care services consumption, see U.S. Department of Health, Education, and Welfare, *Expenditures for Personal Health Services: National Trends and Variations, 1953–1970* (Washington, D.C.: U.S. Government Printing Office, 1973), DHEW pub. no. (HRA) 74-3105; and Lee Benham and Alexandra Benham, "Utilization of Physician Services Across Income Groups, 1963–1970," in *Equity in Health Services,* ed. Ronald Andersen, Joanna Kravits, and Odin Andersen (Cambridge, Mass.: Ballinger, 1975), pp. 97–103.

7. "Economic Class and Differential Access to Care: Comparisons Among Health Care Systems," *International Journal of Health Services,* 5, no. 3 (Summer 1975):377.

8. In brief, economic efficiency means securing the maximum amount of goods and services from a fixed amount of scarce resources—land, raw materials, capital, and labor. The relationship between waiting time and economic efficiency is developed in Frank Sloan and John Lorant, "The Role of Waiting Time: Evidence from Physicians' Practices," *Journal of Business,* 50, no. 4 (October 1977):486–507. It is discussed more indirectly in Barry Schwartz, *Queuing and Waiting: Studies in the Social Organization of Access and Delay* (Chicago: University of Chicago Press, 1975).

9. See Victor Fuchs, *Who Shall Live? Health, Economics, and Social Choice* (New York: Basic Books, 1974).

10. Aday, "Economic and Noneconomic Barriers to the Use of Needed Medical Services," *Medical Care,* 13, no. 6 (June 1975):447–56; Aday and Andersen, *Development of Indices of Access to Medical Care* (Ann Arbor: Health Administration Press, 1975).

11. "Utilization of Physician Services."

12. "Economic Class and Differential Access to Care."

13. See, for example, Aday and Andersen, *Development of Indices.*

14. "Effects of Insurance on Demand for Medical Care," in *Empirical Analyses in Social Policy,* ed. Ronald Andersen, Joanna Kravits, and Odin Andersen (Cambridge, Mass.: Ballinger, 1975), p. 108.

15. Frank Sloan and Bruce Steinwald, "Variations in Appointment Delays for Ambulatory Services," *Policy Sciences,* in press.

16. Frank A. Sloan, "Access to Medical Care and the Local Supply of Physicians," *Medical Care,* 15, no. 4 (April 1977):341–43.

17. Estimate of the proportions of physicians not willing to accept new patients are presented in Charles Berry, Rachel Feilden, Philip J. Held, and Judith Woolridge, *Report on the Physician Capacity Utilization Telephone Surveys* (Princeton: Mathematica, 1976).

18. These points are discussed more fully in Alberta Parker, "The Dimensions of Primary Care: Blueprints for Change," in *Primary Care: Where Medicine Fails,* ed. Spyros Andreopoulos (New York: John Wiley, 1974), pp. 15–77.

19. Aday and Andersen, *Development of Indices,* shows that responses to attitudinal questions in the CHAS survey are related to responses to the more objective questions. Apparently these relationships are not sufficiently strong to be reflected in the tables prepared for this essay.

20. "Economic Class and Access to Physician Services Under Public Medical Care Insurance," *International Journal of Health Services,* 3, no. 3 (Summer 1973):341–55.

21. William Stewart and Philip Enterline, "Effects of the National Health Service on Physician Utilization and Health in England and Wales," *New England Journal of Medicine,* 265, no. 24 (1961):1187–94.

22. Kauko Nyman and Esko Kalimo, "National Sickness Insurance and the Use of Physicians' Services in Finland," *Social Science and Medicine,* 7, no. 7 (1973):541–43; T. Purola, E. Kalimo, K. Nyman, and K. Sievers, "National Health Insurance in Finland: Its Impact and Evaluation," *International Journal of Health Services,* 3, no. 1 (Winter 1973):69–80.

23. Sloan and Lorant, "Role of Waiting Time."

24. Sloan, "Access to Medical Care."

25. Frank Sloan and John Lorant, "The Allocation of Physicians' Services: Evidence on Length-of-Visit," *Quarterly Review of Economics and Business,* 16, no. 3 (Autumn 1976):85–103.

CHAPTER 9

The Uses of a Diagnosis:
Doctors, Patients, and Neurasthenia

Barbara Sicherman

Of all the charges that have been brought against the U.S. medical profession by its contemporary critics, one of the most inflammatory is the claim that the profession is responsible for the "medicalization" of American life. From birth to death, the charge reads, social, moral, political, and religious frames of reference are being usurped by a medical mind set that sees a decisive role for the physician in every possible aspect of living, and is prepared to designate as "disease" any form of behavior that the dominant cultural groups find disagreeable or disruptive. It can be argued, from this point of view, that the preceding essays flagrantly abet this medical imperialism. After all, responsibility for personal agency and the construction of meaning, attention to moral, political, and economic dimensions of patients' (and physicians') lives, and involvement in potential transformation of the very nature of the human hardly constitute norms for professionally expert medical care.

These arguments, however, frequently make one hazardous assumption: that it is possible to empty out of the medical encounter all extraneous concerns, until what remains is readily identifiable as a specifically medical matter, calling for the legitimate application of specifically medical procedures and expertise. Corollary to this assumption is the value orientation of professional restraint, which is often expressed in a reluctance to engage patients on any but physiological or organic (and, presumably, morally and personally neutral) grounds. The support for this assumption is often couched either in highly technical and philosophical terms, so that the matter ends up appearing like a question of epistemology, or as part of a full-scale ideological broadside. Few treatments of the question deal concretely and sympathetically with the actual clinical and human aspects of the meeting between a suffering individual and a caring physician.

In the following essay, Barbara Sicherman goes beneath the epistemological or ideological level to reach the human core of the medical encounter. Her account of the vicissitudes of "neurasthenia" as a diagnostic category in turn-of-the-century U.S. medicine brings home the liberating potential of a negotiated diagnostic process that is centered in the daily realities of both patients and physicians. In this case, patients are liberated from the stigma and despair of perplexing symptoms and behavior, and physicians are freed to express their empathy and desire to help in the absence of "standard" remedies. The essay demonstrates in vivid and personal terms that medicine is not a logic-tight, self-sufficient discipline, snugly insulated from individual personalities and historical circumstances. And, although not necessarily contradicting the value of professional restraint, this perspective is a reminder that, for all its scientific and intellectual rigor, medicine always has a human use.

In 1869 George M. Beard suggested a common origin and the designation "neurasthenia" for a staggering variety of symptoms that had long taxed the ingenuity and the patience of physicians. A pioneer specialist in neurology, Beard made his reputation in New York City by treating the functional nervous disorders, that is, those for which no gross pathology could be found.[1] Neurasthenia was one of these, a disease characterized by profound physical and mental exhaustion. It was also a protean condition that might attack any organ or function. Its characteristic symptoms included sick headache, noises in the ear, atonic voice, deficient mental control, bad dreams, insomnia, nervous dyspepsia, heaviness of the loin and limb, flushing and fidgetiness, palpitations, vague pains and flying neuralgia, spinal irritation, uterine irritability, impotence, hopelessness, and such morbid fears as claustrophobia and dread of contamination.[2]

To a modern observer, as to a contemporary critic, Beard appears to have "greatly overloaded his subject."[3] But by suggesting a common pathology, prognosis, history, and treatment for such varied behavioral attributes, Beard was attempting to bring order to the chaotic field of the functional nervous disorders. In the absence of clear anatomical changes, or hard and fast tests, such conditions not only tested the physician's diagnostic skills, but invited the disbelief of friends and relatives. Beard acknowledged that neurasthenia was subjective, its symptoms "slippery, fleeting, and vague." But he insisted that it was as real a disease, with as genuinely somatic a course, as smallpox or cholera. "In strictness," he wrote, "nothing in disease can be imaginary. If I bring on a pain by worrying, by dwelling on myself, that pain is as real as though it were brought on by an objective influence."[4]

Beard had not discovered a new disease, as even he acknowledged. But until his premature death in 1883, he labored to secure for neurasthenia an honored place in the medical lexicon. Motivated in part by personal need—he had wrestled with the symptoms of the disease in his youth—Beard was able to transform his own struggles into a disease syndrome that struck a responsive chord among his contemporaries. By interpreting diverse physical and mental symptoms as the common consequence of an excessive expenditure of nervous energy, he brilliantly blended scientific theories about the nature of the nervous impulse, the conservation of energy, and biological evolution into a plausible disease entity.

Beard defined neurasthenia as an "impoverishment of nervous force. . . . 'Nervousness' is really nervelessness." Physicians in the late nineteenth century believed that each individual possessed a fixed amount of nervous energy, determined mainly by heredity, which acted as a messenger between various parts of the body. Neurasthenia resulted when demand exceeded supply; even a tiny excess could cause the entire system to break down. Immoderate toil or worry, lack of food or rest, could induce an acute attack or even a chronic condition. The exhaustion of any one bodily system—the brain, for instance—could by the principle of reflex irritation spread to the reproductive and digestive systems, causing a total breakdown. Two popular metaphors—the overloaded electrical circuit and the overdrawn bank account—graphically illustrated the process for layman and physician alike.[5]

Just as physicians considered nervous energy limited, they believed that contemporary society placed inordinate demands on that supply. The dynamism of the Gilded Age, so welcome in other respects, thus became a source of social and psychological as well as physical stress. Beard drew on evolutionary theory to support his belief that nervousness was peculiarly an American phenomenon. In his long list of causes, he gave special attention to the periodical press, steampower, the telegraph, the sciences, and the increased mental activity of women. By encouraging men and women to experience life more fully, these five characteristic features of nineteenth-century civilization—most advanced in

America—placed too many demands on their limited supplies of nervous energy. Civilized society also demanded repression of the emotions, a refinement from which savages were exempt, and thus additionally drained human energies.[6]

Beard thought his work had initially been ignored, but by 1880 he contended that the subject "after long standing and waiting at the doors of science, has, at last, gained admission." A large popular and technical literature supported his claim. A tract by S. Weir Mitchell, the Philadelphia neurologist who developed the rest cure for neurasthenia, choicely titled *Wear and Tear,* sold out in ten days and went through five editions between 1871 and 1881; his *Fat and Blood* did even better. In the late 1880s a *Journal of Nervous Exhaustion* appeared briefly. And in the 1890s, two Shattuck lecturers, charged with enlightening members of the Massachusetts Medical Society on diseases prevalent in the Commonwealth, chose neurasthenia as their subject. When Beard's one-time partner, A. D. Rockwell, brought out a new edition of Beard's treatise for physicians in 1901, he noted that "neurasthenia is now almost a household word." Whether accurate or not, he continued, the diagnosis proved "often as satisfactory to the patient as it is easy to the physician."[7]

Even as Rockwell wrote, Beard's classic formulation of neurasthenia as a syndrome characterized by a deficiency of energy had begun to break down. The diagnosis had become so widespread, its use so imprecise, that many physicians believed it had outlived its usefulness. One called it the newest garbage can of medicine.[8] No longer able to provide a coherent explanation for the symptoms it had once readily encompassed, neurasthenia lost ground in the first two decades of the twentieth century both to demonstrably organic ills and to conditions increasingly assumed to be of psychological origin. New diagnostic tests made it possible to distinguish a number of conditions characterized by exhaustion, among them anemia, pulmonary tuberculosis, incipient paresis, lead poisoning, and Addison's disease together with other endocrine disorders.[9] Just as the diagnosis fever had earlier given way to more precise formulations, so exhaustion came to be viewed less as an essence than as a symptom.

A preference for psychological interpretations of the psychoneuroses was also apparent by 1900, a consequence mainly of the discovery of unconscious mental states. Pioneer psychopathologists like Pierre Janet and Sigmund Freud proposed psychodynamic interpretations of many physical and psychological symptoms formerly assumed to be of somatic origin. Thus Janet substituted the term *psychasthenia* for neuroses in which obsessions and phobias predominated. He attributed these to reduced psychic energy and discarded neurasthenia because he found no evidence of any physiological etiology. Freud retained the term, but wished to limit it to the relatively infrequent cases of physical exhaustion brought on by masturbation or nocturnal emissions. He considered it an actual neurosis as distinct from the more common psychoneuroses that psychoanalysis did so much to elucidate.[10] American physicians debated these concepts and, although some still accorded neurasthenia a limited place, Beard's earlier synthesis was effectively demolished by 1920.[11]

In retrospect it is clear that what was called neurasthenia actually comprehended a range of conditions that included depressive, obsessive, and phobic states later classified as psychoneuroses; mildly psychotic and borderline states; palpable physical ills that could not then be adequately diagnosed; and a host of symptoms that are today considered psychophysiological. Leonard Woolf was quite correct when he called neurasthenia "a name, a label, like neuralgia or rheumatism, which covered a multitude of sins, symptoms, and miseries."[12]

This modern diagnostic nemesis has recently attracted the attention of historians precisely because it so neatly illustrates the interplay of scientific theory and cultural values in the fashioning of a disease entity. Concentrating on physicians' generalizations about the disease, scholars for the most part have considered neurasthenia within the framework of intellectual history. The best of these studies securely anchors Beard's work in the medical and social structures of the Gilded Age, taking seriously his now dated explanatory model as a measure of the intellectual temper of the time.[13] Others, unable to see past the colorful etiology of the disease, have claimed that the term *neurasthenia* "stood for conflicting . . . ideologies," and, on the patient's part, was "a reservoir of class prejudices, status desires, urban arrogance, repressed sexuality, and indulgent self-centeredness."[14]

However imprecise the label *neurasthenia* now appears, it is surely unfair to doctors and especially to patients to view illness purely as an intellectual construct. To ignore the clinical context in which disease is identified is to miss the distinguishing feature of medical practice. For it is in the consulting room, the hospital clinic, and at the bedside that the daily drama of diagnosis and treatment takes place. There the patient offers up the symptoms that have already caused sufficient distress to prompt the encounter. As a psychoanalyst reminds us: "For the patient illness is always an uncanny experience. He feels something has gone wrong with him, something that might, or certainly will, do him harm unless dealt with properly and swiftly. What 'it' is, is difficult to know."[15]

In what is frequently a highly charged atmosphere, the physician's primary task is to identify "it," to transform the diffuse symptoms of his patient into a condition that can be rationally understood and treated. To such an encounter each party brings his own preconceptions about illness, expectations of the other, and more or less enduring personality traits, shaped by class and social position as well as individual need. If the physician fails to make sense of the patient's troubles—or to relieve them—neither he nor his patient will retain much confidence in his skill. If the interpretation is unacceptable, the patient may take his business elsewhere.

In the late nineteenth century, neurasthenia proved a satisfactory label to doctors and patients alike. By incorporating into a disease picture a host of behavioral symptoms, many of which would otherwise have been deemed self-willed and thus deviant, the diagnosis legitimized new roles for physicians and their patients. For patients, it provided the most respectable label for distressing, but not life-threatening, complaints, one that conferred many of the benefits—and fewest of the liabilities—associated with illness. Certainly it was preferable to its nearest alternatives—hypochondria, hysteria, and insanity, not to mention malingering.

At a time when psychiatry was limited to the institutional care of psychotic patients, those who specialized in the functional nervous disorders were actually providing psychiatric services for many patients. Thoughtful clinicians understood that deep-rooted personality needs often influenced the onset of an illness, and that the relationship between doctor and patient affected the patient's capacity to recover. Although their suspicion of psychology kept them from exploring this relationship fully, physicians sometimes acknowledged that they ministered to the soul as well as the body. As confessors, they concerned themselves with all aspects of the patient's behavior. Neurasthenia was thus an important chapter in the expansion of the medical sphere that has characterized modern American society.

As a diagnosis on the borderland of medicine and psychiatry, neurasthenia augmented therapeutic approaches in both fields. Medicine had reached an ambiguous stage when the disparity between actual achievement and future promise was especially great. Scientists, by correlating clinical and pathological data, had identified the basic diseases in modern form by mid-century. As typhus and malaria replaced the symptomatic designation fever, it became possible to search for pathogenic microorganisms. The first such organism was identified in 1876, but two decades elapsed before the great medical discoveries yielded practical results. In the meantime, death rates remained high and the art of therapeutics perilously low. Recognizing that there were few specific remedies, medical leaders repudiated many traditional therapies as unavailing or positively harmful. This therapeutic nihilism, although an advance over the heavy drugging of the past, left the practitioner in a peculiarly vulnerable position. For, as the authors of guides for aspiring physicians noted, patients expected medicines and even specific courses of treatment. If they did not receive them from members of the regular profession, they might patronize adherents of medical sects who still offered a holistic view of disease, or one of the numerous vendors of patent medicines.[16]

The laboratory cast of mind of professional leaders at the end of the century further highlighted the practitioner's impotence. In this era of extreme somaticism, a respectable disease required a specific and identifiable etiology, pathology, and therapy. The discovery that microorganisms caused specific diseases contributed to this outlook. So did insistence on a localized pathology exemplified in Rudolf Virchow's famous dictum: "There are no general diseases . . . only diseases of organs and cells." In their efforts to make medicine an exact science the most prominent physicians often overlooked—and certainly underrated—the importance of clinical medicine. Their emphasis on basic research in chemistry, bacteriology, and anatomy, so productive in other respects, did little to help either the ambitious practitioner or the anxious patient in their mutual quest.[17]

Neurasthenia offered the practitioner a way out of this therapeutic dilemma. The new label, with its implied precision, emphasized what physicians could do for their patients rather than their impotence. At a time when physicians felt comfortable only with clearly organic disorders, a diagnosis of neurasthenia permitted some to address themselves to less tangible clinical issues and to provide an essentially psychological therapy under a somatic label. The diagnosis and its treatment helped physicians to justify a traditional role, threatened by the one-sided emphasis on science, of providing advice and comfort to patients and their families. In view of the impoverished state of medical therapeutics in the late nineteenth century, this was by no means an insignificant achievement.[18]

Conditions of weakness had long been known to physicians by a variety of names, among them debility. But the emphasis on weakness of the nerves coincided with the rise of neurology as a medical specialty in the years after the Civil War. Knowledge of the brain and nervous system advanced rapidly in Europe after 1860 as experimental physiologists demonstrated that fixed parts of the brain controlled specific motor activities. Important clinical advances, especially J. Hughlings Jackson's work on epilepsy and Jean-Martin Charcot's delineations of several classic neurological disorders, followed. By the late 1860s, important teaching and hospital positions in neurology had been established in England, France, and the German-speaking world, a sign that the specialty had come of age.[19]

Beard and Mitchell belonged to the pioneer generation of physicians who established neurology on a firm professional footing in the United States. Concentrated in large cities on the eastern seaboard and Chicago, they began in the 1870s to found the journals and societies that constitute the core of a professional identity. In their bid for recognition, the neurologists encountered resistance from general practitioners opposed to specialization of any kind, and outright hostility from the medical superintendents of asylums for the insane who since the 1840s had claimed exclusive authority over the care of the mentally ill. At a time when all experts considered insanity a disease of the brain, neurologists legitimately claimed competence in the field of mental as well as neurological disorders. But because the two fields had developed separately in the United States, ambitious young specialists like Beard found it necessary to challenge what amounted to the superintendents' monopoly in caring for the mentally ill. Rivalry between competing specialists was particularly intense during the 1870s and 1880s. In the struggle for professional status and monetary rewards, neurasthenia helped the neurologists build up their clienteles. Since the organic nervous disorders were relatively rare, specialists welcomed patients with less tangible ills who crowded their waiting rooms. Some earned sizable fees for this work; Weir Mitchell reputedly made $70,000 in a good year, much of it in consulting fees.[20]

Professional needs help to explain the advantage of a new diagnosis. But to discern how and why neurasthenia was used, one must turn from the institutional to the clinical setting. The typical neurasthenic patient presented the physician with a rich variety of symptoms. A diagnosis by exclusion, neurasthenia could be established only after a thorough physical examination and appraisal of the patient's actual, as distinct from stated, discomfort had ruled out any other condition. (Beard once listed forty-eight ailments with which it might be confounded.)[21] Once satisfied that the patient had no organic disease, the physician must decide what label to attach to the condition.

Neurasthenia had most often to be distinguished from hysteria and hypochondria, the other major functional nervous disorders.

Hysteria, long the most frequent nervous disease of women, had become in Weir Mitchell's view "the nosological limbo of all un-named female maladies. It were as well called mysteria." The typical hysteric manifested bizarre symptoms—convulsive fits, trances, choking, tearing the hair, and rapid fluctuations of mood. Where languor characterized the neurasthenic, Beard considered "acuteness, violence, activity, and severity" the essence of hysteria. Moral considerations as well as the physician's empathy for particular patients undoubtedly influenced diagnostic decisions in ambiguous cases. Where neurasthenics seemed deeply concerned about their condition and eager to cooperate, hysterics were accused of evasiveness—*la belle indifférence*—and even intentional deception. Physicians sometimes contrasted the hysteric's lack of moral sense with the neurasthenic's refined and unselfish nature. "The sense of moral obligation [in the hysteric] is so generally defective as to render it difficult to determine whether the patient is mad or simply bad." By contrast, patients suffering from "impaired vitality" were "of good position in society . . . just the kind of women one likes to meet with—sensible, not over sensitive or emotional, exhibiting a proper amount of illness . . . and a willingness to perform their share of work quietly and to the best of their ability." [22]

Hypochondria had been the most common diagnosis for men with ill-defined complaints. Once a medically respectable disease, by the 1870s hypochondriasis had acquired the connotation of an imaginary illness. Neurasthenics and hypochondriacs both displayed inordinate interest in the vagaries of their bodies, but physicians considered the former more often the victims of circumstances, or lack of prudence, while the difficulties of the latter, if not dismissed entirely, appeared to be distinctly self-induced. [23]

Although nineteenth-century physicians and historians alike have written at length about women's ill health, the subject of illness in men has been neglected. [24] Yet neurasthenia seems to have been a particularly useful label for men. If women were sometimes expected, and perhaps even encouraged, to be weak and sickly, an ethos of fortitude made it difficult for men to exhibit weakness of any kind. Illness, in all its presumed objectivity, was one of the permissible exceptions. It is significant, therefore, that several physicians—mistakenly—considered neurasthenia a male disease, a striking assertion at a time when the profession rarely lost an opportunity to decry the ill-health of American women.[25] While acknowledging that neurasthenia afflicted women more often than men, Beard was especially eager to legitimize it as a diagnosis for men. He insisted that hypochondria, which he defined as "groundless fear of disease," was extremely rare; the label too often covered the diagnostician's failure to detect the real trouble.[26]

Neurasthenia then was the diagnosis of choice for men and women whose diffuse symptoms might otherwise have been dismissed as hypochondria or hysteria. As a new diagnosis, neurasthenia escaped the pejorative connotations associated with its nearest alternatives. Doctors had often suffered from neurasthenia themselves—Beard estimated that physicians constituted one-tenth of his clientele—and empathized with similarly distressed patients.[27] Certainly many of its putative causes—overwork or the too solicitous care of sick relatives—resulted from an excess of essentially admirable traits.

Neurasthenia was also preferable to a diagnosis of insanity, then considered an incurable disease. Despite their rivalry, American neurologists and superintendents agreed with Beard that neurasthenia was "the door that opens into so many phases of mental disease." It was a warning signal, which, if unheeded, might lead from a temporary physical breakdown to a permanent state of melancholia. Edward Cowles, the influential superintendent of McLean Asylum, went so far as to suggest in his Shattuck lecture of 1891 that "all people of previously sound health and constitution, who become insane with ordinary functional mental disorders, have their psychoses dependent upon neurasthenic conditions of the organism."[28]

Neurasthenics suffered from many of the symptoms of those hospitalized for insanity, including loss of mental control, depression, morbid fears, and obsessions. Presumably the persistence and severity of these symptoms helped to separate the insane from the neurasthenic, but diagnostic criteria were by no means clear. Class considerations, the tolerance of physicians for particular symptoms, and the ability of family members to care for patients undoubtedly influenced diagnostic decisions, then as now. Like Virginia Woolf, an upper-class patient suffering from hallucinations and severe feeding disorders might frequently be diagnosed as neurasthenic.[29] An individual with similar problems, but fewer financial resources and less loyal family and friends, might have been declared insane and placed in an asylum. Given the importance of the therapist's expectations on the patient's chances of recovery, the more optimistic diagnosis may have kept some individuals who would today be considered schizophrenic or borderline from long hospital stays and possible deterioration.[30]

Class prejudice undoubtedly influenced the attitudes of upper- and middle-class patients and their physicians toward the asylums, as the rhetorical query of one neurologist suggests: "Should the psychical symptoms of instability, distrust, and confusion of mind be used as an excuse for, and can such a condition be most effectively combated by, sending such a delicate, sensitive, nervous invalid to an insane asylum? We think not." But at a time when public hospitals suffered from overcrowding, understaffing, and low recovery rates, treatment at home or in one of the new nerve retreats was the rational choice for those who could afford it. Such individuals could also escape the stigmatizing label of insanity. For even after recovery, formerly hospitalized patients often continued to be reminded that they had been "crazy a number of years ago."[31]

Many late-nineteenth-century physicians accepted Beard's generalization that neurasthenia was principally a disease of the "comfortable classes." Like Beard, their patients were probably drawn largely from the business and professional classes in large cities. Those with diverse clienteles reached other conclusions. In 1869, the year Beard published his first article on the subject, a superintendent in Michigan independently discovered neurasthenia—and so labeled it—in the hardworking farm women near his hospital. To his surprise, Weir Mitchell diagnosed it in such unlikely victims as working-class male clinic patients. By the early years of the twentieth century, neurasthenia had become the most frequent diagnosis of the working-class patients who attended the neurological outpatient clinics at Boston City and Massachusetts General Hospitals. The deficient-energy syndrome could be applied to the most varied individuals, and was not just a euphemism for serious mental illness in middle-class patients.[32]

It would appear that age and marital status had more to do with the disease, or at least with the diagnosis, than either class or sex. Many neurasthenic patients were young and single. In one study of 333 neurasthenics, two-thirds were between the ages of 20 and 40, with the incidence highest among those 20 to 30 and the average age 33.3. Almost one-third of the women and over two-fifths of the men were single, a figure no doubt partly related to their age.[33] Observing the relationship between neurasthenia and young adulthood, Beard noted that the "dark valley of nervous depression" often disappeared between the ages of twenty-five and thirty-five. Once cured, the former sufferer went on to a "healthy and happy maturity."[34]

Beard spoke from personal experience. Between the ages of seventeen, when he completed his preparatory course at Phillips Andover Academy, and twenty-three, when he graduated from Yale, Beard suffered from ringing in the ears, pains in the side, acute dyspepsia, nervousness, morbid fears, and "lack of vitality." His journal reveals a young man beset by religious and vocational indecision. Reared in an austere and religious family that rejected drinking and smoking and warned its children of the snares of worldly success, Beard chastised himself for his coldness and "hanging back" in religious matters. Health and joy finally came with his decision to become a physician (which was equally a rejection of the ministry, the occupation of his father and two brothers). Beard entered medicine with a passionate commitment to medical and hygienic reform. By this time, too, he had begun to enjoy the worldly pleasures of champagne and Turkish tobacco, and soon after became engaged. His recovery seems to have been permanent. A minister who knew Beard in later life described him as a man who "put courage, hope, strength into one's heart, and his atmosphere was always healthy. He did not gush with over-warmth, or freeze with over-cold."[35]

In conjunction with other case materials, Beard's experience

suggests that for many middle-class men and women neurasthenia incorporated elements of today's fashionable identity crisis.
Clearly individuals reaching maturity in the second half of the
nineteenth century had no monopoly on the trials of establishing
a satisfactory adult identity. But cultural imperatives may have
made the task particularly problematic. Intellectuals who struggled to emancipate themselves from the introspective and gloomy
religious teachings of their childhood often suffered acutely from
the loss of faith that accompanied Darwinism, higher criticism of
the Bible, and the growing authority of science. In a society of
changing and often conflicting values, the decline of spiritual cer-
titude intensified feelings of isolation. Educated women struggled
to reconcile their desire for independence with still potent family
expectations that they would live out traditional female roles. For
men, longer professional training and the desire to achieve a
higher standard of living necessitated later marriages; prescriptions for "masculinity" often meant disavowing "feminine" emotional impulses. Both men and women encountered a sexual code
that demanded purity in thought as well as in deed, restraint
within marriage as well as abstinence outside it. But men were
sometimes also expected to be rough and ready.[36]

William James is a good example of a Victorian incapacitated by
psychosomatic ills, mental anguish, indecision, and an inability to
believe. As a young man he developed digestive and eye troubles,
weakness of the back, and a "feeling of loneliness and intellectual
and moral deadness." He feared being alone in the dark, had
morbid obsessions, and for a time felt continually on the verge of
committing suicide. His family considered his condition
hypochondriacal, but James claimed he was "a victim of neurasthenia, and of the sense of hollowness and unreality that goes with
it." Relief first came with his decision to believe in free will. Of the
same generation as Beard, James tried to reconcile science and
religion, resisted determinism in both, and struggled to find a
genuine vocation. He successively tried art, natural history,
medicine, and psychology and did not commit himself to
philosophy, his first love, until the age of fifty-seven. It has recently been suggested that James's intense relationship with his

domineering Swedenborgian father complicated this struggle, and that his illness gave him a psychic moratorium and a legitimate reason for disobeying parental wishes. His symptoms subsided following his first professional position (at thirty) and marriage (at thirty-six).[37]

If men sometimes found it difficult to choose the right profession, educated women faced a dilemma merely by wanting to have a vocation. Those who chose to defy convention as well as those who gave up their aspirations might find life equally intolerable. Jane Addams has described the years of backaches, depression, and purposelessness that followed her graduation from college. She even consulted Weir Mitchell, with little benefit. She diagnosed her problem as an inability to find a practical way to fulfill the ideals she had acquired in college and a disinclination to follow the course favored by her stepmother, including marriage and the dilettantish pursuit of culture. For Jane Addams and, she believed, for others like her, the decision to found a social settlement and create a new kind of community proved immensely liberating.[38] Charlotte Perkins Gilman experienced a more severe breakdown following her marriage and birth of a daughter. Her vague but exalted hopes of helping mankind seemed threatened by these events, so inescapable a part of most women's lives. In her case, Mitchell's advice compounded her difficulties and reduced her to playing with a rag doll on the floor. Her symptoms finally abated when she separated from her husband and began to pursue an independent course as a writer and lecturer.[39]

Because evidence about sexual behavior is harder to come by than information about vocational and religious conflict, it is difficult to assess its role in neurasthenia. Beard for one was acutely sensitive to the difficulties that contemporary sexual mores posed for his patients. It is possible that he had personally experienced such stress, for shortly after his engagement he asked God's blessing for his spiritual interests. He went on to declare: "The most solemn and weighty of any experience with the exception of religious experience is the love life of a man."[40]

In his posthumously published *Sexual Neurasthenia*, Beard insisted that sexual complaints had been vastly underestimated as a cause of nervousness, in men especially. He believed that sexual desire, like neurasthenia itself, plagued the sensitive men and women of the middle classes more than those of phlegmatic temperament who lived and worked outdoors. Masturbation he viewed as a nearly universal practice, for women as well as men, and did not think it invariably harmful if not begun too early in life or indulged in too often. As for other sexual difficulties, such as impotence and nocturnal emissions, Beard advised his patients not to worry about them: "Live generously. Work hard. . . . As soon as convenient, get married, but at all events keep diligently at work." Most important, he offered reassurance: *"I have known personally of very many young men who have passed through difficulties of the kind and are now well and the fathers of healthy families."* Perhaps it was advice of this sort that prompted the comment, by a minister-friend at the memorial service for Beard, that "many joy children were born of his kindly words and kindly deeds, while of sad ones there were none to moan."[41]

The self-study of a neurasthenic patient, herself a specialist in mental and nervous disorders, suggests some of the conflicts that must have been central to many neurasthenic individuals, particularly those who resigned themselves to lives of partial nervous invalidism. Written in 1910 with pre-Freudian innocence, *The Autobiography of a Neurasthene* by Margaret Cleaves is a classic study of unresolved dependency needs that were at least partly met by her long-term relationship with her physician.[42]

Dr. Cleaves describes herself as hardworking to a fault, so completely devoted to her patients that "they are my family and my friends. I have none other, and science is my mistress." Overwork led first to a "sprained" brain and later to a "complete crash," accompanied by the sensation of hot blood pouring into her ears, an inability to concentrate or to "bear a touch heavier than the brush of a butterfly's wing," depression, copious weeping, fears of going insane, and other typical neurasthenic symptoms. Learning to live within the margin of her slender nervous endowment proved difficult, but essential, for she suffered "utter lassitude of body," "weariness of mind," and a "sense of physiologic sin" from the slightest indiscretion, even an excess in diet. Social events proved particularly tiring, for she could not control them. Always she fought against her illness, which she took pains to distinguish from hysteria.

Between acute attacks she carried on her work. But even as she took pride in her ability to care for her patients, it is clear that she resented her responsibilities, particularly because there "was no one to look after [her] needs." She attributed her illness (which she considered constitutional) to feeding insufficiencies in infancy, aggravated by the death of her father when she was fourteen. Thus she notes that the too early arrival of a younger sister interfered with her babyhood by depriving her of milk. Upbraided throughout her life for her failure to eat, she attributed her later preference for milk products to this early deprivation. When she was acutely ill, milk was often her only source of nourishment. She thought of her father, a physician after whom she seems to have modeled herself, as her best friend and, following the death of the family's only son, tried to become her "father's boy." She must bitterly have resented his death, even as it devastated her, for she insisted that he would have protected her against the stresses and strains she encountered in later life. For years she had a recurrent dream of being a child cradled in her father's arms. The dream disappeared after her most severe breakdown, and she missed the comfort it had afforded her.

The patient was fortunate enough to find a sympathetic physician who cared for her for many years, often visiting her daily during her acute attacks. If he did not completely understand her condition—at least until he had himself suffered a neurasthenic breakdown—he was compassionate: "I told him all this tale of woe, of my past life . . . [and] laid bare my soul to my professional confessor." She depended on her physician greatly, and in times of special need on a trained nurse as well. When others responded to her needs, she reported: "It seemed worthwhile to have suffered for the sake of all this comfort." Her course of treatment— rest, limitation of activities, tonics, massage—was designed to replenish her meager supply of "neuronic energy." But given this patient's personality and her isolated life in New York City, the close relationship with her physician-confessor, by providing a substitute for other forms of intimacy, was obviously the crucial element.

The patient's struggles with her propensity toward invalidism were familiar enough to therapists, who insisted that each case required individualized treatment. Prescribing rest for one patient might be restorative, while for another with similar symptoms, it could be completely wrong. Clinicians thus recognized that the relationship between doctor and patient was often the most potent agency in effecting a cure. Given contemporary insistence that disease was an entirely objective phenomenon, they could not pursue such insights very far. Beard, for example, outraged fellow members of the American Neurological Association when he reported a series of experiments with "definite expectation"—what a later generation called suggestion—in which he cured patients of rheumatism and neuralgic sleeplessness by prescribing placebos. One colleague denied the existence of mental therapeutics entirely, a second considered it more dangerous than handling the most powerful drugs, while still another claimed that doctors had known about royal touch cures for centuries, but before practicing such deceits should "give up our medicines and enter a convent." [43]

The therapeutic guidelines of S. Weir Mitchell, member of Philadelphia's upper class and a popular novelist, proved less controversial. Mitchell first tried out the rest cure on Civil War soldiers suffering from acute exhaustion brought on by marching. He did not repeat it until 1874 when, despairing of any other treatment, he ordered an exhausted invalid to bed. He carried the principle of rest to what he later admitted was "an almost absurd extreme." The patient—a ninety-five-pound invalid who had tried every available cure—was fed and washed by others, forbidden to read, use her hands, or talk. At first a maid even turned her when she wished to move. Mitchell subsequently systematized the treatment to include total isolation of the patient from the family, a trained nurse, a carefully regulated diet (often limited initially to milk), tonics for the nerves, rest, and massage. The treatment's success could be explained in the somatic terms so appealing to this generation, and Mitchell emphasized the benefits of building up the patient's fat and blood by this method.[44]

But Mitchell also appreciated the moral aspects of the rest cure. The separation of patients from the moral poison of their accustomed environments, especially the attentions of too solicitous relatives, was often an essential condition for recovery. Isolation also enhanced the physician's influence over the patient, which Mitchell considered of supreme importance: "The man who can insure belief in his opinions and obedience to his decrees secures very often most brilliant and sometimes easy success." Confidence in the physician produced "that calmness of trustful belief which alone will secure the rest of mind we want." At first he found it surprising "that we ever get from any human being such childlike obedience. Yet we do get it, even from men."[45]

The similarity between the rest cure—with its bland diet, lack of external stimuli, and complete dependence on the physician—and infancy is apparent. Indeed, the enforced regression may well account for its success. The rest cure permitted individuals who ordinarily survived only by desperate effort to remove themselves from daily life and to submit for a time to the attentions of a charismatic physician like Mitchell. The physician in turn imposed reciprocal obligations. During convalescence, Mitchell lectured patients on the value of self-control and used his by then considerable influence to exact a "promise to fight every desire to cry, or twitch, or grow excited."[46] The paternalism of this therapy may help to explain why Charlotte Perkins Gilman and Jane Addams—women who temperamentally rejected the subordinate role assigned to their sex—were among Mitchell's most conspicuous failures.

Clearly there was often a therapeutic fit between physicians like Beard and Mitchell who had mastered their own nervous crises and their neurasthenic patients, many of whom—like the doctors themselves—were from the middle and upper classes. But class was not the sole determinant of a physician's response to patients. A. A. Brill, one of Freud's earliest American disciples, described the rapt attention with which as a medical student he attended the clinic on neurasthenia: "In contrast to the psychotics, the neuras-

thenics inspired one with a sympathetic interest; they spoke feel-
ingly about their symptoms and apparently wanted to be
helped."[47] What more could a young physician, eager to be of
service, ask of a patient?

The perception of pain, the significance attached to symptoms,
even the symptoms themselves vary greatly, depending not only
on individual personality needs but on class and ethnic patterns.
Today middle-class individuals are more willing to consult psychiatrists and to discuss emotional problems. And, despite the
somatic orientation of medicine in the late nineteenth century,
articulate individuals like William James often considered their
illness in the context of their search for a meaningful personal
identity.[48]

Although working-class men and women may lack a vocabulary
of psychological distress, they are by no means immune from the
effects of emotional stress; indeed, today they tend to be more
subject to psychophysiological illnesses than members of other
social groups. Recent clinical and sociological studies also indicate
that visits to physicians for minor symptoms are often prompted
by such needs as a desire for reassurance, for a close relationship
with someone, for sanction to escape onerous duties or
conflicts—needs which are often intensified during periods of
severe psychological stress.[49]

It is likely that in the late nineteenth century many of the conflicts of less articulate individuals manifested themselves in the
myriad of physical symptoms that constitute the central clinical
picture of neurasthenia. Not only were working-class patients
treated for neurasthenia in outpatient clinics, but they sometimes
entered Massachusetts General Hospital (then primarily an institution for charity patients) for extended periods. Nor were
physicians unsympathetic to such patients. Hospital case records
were not devoid of moral judgments, but the individuals described as "stupid," "lacking gumption," or "intent on deception"
were more often diagnosed as hysterical than as neurasthenic.
Doctors carefully recorded the complaints of individuals who
were run down or "unable to keep about" after overworking or an
imperfect recovery from an illness. Patients might complain of
sinking feelings about the heart, an inability to bear the weight of

their own hands, seeing stars, sensations of smothering, and "bearing down" pains. Their physical symptoms included palpitations and shortness of breath and a rich variety of gastric complaints (anorexia, vomiting, belching, constipation). The interpretation of these symptoms was entirely somatic. An occasional entry reported a recent death in the family, but attributed the breakdown to excessive exposure to cold or rain at the funeral rather than to the psychological effects of the loss.[50]

What is most surprising is that cigarmakers, millworkers, seamstresses, and housewives received modified versions of the rest cure for weeks and even months. Like the middle-class patients seen in private practice, they received a variety of physical therapies—including tonics, bromides, cannabis, massage, and blisters over tender spots. Special diets ranged from milk, cream toast, and eggnogs to oysters, whiskey, sherry, and beer. The entry for a particularly frail woman read, "Keep her quiet and stuff with food." The treatment seemed to work, for within three weeks the patient left the hospital "much relieved," with the notation that "rest was apparently all that she needed." Many patients seemed to enjoy their hospital stays—one entry recorded a patient "seemed disposed to remain indefinitely"—and a few kept their physicians informed of their latest symptoms after discharge. Since so many of these patients were single, it is likely that their illness and hospital sojourns provided some with psychological as well as physical care that they could obtain in no other way.[51]

During its brief reign as the national disease, neurasthenia gave physicians a rationale for diagnosing and treating many types of stress. Whatever the limitations of their construct, physicians like Beard and Mitchell pioneered in developing respectable therapies for patients with problems otherwise excluded by medicine and psychiatry. Although asylum superintendents maintained that neurasthenia might lead to insanity if not treated early enough, their isolation from general medicine and their restricted conception of their role gave them no way of reaching men and women before serious trouble occurred. The rest cure and related therapies provided individuals with alternatives to inaction or incarceration.

During the first two decades of the twentieth century the scope of psychiatry expanded almost beyond recognition. Physicians openly practiced psychotherapy in offices and in outpatient clinics in general and psychiatric hospitals. Some participated in prophylactic programs in schools, prisons, and industry. Most practitioners still worked in mental hospitals, but professional spokesmen insisted that psychiatry must concern itself not only with the psychoses but with "the smallest diseases and the minutest defects of the mind" and even with the efficiency of normal individuals. The new practitioner was "educator, preacher, sociologist" as well as asylum superintendent and dispenser of drugs.[52]

Specialists in the functional nervous disorders had pioneered in the expansion of the physician's social role. Even by diagnosing neurasthenia, they were interpreting behavioral symptoms that some found morally reprehensible (an inability to work for no apparent cause, compulsive or phobic behavior, bizarre thoughts) as signs of illness rather than wilfulness. They thus legitimized the right of individuals with such difficulties to be considered, and to consider themselves, victims of disease, and their own right as healers, to treat them.

Beard went further than most in asserting the physician's obligation to become a power in society. He not only insisted that neurasthenia be taken seriously, but urged that the categories kleptomania, inebriety, and pyromania—all safely medical— replace the traditional moralistic designations of stealing, drunkenness, and arson. A rebel against the evangelical faith of his childhood, Beard relished the substitution of physician for priest as arbiter of social and personal mores. Mitchell, noting the similarity between the physician's role and that of the priest, also thought members of his profession more fitted to probe human character: "The priest hears the crime or folly of the hour, but to the physician are oftener told the long, sad tales of a whole life."[53]

So much attention to a disease that could easily have been dismissed as minor also reveals a changed attitude toward health and disease. Long before the popularization of psychoanalysis, physicians interested in mental and nervous disorders proclaimed the relativity of health and illness. One superintendent declared that "perfect health of mind is probably . . . exceptional." And an influential lay philanthropist went so far as to claim: "The question to be considered is, not whether such and such a person is insane—that is, indisposed mentally: of course he is, more or less, like the rest of us—but, *How much* out of health is he?" Many no doubt reached such conclusions on the basis of personal experience. A fictional physician drawn by Weir Mitchell—a self-portrait—noted that even "to the most healthy nature, at times [come] inexplicable desires, moments of unreason, impulses which defy analytic research, even brief insanities." To the extent that individuals considered such conditions mental aberrations rather than sinful thoughts, they would consult physicians rather than ministers.[54]

The relationships between symptoms and diagnosis, disease and culture, doctors and patients are inevitably complex. Any attempt to understand them historically must take account of the clinical context in which doctors and patients interact; certainly this must be the case for a disease as subjective as neurasthenia. The available clinical materials suggest that neurasthenia was a complex reality for the doctors and patients charged with interpreting puzzling mental and physical difficulties they did not fully understand. If the particular insights of late-nineteenth-century physicians into the psychological and psychophysiological aspects of illness disappoint us, it is not altogether certain that we have, even today, found satisfactory solutions to conditions of this sort.

NOTES

Work on this article was greatly assisted by fellowships from the Radcliffe Institute and the Peter B. Livingston Fund. I am indebted to Phyllis Ackman, Martin Duberman, Nathan G. Hale, Jr., Dolores Kreisman, Charles E. Rosenberg, Barbara G. Rosenkrantz, Bennett Simon, and Martha Vicinus for their comments on earlier drafts and to Catherine Lord for research assistance. I also want to thank Dr. G. Octo Barnett and James Vaccarino for permission to use the medical records of the Massachusetts General Hospital, 1875-1900.

1. The best analysis of Beard's career is Charles E. Rosenberg, "The Place of George M. Beard in Nineteenth-Century Psychiatry," *Bulletin of the History of*

Medicine, 36 (May–June 1962):245–59. See also Henry Alden Bunker, Jr., "From Beard to Freud: A Brief History of the Concept of Neurasthenia," *Medical Review of Reviews,* 36 (March 1930):108–14.

2. George M. Beard, *A Practical Treatise on Nervous Exhaustion (Neurasthenia): Its Symptoms, Nature, Sequences, Treatment,* 2nd ed., rev. (New York, 1880), pp. 11–85. See also George M. Beard, *American Nervousness: Its Causes and Consequences* (New York, 1881), pp. 7–8.

3. "The Question of the Existence of Neurasthenia," *Medical Record,* 29 (February 13, 1886):185–86.

4. *Nervous Exhaustion,* pp. 85, 80.

5. George M. Beard, *Sexual Neurasthenia (Nervous Exhaustion): Its Hygiene, Causes, Symptoms, and Treatment, with a Chapter on Diet for the Nervous,* ed. A. D. Rockwell (New York, 1884), p. 36. Cf. Beard, *Sexual Neurasthenia,* pp. 61–62, and *American Nervousness,* p. 9.

6. Beard, *American Nervousness,* pp. 96–192.

7. Beard, *Nervous Exhaustion,* p. xix; Edward Cowles, "Neurasthenia and Its Mental Symptoms," *Boston Medical and Surgical Journal,* 125 (July–August 1891):49–52, 73–76, 97–100, 125–28, 153–57, 181–86, 209–14; Robert T. Edes, "The New England Invalid," *Boston Medical and Surgical Journal,* 133 (July 1895):53–57, 77–81, 101–07; Beard, *Nervous Exhaustion,* 4th ed., rev. and enl. by A. D. Rockwell (New York, 1901), p. 3. Numerous references to neurasthenia may be found in the several series of the *Index-Catalogue of the Library of the Surgeon General's Office.*

8. Quoted in A. A. Brill, "Diagnostic Errors in Neurasthenia," *Medical Review of Reviews,* 36 (March 1930):123.

9. I. S. Wechsler, "Is Neurasthenia an Organic Disease?" *Medical Review of Reviews,* 36 (March 1930):115–21; idem, "The Psychoneuroses and the Internal Secretions," *Neurological Bulletin,* 2 (May 1919):199–208; Edes, "The New England Invalid," pp. 78–80.

10. On the shift in diagnostic styles, see Henri F. Ellenberger, *The Discovery of the Unconscious: The History and Evolution of Dynamic Psychiatry* (New York: Basic Books, 1970); and Nathan G. Hale, Jr., *Freud and the Americans: The Beginnings of Psychoanalysis in the United States, 1876–1917* (New York: Oxford University Press, 1971), esp. pp. 71–173.

11. See, for example, Charles L. Dana, "The Partial Passing of Neurasthenia," *Boston Medical and Surgical Journal,* 150 (March 31, 1904):339–44; and G. Alder Blumer, "The Coming of Psychasthenia," *Journal of Nervous and Mental Diseases,* 33 (May 1906):336–53. Widely used in World War I, the term *neurasthenia* largely disappeared in the United States by the 1930s and reappeared in the 1968 diagnostic manual of the American Psychiatric Association. See John C. Chatel and Roger Peele, "A Centennial Review of Neurasthenia," *American Journal of Psychiatry,* 126 (April 1970):1404–13.

12. *Beginning Again: An Autobiography of the Years 1911 to 1918* (New York: Harcourt Brace & World 1964), pp. 75–76.

13. Rosenberg, "The Place of George M. Beard." Cf. Chatel and Peele, "A Centennial Review of Neurasthenia"; Bunker, "From Beard to Freud"; and S. P. Fullinwider, "Neurasthenia: The Genteel Caste's Journey Inward," *The Rocky Mountain Social Science Journal*, 2 (April 1974):1–9.

14. John S. Haller, Jr., and Robin M. Haller, *The Physician and Sexuality in Victorian America* (Urbana and Chicago: University of Illinois Press, 1974), pp. 5–43.

15. Michael Balint, *The Doctor, His Patient and the Illness*, 2nd ed., rev. (London: Pittman Medical Publishing Co., 1964), p. 41. This work is an excellent introduction to the psychological aspects of general medicine.

16. Richard Harrison Shryock, "The Interplay of Social and Internal Factors in Modern Medicine: An Historical Analysis," in his *Medicine in America: Historical Essays* (Baltimore: Johns Hopkins University Press, 1966), pp. 307–32; idem, *The Development of Modern Medicine: An Interpretation of the Social and Scientific Factors Involved* (New York: Hafner, 1947), pp. 248–303.

17. Cf. Erwin H. Ackerknecht, *Rudolf Virchow: Doctor, Statesman, Anthropologist* (Madison: University of Wisconsin Press, 1953). For a critical view of the laboratory approach to medicine, see Knud Faber, *Nosography: The Evolution of Clinical Medicine in Modern Times*, 2nd ed., rev. (New York: Hoeber, 1930), esp. pp. 68–71, 76, 87.

18. On the ambiguities of medical practice in the late nineteenth century, see Charles Rosenberg, "The Practice of Medicine in New York a Century Ago," *Bulletin of the History of Medicine*, 41 (May–June 1967):223–53.

19. There is no adequate history of neurology in English. But see Erwin Ackerknecht, *A Short History of Psychiatry*. Trans. from the German by Sulammith Wolff (London and New York: Hafner, 1959).

20. On early American neurology, see Charles L. Dana, "Early Neurology in the United States," *Journal of the American Medical Association*, 90 (May 5, 1928), pp. 1421–24; Louis Casamajor, "Notes for an Intimate History of Neurology and Psychiatry in America," *Journal of Nervous and Mental Diseases*, 98 (December 1943):600–08; and Barbara Sicherman, "The Quest for Mental Health in America, 1880–1917" (Dissertation, Columbia University, 1967), pp. 35–45, 231–39.

21. *Sexual Neurasthenia*, pp. 32–33, and *Nervous Exhaustion*, pp. 86–117. For contemporary views on this type of illness, see Gerald Chrzanowski, "Neurasthenia and Hypochondriasis," in *Comprehensive Textbook of Psychiatry*, ed. Alfred M. Freedman and Harold I. Kaplan (Baltimore: Williams & Wilkins, 1967), pp. 1163–68; and David Mechanic, "Social Psychological Factors Affecting the Presentation of Bodily Complaints," *New England Journal of Medicine*, 286 (May 25, 1972):1132–39.

22. S. Weir Mitchell, *Rest in Nervous Disease: Its Use and Abuse*, in *A Series of American Clinical Lectures*, ed. E. C. Seguin (New York, 1875), I, 94; Beard, *Nervous Exhaustion*, p. 103; A. S. Myrtle, "On a Common Form of Impaired Vitality," *The Medical Press and Circular*, 17 (May 6, 1874):375–76. Cf. Carroll

Smith-Rosenberg, "The Hysterical Woman: Sex Roles and Role Conflict in 19th-Century America," *Social Research,* 39 (Winter 1972):652–78; and Ilza Veith, *Hysteria: The History of a Disease* (Chicago: University of Chicago Press, 1965).

23. Esther Fischer-Homberger, "Hypochondriasis of the Eighteenth Century—Neurosis of the Present Century," *Bulletin of the History of Medicine,* 46 (July–August 1972):391–401.

24. Cf. Ann Douglas Wood, "'The Fashionable Diseases': Women's Complaints and Their Treatment in Nineteenth-Century America," *Journal of Interdisciplinary History,* 4 (Summer 1973):25–52; Carroll Smith-Rosenberg and Charles Rosenberg, "The Female Animal: Medical and Biological Views of Woman and Her Role in Nineteenth-Century America," *Journal of American History,* 60 (September 1973):332–56; and Regina Morantz, "The Lady and Her Physician," in *Clio's Consciousness Raised: New Perspectives on the History of Women,* ed. Mary S. Hartman and Lois Banner (New York: Harper & Row, 1974), pp. 38–53.

25. See Joseph Collins and Carlin Phillips, "The Etiology and Treatment of Neurasthenia. An Analysis of Three Hundred and Thirty-Three Cases," *Medical Record,* 55 (March 25, 1899):413–22; and Paul Schilder, "Neurasthenia and Hypochondria: Introduction to the Study of the Neurasthenic-Hypochondriac Character," *Medical Review of Reviews,* 36 (March 1930):165.

26. *Nervous Exhaustion,* pp. 96–98.

27. Ibid., p. 80. Mitchell too suffered from neurasthenia. See Margaret C.-L. Gildea and Edwin F. Gildea, "Personalities of American Psychotherapists," *American Journal of Psychiatry,* 101 (January 1945):464–66; and Anna Robeson Burr, *Weir Mitchell: His Life and Letters* (New York: Duffield & Co., 1929).

28. "The Problems of Insanity," *The Physician and Bulletin of the Medico-Legal Society,* 13 (March 1880):244; Cowles, "Neurasthenia and Its Mental Symptoms," p. 50.

29. *The Letters of Virginia Woolf,* Vol. I: 1888–1912, eds. Nigel Nicolson and Joanne Trautmann (New York and London: Harcourt Brace Jovanovich, 1975), pp. 141–42.

30. The classic work on the relationship between social class and the diagnosis and treatment of psychiatric illness is August B. Hollingshead and Frederick C. Redlich, *Social Class and Mental Illness: A Community Study* (New York: John Wiley & Sons, 1958). Gerald N. Grob discusses the ways class, race, and ethnicity influenced treatment in mental hospitals. See *Mental Institutions in America: Social Policy to 1875* (New York: Free Press, 1973), esp. pp. 221-56.

31. Edward C. Mann, "A Plea for Lunacy Reform," *The Medico-Legal Journal,* 1 (1884):159; discussion of William A. Hammond, "The Non-Asylum Treatment of the Insane," *Transactions of the Medical Society of New York* (1879), p. 297.

32. E. H. van Deusen, "Observations on a Form of Nervous Prostration (Neurasthenia), Culminating in Insanity," *American Journal of Insanity,* 25 (April 1869):445–61; S. Weir Mitchell, "Clinical Lecture on Nervousness in the Male,"

The Medical News and Library, 35 (December 1877):177–84. See also Cecil Mac-Coy, "Some Observations on the Treatment of Neurasthenia at the Dispensary Clinic," *Brooklyn Medical Journal,* 17 (September 1903):399–401; and annual reports of Boston City and Massachusetts General Hospitals.

33. Collins and Phillips, "The Etiology and Treatment of Neurasthenia," pp. 413–22. My own research in Massachusetts General Hospital records reveals a similarly high proportion of neurasthenic patients between the ages of twenty and forty and an even higher proportion of single patients.

34. *American Nervousness,* pp. 282–84.

35. Beard's case is discussed in Barbara Sicherman, "The Paradox of Prudence: Mental Health in the Gilded Age," *Journal of American History,* 62 (March 1976):890–912. The quotation from the minister appears in J. L. Willard, *Sermon by the Rev. J. L. Willard, of Westville, Connecticut at the Funeral Services of Elizabeth A. Beard. Together with Comments upon the Life and Career of the Late Dr. George M. Beard* (Grand Hotel, New York, [1883]), p. 4, in George M. Beard Papers, Yale University Library, New Haven, Conn.

36. In addition to works discussed in nn. 22 and 24, see Hale, *Freud and the Americans,* pp. 24–46; and Charles E. Rosenberg, "Sexuality, Class and Role in 19th-Century America," *American Quarterly,* 25 (May 1973):131–53.

37. Cushing Strout, "William James and the Twice-Born Sick Soul," in *Philosophers and Kings: Studies in Leadership,* ed. Dankwart A. Rustow (New York: Braziller, 1970), pp. 491–511; Erik H. Erikson, *Identity: Youth and Crisis* (New York: W. W. Norton, 1968), pp. 19–22, 150–55. Compare the similar case of G. Stanley Hall, the psychologist who later formulated the modern concept of adolescence, in Dorothy Ross, *G. Stanley Hall: The Psychologist as Prophet* (Chicago: University of Chicago Press, 1972), pp. 309–40.

38. Jane Addams, *Twenty Years at Hull-House. With Autobiographical Notes* (New York, 1911), pp. 64–88, 113–27. Cf. Allen F. Davis, *American Heroine: The Life and Legend of Jane Addams* (New York: Oxford University Press, 1973), pp. 24–37.

39. Charlotte Perkins Gilman, *The Living of Charlotte Perkins Gilman: An Autobiography* (New York: Harper & Row, 1975; originally published in 1935), pp. 78–106. See also her short story about the same events, "The Yellow Wall-Paper," reprinted in *The Oven Birds: American Women on Womanhood 1820–1920,* ed. Gail Thain Parker (Garden City, N.Y.: Doubleday, 1972), pp. 317–34.

40. George M. Beard, "Private Journal," p. 217, in George M. Beard Papers, Yale University Library.

41. pp. 102–03, 122, 119–20; Willard, *Elizabeth A. Beard and Dr. George M. Beard,* p. 4.

42. *An Autobiography of a Neurasthene. As Told by One of Them and Recorded by Margaret A. Cleaves* (Boston, 1910). Although presented as an as-told-to autobiography, this work is probably the story of Margaret Cleaves herself. Insofar as they are known, the facts of Margaret Cleaves's family background, early life, and professional career closely resemble those of the subject of the autobiography.

43. "American Neurological Association," *Journal of Nervous and Mental Diseases*, 3 (July 1876):429–37.

44. S. Weir Mitchell, "The Evolution of the Rest Treatment," *Journal of Nervous and Mental Diseases*, 31 (June 1904):368–72; *Rest in Nervous Disease*, esp. pp. 94–96; *Fat and Blood: An Essay on the Treatment of Certain Forms of Neurasthenia and Hysteria*, 5th ed. (Philadelphia, 1888); and *Lectures on Diseases of the Nervous System: Especially in Women*, 2nd ed., rev. (Philadelphia, 1885), esp. pp. 265–83.

45. *Fat and Blood*, pp. 40–42, 47–49, 55–62; *Rest in Nervous Disease*, p. 84.

46. *Rest in Nervous Disease*, p. 94; *Diseases of the Nervous System*, p. 38. For a discussion of regression as a psychoanalytic technique, see Karl Menninger, *Theory of Psychoanalytic Technique*, (New York: Basic Books, 1958), esp. pp. 43–76.

47. "Diagnostic Errors in Neurasthenia," p. 122.

48. Cf. Dewitt L. Crandell and Bruce P. Dohrenwend, "Some Relations Among Psychiatric Symptoms, Organic Illness, and Social Class," *American Journal of Psychiatry*, 123 (June 1967);1527–38; and Mechanic, "Social Psychological Factors Affecting the Presentation of Bodily Complaints," pp. 1132–39. See also William James's letters to James Jackson Putnam in the James Jackson Putnam Papers at The Francis A. Countway Library of Medicine, Boston.

49. Cf. John D. Stoeckle, Irving K. Zola, and Gerald E. Davidson, "The Quantity and Significance of Psychological Distress in Medical Patients: Some Preliminary Observations About the Decision to Seek Medical Aid," *Journal of Chronic Diseases*, 17 (October 1964):959–70.

50. The material in the next two paragraphs is drawn from Massachusetts General Hospital, Medical Records (East and West Wings), 1880–1900. See, for example, vol. 381 (1885), p. 82, and vol. 455 (1893), p. 124. For judgmental comments, see vol. 349 (1880), p. 198, and vol. 381 (1885), p. 250. Charles Rosenberg informs me that he found similar material on working-class patients at Pennsylvania General Hospital.

51. Ibid., vol. 487 (1897), p. 42. One of these letters appears in vol. 451 (1893), p. 56. The comment about wanting to stay refers to the same patient during a second hospitalization. Cf. vol. 457 (1894), p. 306.

52. E. E. Southard, "Cross Sections of Mental Hygiene, 1844, 1869, 1894," *American Journal of Insanity*, 76 (October 1919):109; Charles L. Dana, "The Future of Neurology," *Journal of Nervous and Mental Diseases*, 40 (December 1913):753–57.

53. George M. Beard, *Our Home Physician: A New and Popular Guide to the Arts of Preserving Health and Treating Disease* (New York, 1870), pp. xxi, 672; Mitchell, *Doctor and Patient*, 3rd ed. (Philadelphia, 1889), p. 10; cf. p. 6.

54. Peter Bryce, "The Mind and How to Preserve It," *Transactions of the Medical Association of the State of Alabama* (1880), p. 260; Philip Garrett, "President's Address," *National Conference of Charities and Correction Proceedings*, 12 (1885):20; *Dr. North and His Friends* (New York, 1900), p. 389.

CHAPTER 10

The Diagnostic Process:
Touchstone of Medicine's Values

Paul W. Pruyser

Extending the discussion of diagnosis from the uses of a particular nosological category to fundamental implications of the diagnostic process itself, Paul Pruyser finds important clues to the value system in medicine. This chapter also moves us from the nineteenth into the twentieth century, and formulates some surprising but serious new alternatives in diagnosis—namely, that patients might be considered the leaders of their own diagnostic teams.

Interestingly enough, the very word diagnosis contains the root gnosis, a term for knowledge but, in the usage of the ancient Gnostics, implying secret knowledge controlled by the initiated priests and preserved as instrumental to their power from the gods. Especially in medical practice, to relinquish such power, to "give away" knowledge, to act as consultant rather than as primary decision maker, could appear flagrantly irresponsible to some physicians. But Pruyser indicates how this might very appropriately occur, given some possible limiting conditions.

Drawing explicitly on the psychoanalytic model of partnership and on a deep respect for the fostering of autonomy and respect for persons, he gives an innovative picture of how professional competence could be maintained without the earlier abusive implications that patients are incompetent, passive, and dependent.

Worsened by healing
—Vergil,
The Aeneid 12:46

The following episode recently came to my attention: A sixty-year-old married woman made a routine annual examination visit to her gynecologist's office, a group practice in which she had been a registered patient for many years. This time she was to be seen by a new partner, a man in his upper thirties. After having

waited in the reception room for a considerable time, the patient
was ushered by the nurse into an examination room and, after
disrobing, positioned on the examination table. She had been
lying there alone, in an awkward posture, for ten minutes, when
the physician came in with the nurse. Leafing through the patient's chart, he said, "Well, ____ (grossly mispronouncing her first
name) . . . let me see. . . . We had a little bleeding last time." The
patient flared up with: "What? *We*? *I* had some bleeding. *You*
didn't."

Common as this type of encounter appears to be, one can
hardly imagine a more ludicrous or gruesome start for a doctor-
patient relationship. The patient is first rendered supine, physically immobilized, and then insulted. The doctor takes it upon
himself to address her by her first name, and that incorrectly; he
does not really greet her, but falteringly reads her name from the
chart; he disregards her matronly age; naively, he lets slip a "let
me see," that dangerous giveaway of a profession always accused
of voyeurism. And in his phraseology he identifies himself with
the patient to the point of assuming her gender and sharing her
symptom. What seems to be uppermost in his mind is not the
person before him, but "the complaint"—a rubric that professionally, and in all likelihood habitually, prestructures his approach to and conversation with all his patients. Casting about for
something under that rubric, he settles on last year's item, as
charted. The implication is that he, the doctor, always wants a sign
or symptom to legitimate a patient's presence in his office, even
for periodic preventive check-ups! Everything else is subordinate
to that rubric, in which his expertise is vested; and conceptual
subordination spreads to become social subordination when, by
using her first name, he puts the patient in the role of a little girl
or an underling.

I want to use this brief initial phase of a visit to the gynecologist
as a point of departure for some reflections about diagnosis. I
take diagnosing as the heart of medicine, the single most important task of physicians and the most frequent functional activity in
medical practice. Although it is true that some physicians, for
example, surgeons, spend a great deal of time in specialized

therapeutic interventions, many general practitioners, pediatricians, family physicians, and psychiatrists find the bulk of their work to consist of diagnostic explorations. They tease out and formulate problems, preliminary to writing prescriptions that initiate some therapeutic intervention. Much of the therapy is done by other parties, including impersonal, unseen drug action.

For my reflections I shall use a determinate vantage point: the precepts and body of knowledge that have accumulated in psychoanalysis, been more or less appropriated by dynamic psychiatry, and begun to hold clues for medicine in general. My contention is that psychoanalysis has most forthrightly raised some crucial questions about the diagnostic process and, in trying to answer these, provoked a cardinal shift in the whole *ethos* of diagnosing. To put this shift in a nutshell, anticipating the reflections that will form the bulk of this essay, psychoanalysis has changed diagnosing from a unilateral, often authoritarian, procedure in which a physician interrogates, inspects, palpates, and variously tests patients, and then pronounces "his" diagnosis (which is seen as the physician's professional and intellectual property), into a bilateral process in which patients, soliciting help from an expert, come to diagnose themselves. The diagnostic ethos has moved by some Copernican revolution from an *allogenic* to an *autogenic* center; *iatric* dominance has given way to the *patient's* initiative, and medical investigation has been restyled to maximize the patient's power for self-assessment.

Having summed up my contention thus decisively, I should enter the caveat that I am exposing a principle rather than describing a prevalent practice. Despite its anchorage in the humane tradition in medicine, the psychoanalytic principle goes so much against the grain of established views, habits, and prerogatives in the healing arts that there is a wide gap between the principle and the observable facts of practicing. Many psychiatrists fail to acknowledge the principle, find it noble but unworkable, or have great difficulty living up to it; and among psychoanalysts, backsliders are proportionately as numerous as in other high-minded movements. Nevertheless, the principle retains its revolutionary power and teaching value, and although its psychoanalytic origin is rarely acknowledged, it seems to be emulated implicitly today by quite diverse groups of health workers and consumers of medical science who find much to criticize in the prevailing ethos, style, and forms of health services. Many medical schools and hospitals are groping toward a change, not merely in curriculum and techniques, but in the very philosophy that should guide their enterprises; and if faculty or hospital staff members prove unwilling or slow to change, the students and "lower-echelon" health workers will exert relentless pressure, or face them with de facto alternatives of practice. Similarly millions of patients or prospective patients are demanding a change in medical attitudes, all groups arguing in one way or another for a much needed *humanizing* of medical practice, in which the patients' (and the doctors') dignity and modes of decision-making will be vouchsafed. Reflections on the spirit of health care are in the air, raising issues beyond those of medical ethics and forensics. That is why I am speaking of changes in the *ethos* of medicine, illuminated by thoughts on the diagnostic process.

Who Is to Know What in the Diagnostic Process?

Although medical diagnosing is typically seen as a two-party transaction, a great many disturbances in well-being are diagnosed by one party. After repeated instances of a burning sensation in the stomach, one says to oneself "heartburn" and buys antacids. A critical (but culturally and personally highly variable) point must be reached for simple self-assessment to give way to a desire for a two-party diagnostic transaction. In that transition, the ailing person assumes a new, provisional role—patienthood—for the time being, until he or she can be released from that role by cure, talked out of it by being denied the privilege, or hardened into it by chronicity, incurability, or further mishaps. Assuming patienthood is an ambiguous thing, conferring rights, duties, and exemptions from duties, and usually verified, certified, or legitimated by a second party, the physician, who is granted some influence over a third party, the relevant public, on the patient's behalf. In the patient's role, once assumed and certified, one must manifest two contrary series of convictions: on the one hand, there must be signals of impediment, pain, dysfunction, and so forth; on the other hand, there must be a desire for health, signs of betterment if possible, and at least some willingness to entertain contracting for certain interventions or ministrations that are not standard procedures in normal life.

In a medical two-party transaction, who makes the diagnosis and how is it formulated? The first answer is, of course, the doctor, in the vocabulary of the medical profession. Doctors are trained to know what to look for, what to ask, what tests to run, and to put the result of their searches and cogitations in a verbal formula commensurate with the nosology to which their profession subscribes. Apparently, the diagnostic formulation, although ostensibly made for the patient's benefit, is owed primarily to the physician and his or her colleagues, for there are arguments whether or not the diagnosis is to be shared with the patient, particularly when it has ominous prospects. As the phrase has it: "Should the doctor *tell* the patient he has cancer?" This phrase itself implies that at least some diagnoses are shrouded in professional secrecy. The formulation and its occasional secrecy also imply that the patient is not a full partner in the diagnostic process, but is in some sense only its subject, and that he or she is kept at bay while the doctor does the probing and thinking. To put it starkly: The diagnostician is the knower, the patient is an ignoramus; the diagnosis is written in the chart to which the patient has no access; and the diagnostician may or may not propound the ailment's name or description to the patient after the latter has offered himself or herself for inspection and study. It requires benevolent wisdom or art rather than science to decide whether sharing the diagnosis with the patient will have a soothing or scaring effect, and which of these is therapeutically desirable in a given case. In this sense, the diagnosis does not stand alone, but is caught up in curative efforts, in which indeed the whole diagnostic process may be embedded from the start. I will say more about the relation between therapy and diagnosis shortly.

I have described a prevalent model of medical transaction so as to tease out its underlying principle: that diagnosing is the doctor's duty and prerogative. I am not insinuating that these are acquired by medical usurpation; it may well be that both the duty and the prerogative have been granted to doctors by patients through centuries of evolving mores and legislation. My sole point is that, in this conception of diagnosis, the parties are unequal— the doctor's position elitist, the patient's role passive and submissive—and the diagnostic outcome is likely to be skewed by the selective attentions and inattentions of the diagnostician, particularly when she or he is a specialist in a particular branch of medicine.

A second answer to "Who makes the diagnosis?" is given by psychoanalysis. At its inception, psychoanalysis was practiced in a medical subculture suffused with diagnostic terms and labels that had arisen from nosological ignorance: hysteria, neurasthenia, psychasthenia, neurosis, and so on. At the end of the nineteenth century, these medical terms were only hapless words, pretentious ones to be sure, that stood for mysterious, poorly understood disorders that could be delimited only as vague clinical pictures, overlapping both with each other and with a few better-known disorders such as epilepsy and toxic states. Recognizing their scientific ignorance about these clinical pictures, Breuer and Freud took the poor diagnostic labels only as a starting point for a new kind of diagnostic process in which patients, speculatively held to be suffering from "reminiscences," were offered the opportunity for an astute self-assessment with the help of a mentor. Moreover, the crucial shift that Freud managed to introduce in the doctor-patient relation was for the doctor to abandon the authoritarian technique of hypnosis to become a good and sympathetic listener, and for the patient to abandon passivity and become the diagnostician (and by implication the nosologist) of his or her own case. By freely subscribing to a rule of ruthless honesty, the patient comes to discover the psychological rationale and psychohistorical origin of his or her symptoms or complaints and thereby to see alternative modes of problem-solving. And the diagnosis at which the patient arrives, after much soul-searching and interaction with the analyst, is not a nosological noun, such as "hysteria," but a personal or existential action phrase, such as: "When I seemed so cool on that occasion, I was really terrified by my mother's stern demand."

At this point, the reader may object that I am comparing apples and oranges. After all, physical symptoms and psychic complaints require very different approaches, stylized in the differences between "medical" and "psychiatric" diagnoses. The fact is, however, that in a doctor's office the distinction between physical and psychic is quite academic and can at best be made only at the end, not the beginning, of a diagnostic process. Thousands of general practitioners assert that between one-half and two-thirds of their patients come with unclassifiable complaints; many patients talk with psychiatrists about body dysfunctions; and pediatricians are frequently presented with phenomena that can at first be described only as undesirable conduct or behavior disorders. Sedatives, tranquilizers, and mood-altering drugs are widely prescribed in response to mere complaints that have not been properly diagnosed; this is paradoxical, for it means that precisely when doctors think "It's emotional," they decide to intervene physically by chemical action. If the practice of medicine yields any practical precepts, it is that in clinical situations the physical and the psychic are rarely distinguishable.

The psychoanalytic advice to the doctor is: "Don't rush to alter, except when life is acutely endangered. Don't take symptoms immediately away, for the patient probably needs them for the time being. The vaguer the complaint, the more likely are its adaptive value, its psychoeconomic utility, and its psychodynamic necessity." The psychoanalytic advice to the patient is: "I am not sure that you really want to be relieved right away, although you seem to say so. Try to understand why you have this symptom. Maybe you yourself can best figure out what brought it on and what makes it persist. It would be flippant to name your ailment, as if we knew what we were dealing with. Actually, you have to take the lead in making the diagnosis, and chances are that such a self-study will itself give you some relief."

These propositions round off to a very different diagnostic process, involving an ethos that advocates a diagnostic *partnership*. The doctor-patient relation in this partnership is egalitarian, not elitist or authoritarian. The patient can see in the doctor an expert who can provide counsel in the medical aspects of intended (and granted) self-explorations. Analogous to the designation of attorneys as "counselors at law," physicians may be seen as "counselors in medicine," assisting their patients in getting hold of their troubles and putting them in medical perspective. Humanistic values are thus being brought to bear upon diagnosis—that is, precisely at the point where the patient can reasonably make the greatest claim on assistance from the medical profession. For although the profession may not be able to offer a cure, or alleviation of suffering, it can always assist in teasing out what the trouble is.

From the Diagnostic Partnership to Diagnostic Teamwork

Today, in hospitals, clinics, and certain types of group practice, the relationship between doctor and patient tends to be only one part—the center if one wishes—of a whole network of diagnostic relations. The patient's trouble is assessed by a diagnostic team comprising several disciplines whose members engage in their own transactions with the patient, eventually compiling their observations, test data, and interview material. It usually falls to the physician to head such a team, to draw inferences from the diverse data, and to formulate a diagnosis that is allegedly a synthesis of all team members' contributions to the diagnostic process. The social worker, the nurse, various laboratory technicians, consulting specialists, maybe a psychologist, a chaplain, or a physiotherapist, and of course the physician "in charge"—all have asked the patient some questions, assigned some task, or secured cooperation in some laboratory or testing procedure. In the course of these investigations, the patient visited different offices, was addressed in different vocabularies, met people of different moods and manners, and made some discerning observations about the efficacy of team functioning. When the studies have been completed, the patient sits beside the physician's desk to be informed about the diagnosis—if he or she is lucky. The patient is likely to have already received some provisional or definitive treatment and may even be ready to be discharged, without ever having heard a word about the diagnosis!

What I am trying to sketch is a "low" form of team diagnosis that is liable to repeat all the indignities, elitism, authoritarianism, and disregard for patients' right to understand their condition that we have found in some single doctor-patient relationships. Such a diagnostic team can add terrible feelings of being fragmented to patients' already sorry plight. They may feel poked at and analyzed into minutiae by so many people, each of whom begs questions by deferring to a rarely seen doctor, that they may despair of ever understanding anything about their ailments. They are glad to go home, possibly with the illness unchanged, but delivered from the nightmare of diagnostic investigations.

In reaction to this picture, we all seek to pride ourselves on being members of a superior diagnostic team. Our team consists of top-notch professionals, smoothly collaborating in a real team spirit, in which the patient is caught up, as if—be the metaphor permitted—infectiously. Still more humanely, we have organized our clinic or hospital to be like a little community in which the patients help each other to understand themselves, where by example and by conversation, or by guided group processes, they learn from each other to take hold of their condition and grasp something about the reasons behind their symptoms. Moreover, the team members frequently get together to discuss the patient at various stages of their studies, arriving in the end at a diagnosis based on group consensus. And the patient is at all steps fully informed! Even relatives are brought in for discussion and to prepare them for participation in the eventual treatment process.

Undeniably, these progressive features are large gains on the first model. There seems to be some partnership among team members, between each team member and the patient, and even among patients. But the trouble is that diagnostic teamwork cannot live by camaraderie and good spirits alone. If teams are justified by the adage that "two heads are better than one," their performance may amount to mere reduplicative busy work when these heads perceive, feel, think, act, and speak alike. The crucial rationale for a diagnostic team is that its members are *different* and maintain their differences, to give patients the benefit of studying themselves *from different vantage points.* Nor is the diagnostic team merely an organization in which labor is divided for greater efficiency and economy. The good diagnostic team is an interdisciplinary composite in which each member is a specialist maintaining her or his scientific, humanistic, and professional identity, in the conviction that only in this way can patients get hold of all the facets of their problems. The good team has autonomous members, who in turn help patients maintain their autonomy. It recognizes that most medical problems are complex, warranting study in diverse perspectives, each with its own integrity and its own power of resolution.

Interdisciplinary diagnostic teamwork requires many constraints imposed by scientific and humanistic value considerations. In the first place, team members must maintain a delicate balance between disciplinary specificity and dedication to a common goal. Each discipline is a unique perspective (backed by an identifiable combination of a particular basic science, applied science, and theory of technique) in which patients can be understood—or, more desirably, in which patients can come to understand themselves—with the help of an expert. Multiplicity of perspectives is the team's raison d'être. Ideally, this means collaboration of peers, not subordination to a hierarchy in which the disciplines (and their representatives) are ranked in order of alleged importance. It means deliberate maintenance of distinct language games, each germane to a particular discipline. The interdisciplinary team seeks to reach a higher-order synthesis of the compiled diagnostic contributions from the participating disciplines, a diagnosis that not only combines, but rounds off, all the vantage points that have been used.

Second, dedication to the team's common goal (which is explicitly more holistic than any particular discipline can manage to be) should include constraint on the drift toward accommodation to one discipline's dominance. The uniqueness of each perspective must be maintained, or it stops being a perspective. For instance, if a hospital social worker adopts too many medical concepts and accommodates outright to the prevailing medical language, his or her discipline loses its unique moorings and stops being a special vantage point. Its operation in the hospital becomes duplicative, redundant, or worse—a watered-down form of medicine. One profession is sold out to another profession, and the team deteriorates into a management device for the division of labor. And patients are sold short on the promise that their conditions warrant consideration in multiple perspectives; in the end, they will be regarded from only one vantage point.

Third, the interdisciplinary team I am describing requires constraint on answering the question of its leadership. Ideally, its leadership should fall to the profession or person having the greatest synthesizing power in describing and defining the patient's problems and finding workable avenues for intervention. If the diagnostic formulation is to rise above the bits and pieces of the contributing disciplines, synthetic judgment and great integrative capacity are required. Does any discipline have this to an acceptable degree? Does any profession specifically train its members to acquire these capacities? Which discipline can we trust to accomplish this without reverting to the pretentious queen's position of theology or philosophy in the Middle Ages?

Some professionals have answered these difficult questions by vesting their hope, not in any one discipline, but in the team as a whole which, under rotating leadership, strives for a group consensus. But committees are notorious for turning out camels from designs for a horse. Others have answered these questions by subordinating them, often tacitly, to the nature of the institution or organization in which the interdisciplinary team operates. In clinics and hospitals, the team leadership is given to medicine, often to one of its specialties. But can medical thinking transcend its own limits and partialities to do justice to the social, economic, psychological, cultural, existential, and life-situational vantage points in which the patient's predicaments are apprehended by various team members?

In the face of these critical rejoinders, one might toy with the thought that the ideal diagnostic team leader should be *the patient*. If, in each partial diagnostic study, patients were not merely asked to cooperate with or succumb to the various procedures of data-gathering and inference-making, but were fully engaged in self-diagnosis with the help of a particular expert, they themselves might be in the best position to arrive at a synthetic diagnostic formulation. Thought has to be given to the pace at which patients can assimilate diagnostic findings, which may well prove to be quite demanding. But that by itself would not detract from patients' unique suitability for making a diagnostic synthesis attuned to their own life situations. The expected rebuttal to this proposition is, of course, that most patients are too dumb, too illiterate, too invested in their symptoms, and generally too passive to achieve such a synthesis. It will be said that patients, in their perplexity over themselves, turned to the experts in the first place in order to get their answers. How would one dare turn the tables on them?

But this rebuttal is, as we all know today, full of open or subtle denigrations, celebrated in the terms *layman* and *patient*. The layman has always provided an occasion for professional one-upmanship, and not only in medicine. Competence is attributed to professionals, not laymen. The assumption of patienthood is widely seen as an admission of incompetence, helplessness, and weakness. But do these admissions of failure necessarily encroach on judgment? Should they be allowed to truncate the patient's dignity? Should they make the patient a subordinate subject of diagnostic investigations conducted and orchestrated by others? Where does reverence for the patient come in—not just politeness or civility—but reverence? Albert Schweitzer struggled with these questions, and even this towering figure failed to answer them satisfactorily, perhaps precisely because of his toweringness. The questions remain oppressively open, and that is what bespeaks their ethical import. They should not be shoved under the rug or decided by management theory. Nor should they be answered too glibly by sociological clichés which hold that only verbally gifted upper-middle-class patients would have the wherewithal to preside over their own diagnostic exploration, and that lower-class patients are incapable of such self-assessment. If we are concerned with the ethos of medical practice and medical education, these are the kinds of questions we must constantly press upon the mind of the profession's members, particularly the young ones who have not yet succumbed to the routines that feign to have settled them.

Humanistic Values Undergirding the Diagnostic Process

To become a professional implies much more than acquiring the knowledge and skill of one's chosen discipline, to accept peer review, and to uphold technical standards. It demands more than knowing and abiding by the profession's code of ethics which addresses—in the helping and caring professions—such issues as confidentiality, preservation of life, and loyalty to the Hippocratic oath. Whatever peers may demand, professional people in the helping disciplines must put themselves under steady scrutiny for improving the quality of their thoughts and activities, the quality of their interactions with their patients or clients, the quality of their professional and public utterances, the quality of their technical and extracurricular melioristic moves. Most of these self-scrutinies will have to be self-generated, for their subject matter bypasses laws or codes and is not greatly subject to sanctions. To use a psychoanalytic distinction, the "undergirding" values in the diagnostic process I am alluding to in this section have more to do with the professional person's ego ideal than with his or her superego.

For instance, in the helping professions and especially in medicine, thoroughness is a value—a virtue—to be emulated; thoroughness, not from fear of malpractice suits or from ambition to get the institution's top job, but from the humanistic conviction that the patient is entitled to the best, and that anything shoddy is an offense to the patient's and the physician's own dignity. Thoroughness within a collaborative diagnostic process also demands that diagnostic skill include interpersonal skill guaranteeing at all points the patient's human rights. If patients trust themselves to a professional helper, they have a right to that helper's best thoughts, best advice, best understanding. The professional promise to help, with or without fee, obtained in whatever economic system, permits no flippancy. The more we acknowledge that human problems of health and illness are typically complex (witness the inherent difficulties in defining health and illness), the more thorough and comprehensive should be our diagnostic reasoning. I say *reasoning*, not *procedures*, for multiple tests and special studies are sometimes only a foil for poorly directed thought and judgment. Within the limits of the profession and the patient's rights, no stone should be left unturned to foster the patient's (and the doctor's) understanding of the ailment, the condition, or the problem. The patient is worth the effort, and diligence and zest in one's work, now experienced as a collaborative task, are the physician's professional joie de vivre.

Helpers and carers today are the last bastion of respect for the individual in a society that tends more and more flagrantly to trample people underfoot in mass action and mass manipulation. Individuality and personhood are beleaguered from all sides by regimentation and bureaucracy, mass hysteria, and artificially induced low self-regard. The Renaissance made no bones about the grandeur of the individual, and the biblical psalmist considered man "a little lower than the angels." Who today dares echo such positive evaluations of personhood? It seems to me that one social function of professional helpers and carers is to nurture the tender plant of human dignity, and to do so pointedly in relation to all patients or clients if only by providing them with a haven— however limited in space and time—where privacy, tolerance, and reverence can be vividly experienced. This means that no diagnostician can lord it over a patient, and that one should be vigilant to the subtle pseudoprofessional arrogance that relegates the patient to the status of "only a layman." It means adopting a watchful attitude toward the misuses of one's professional language, avoiding inappropriate labeling of individuals by medical class terms such as a carcinoma case, an epileptic, a schizophrenic (not to speak of "schiz"), a mongoloid.

A third set of undergirding values in the diagnostic process centers on the diagnostician's scientific responsibility and identification with a profession and its advance. If one is to be a physician, a nurse, or a psychologist, one had better be a very good one, knowing the basic and applied sciences in and out, always updating, amplifying, correcting, or reworking the knowledge and skills acquired in the past. Although such strivings involve scientific curiosity and perfection of craftsmanship, they partake of a humanistic value orientation when one reflects on their obligatory ethical tenor. One *owes* these strivings to all parties concerned: to patients for their betterment, to the profession for its advancement, to the public which has given this profession a special status, with duties and privileges. And, we should not blush to say, to oneself as a person dedicated to competence and as a creature accepting the biblical challenge of having been made "a little lower than the angels."

Along with these positive values, to be emulated and practiced, there are some "unvalues" to be despised, some cultural or personal penchants to be consciously avoided. Some of these have already been mentioned in the preceding pages. They are more difficult to sum up because they are likely to be time- and culture-bound and imply a degree of corrective reactivity on the part of any professional worker, a watchful counteraction to besetting fads and fashions. Those who pride themselves on performing thorough diagnostic work know all too well that an anti-diagnostic wave is sweeping the country, of diverse origin and with different impetus. Therapeutic furor may ride slipshod over diagnostic patience. Misuse of diagnostic labels (especially in psychiatry) and diagnostic procedures has caused disenchantment or negativism in many people—professionals as well as patients—regarding the uses of diagnosis. Militant diagnostic nihilism is sometimes only a mask for quackery. Belief in patent medicines is close to belief in panaceas, both of which render diagnosis spurious or superfluous. Zealous do-good-ness may foster irrationality and produce antiscientific attitudes. And so on. The main point I wish to make is that in the end, however thoughtful the origins of some of these antidiagnostic penchants may be, patients are sold short on the right to know and understand their predicament and are in addition more likely than ever to be manipulated by somebody's ill-considered activism. However complex the interactions between diagnosis and treatment may be (and they do intertwine and overlap), rationality as well as reverence for troubled people dictate that diagnosis comes before treatment, and that any prescription should logically evolve from diagnostic knowledge.

This bit of medical orthodoxy (literally "right belief") about the logical sequence of steps in the helping process is systematically undermined by some features in modern medicine itself, notably specialization and pharmacotherapy. To put it all too succinctly, when specialists are too numerous, too visible, and overrespectable, a view of the patient as a whole is harder to get. The remaining general practitioners become gatekeepers to the specialists, who are likely to view each patient from one vantage point in which knowledge is on the order of "more and more about less and less." Although I would hold, within the ethos I am considering, that patients are entitled to, if need be, the most specialized knowledge of and interventions in their troubles, I also hold that they should not be truncated from a holistic view of themselves, especially when their problems are complex. By virtue of their specialization, specialists have to leave out many alternative or complementary vantage points and have a hard time considering patients in their personhood, as the opening portion of this essay shows. To boot, in their role as gatekeepers to the specialists, the general practitioners run some risk of becoming triage agents toward patients, allocating them to certain rubrics, referring them to third parties, or "managing" a patient through a succession of referrals. Whatever the intention, such triage and referral work is likely to make patients feel fragmented and unable to gain a comprehensive view of their ailments or predicaments. They will feel sold short again, despite the minutiae of knowledge they may acquire from the specialists to whom they have been referred.

The advances in effective pharmacotherapy, much to be lauded per se, have at times fostered diagnostic sloth in physicians who are otherwise quite thoughtful. A case in point is the prescription of tranquilizers, not after careful diagnostic study, but on the basis of a presenting symptom taken at face value, such as anxiety or agitation. Such overeager symptom treatment can entail tragic results: At times, bereft people who would do well to go through the natural phases of mourning are chemically prohibited from using their natural resources for restoration by these potent, instant tension relievers. The epigraph to this essay alludes to the ever lurking possibility that hasty interventions may make patients worse. A symptom is not a freak happening; it is a determined process that is to be seen in the light of its origin, function, and purpose; in other words, it is to be diagnosed instead of being quickly eliminated. The temptation to do the latter is great when the means are so readily available; worse, the accumulation of such quick symptom removal sets up a dangerous adiagnostic or antidiagnostic backlash that the profession is bringing upon itself.

Finally, if we are identified with the diagnostic ethos whose premises I have sought to outline, we should be wary of conceptions and modes of speaking that threaten to have an opposite tenor. I for one am suspicious of the increasing use of terms such as "health delivery systems," "health maintenance organizations," and other applications of the systems concept to medicine by medical professionals themselves. (This unease on my part does not extend to the heuristic use of general systems theory in the basic sciences of medicine, which has an entirely different aim.) The prevalence of such phrases betrays a penchant for dealing with the problems of medicine in predominantly managerial terms. Borrowed from engineering, industry, political science, or administration, these words are hard to rhyme with the ethos I have stressed. If the individual, particularly the suffering individual, in our society is as beleaguered as I think, I have no hope for an eventual rescue through systems and organizations. On the contrary, we are in dire need of humanizing our existing systems and organizations, not of further bureaucratizing our few remaining persons. Helping and caring require some degree of spontaneity, some feeling of good will, some degree of intimacy, and an enormous respect for individual freedom—all intangibles that cannot be systematized. And just these intangibles, I think, are the deepest wellsprings of our professional ethos. They are the undergirding values of the diagnostic process.

Because of this intimate relation between values and diagnosis, I am tempted to propose a new test: Tell me how you diagnose, and I will tell you what kind of person and what manner of doctor you are.

CHAPTER 11

The Tasks of Care: Humanistic Dimensions of Medical Education

John D. Stoeckle

What are the origins of a physician's professional identity? And how do new professional identities emerge? John Stoeckle is concerned about the way in which that identity since the 1890s and 1900s has been dominated by a particular brand of scientific self-consciousness. The historical background, as developed earlier by Sicherman, leads in Stoeckle's view to some of the dangers of "technicism" as identified by Lifton.

But Stoeckle comes at these problems as a physician and outpatient clinic director. He sees the profound need for a view of care that includes broad sensitivities to the patient as a whole. But while the scientific self-identity of physicians has brought immeasurable progress in the identification and treatment of illness, an overly narrow construction of that identity, especially in the form of dependence on advanced technology, diagnostic intervention, and monitoring procedures, can seriously detract from attending to the broader life issues of the patient. Stoeckle sees the impediments to implementing Pruyser's vision of the patient as convenor of a diagnostic team. How can the physician justify time given to sharing information with the patient, let alone helping the patient make decisions or communicate with the wider network of people who care for the person, when his or her ingrained identity is related to efficiency and scientific exactness? Why go beyond the biological facts?

A shift in professional identity to include the fuller human tasks of care must come about through some altered values and strategies in medical education. For one thing, there must be a challenge to the dominant model of massive urban academic hospitals as primary training sites. In medical practices and neighborhood clinics, for instance, young physicians would see much more quickly the real range of life issues that bear on a person's health or illness. And the rewards and role models would be in the area of patient care.

And beyond this, Stoeckle believes that, historically, real change in medical education has not come so decisively from direct tinkering with the medical school curriculum as from reform in the institutions of care. The leverage for change and innovation may be more powerful in the caretaking operations; as these are altered, the educational programs will begin to shift.

Ample evidence from social science is applicable here–the effects of role modeling, emergence of theory from practice, the dynamics of institutional change, and the resistance to change when academic settings reward and reinforce research over patient care.

In the interests of his strategy, Stoeckle identifies five different tasks of care in modern clinical terms and analyzes their sanctions, priorities, and implementation in a revised medical education.

From experience with ordinary illness (say, the "flu"), going to see the doctor, and attending any school, no one can doubt the enormous human dimensions of illness, care, and education. These facts should hardly require discussion, merely a report of them to remind those who may have forgotten that illness is not merely some objective disease but the patient's distress, discomfort, and disability; that practice is not only technical treatment but the care of patients; and that medical education is not just the transmission of knowledge but teaching and learning for the tasks of care. Both the acts of practice and teaching require a relation—the first between doctor and patient, the second between teacher and student—and in the special circumstances of learning from patients, the doctor becomes a student again. These relations are, above all, *human* relations, with the special "humanistic dimensions" that caring and education have.

Since we all know these plain facts, what is there to discuss? Perhaps the caring tasks and relations need discussion because of nagging doubts that patient care is really as human as it might be. And if it is not, why has not education prepared practitioners for those tasks? The explanations are not simple. They involve complex issues in the direction and organization of medicine and medical education.

Tasks of Care

Medicine's mandate is patient care. Although others might disagree, arguing that its mandate is medical science and technology for medical treatment, medicine's responsibilities are not only the treatment of the patient's disease but the care of his or her distress, discomfort, disability, and dying. In modern clinical terms, these tasks of care are: (1) the diagnosis and treatment of medical and psychological illness; (2) the communication of information about illness, its diagnosis, treatment, prevention, and prognosis; (3) the personal support of patients of all backgrounds, in all stages of illness; (4) the maintenance of the chronically ill; and (5) the prevention, where possible, of the patient's disease and disability through education, persuasion, and preventive treatment. This mandate is part of the history of medicine, as Barbara Sicherman's research shows in chapter 5. Furthermore, these caring tasks—numbered 2 through 5—are themselves crucial to the achievement of a fully informed patient and the construction of a treatment that not only is acceptable to the patient but also promotes his or her adherence. These tasks are equally essential to the goal of respect for the autonomy and initiative of the patient as a person, which, as Wallwork has argued, are crucial humanistic values in medical care and education.

Among these five tasks, that of medical diagnosis and treatment has grown enormously technical and costly. With such technical and costly therapies, it might seem that disease must surely be cured, reducing mortality and morbidity. Indeed, medical therapies are believed to have these important outcomes and therefore to constitute all of what the doctor does or what is really important about the job. But these beliefs about the outcomes of medical care and about the doctor's job as giving medical treatment are misperceptions. It is economic development, not treatment, that has reduced morbidity and mortality.[1] The acts of medical practice are rarely curative. They may, however, be preventive or rehabilitative, provide long-term maintenance, or give simple relief. Nor is the doctor's job as exclusively technical as it may seem. As acts of "doctoring," all the medical tasks contain human dimensions; in each, the *doctor-patient relation,* not technology, is central. Thus, even at their very first encounter, the doctor and the patient negotiate over the diagnosis and treatment of illness, one hopes along some of the lines suggested by Paul

Pruyser in the previous essay. Even if they do not negotiate, at least the doctor is supposed to use "judgment" in applying technique to the individual patient. After diagnosis, the help, if any, that the patient receives depends on the doctor's response to the patient, on his or her supportive, educational, communicative, persuasive, and "caring" behaviors with the patient. Yet nowadays these medical tasks are subject to pressures that may distort their purpose or even eliminate them entirely.

Pressures on Caring Relations

The relation is no longer dominated by the tasks of care but by other imperatives that have become ends in themselves; indeed, the caring relation between doctor and patient no longer seems controlled by the participants themselves. Critics such as Ivan Illich, Jan Howard and Anselm Strauss, and Rick Carlson document this.[2] They argue, in effect, that the expansion of "the health care system"—its technology, specialization, large practice organizations, and more health workers for more "health problems"—has become an end in itself. These forces, regardless of their more basic causes, distort the doctor-patient relation and divert medicine from its tasks. They create, in turn, the modern threats to the relation: its substitution by technology, its subdivision with specialization, its attenuation within larger medical practices, and its increased control over more patients as more social problems are defined as "health problems." And yet none of these forces is really new. They have only grown more powerful as medicine has become more industrialized, technological, specialized, and expansive; they are more apparent because more attention is now being given to their effects on patients—and on health workers as well. Care that *seems* humane enough may really not be. In the provision of highly technical medical therapies, for example, actual caring for the patient may not seem depersonalized, for the staff may truly be concerned. Nonetheless, care can hardly be characterized as humanistic when the decision to use treatment is devoid of ethical concerns as basic as informed consent.

Education: Scientific or for the Medical Tasks?

Often, education is offered as the solution to the diminished effort given to caring tasks. In the increasingly bureaucratic organization of services, the properly educated doctor or other health workers are supposed to "make the difference" in those services by providing personal care. In this case, it is their education that is always supposed to "count," to ensure that they will make care personal even when the organization imposes great odds against such behavior. Indeed, that is the public expectation of professional education expressed in countless surveys about the attributes of a good doctor: "technically competent" and "personally concerned," hence attentive to all the medical tasks. Despite these public expectations of medical education, the pursuit and promise of education have been somewhat different. Medical education has aimed to be scientific, not for the medical tasks.

What is needed now is a realistic assessment of the potential of education—along with reforms of the *direction* and *organization* of medical *practice*—to contribute to medicine's humanistic dimensions. To achieve this, certain historical forces that have diminished such educational efforts should be acknowledged. These include the structure of academic medical centers intended for the preparation of doctors, trends in the ideology (positivistic, factual, specialized) of medical education, and patterns of funding for medical institutions and faculty (research grants, applications for technological support, government and foundation funds for special diseases and treatment "breakthroughs"). As an alternative or complementary effort, the concept of primary care can be advanced as a model for what education and practice might look like if the caring tasks were fully recognized and incorporated into training and practice.

Unlike medical care, medical education has few critics. This is not surprising. First, the academic medical center enjoys such pride and public distinction that it has been above critical examination; second, the center's basic science campus and university hospital are less visible and understandable than the office practices where the public receives most medical aid. As a result, the

structure, ideology, organization, and support of medical education are not widely understood.

Looking at the structure of medical education, it consists not
only of classroom-laboratory teaching but of education in large
treatment institutions such as hospitals and clinics, alongside medical research laboratories. But the public view, for the most part, is
simpler: that of a school for doctors which can limit their number
through highly selective and limited admissions policies. The
more realistic view of medical education is that of a large corporate institution comprising an educational division, the school, but
also organized services, namely, the "teaching hospital," and research laboratories. This complex institution promotes technology, specialization, large-scale medical organizations, and medical
expansion. As a result, it is the academic medical center itself
which ironically exerts the greatest pressures against the learning
of caring tasks. However, it also has the constructive potential of
realigning values in the direction of care. Because of its intellectual traditions, the academic medical center holds promise for the
reexamination and renewed pursuit of the medical tasks that have
been the goals of medical education in the past.

The existing ideology of medical education has been ambiguous with regard to the medical tasks. Most often, educators assert
that medical education is meant to be the start of a lifetime of
learning, a goal not unlike that of liberal education. At the same
time, medical education is to be scientific. Indeed, in an effort to
shed its trial-and-error past and maintain a position of eminence,
medicine, defined as science, has been the dominant theme of
modern professional learning. The ideology has had success.
When the basic sciences became part of medical education, and
when laboratory and clinical science became part of the hospital,
medicine gained enormously in technique. Medical practice was
changed through the technology that research procedures generated. And the research model became fused with the idea of
medicine. Medical education was no longer vocational training for
the tasks of care, but scientific training for scientific hospital
medicine. In a real sense, universities sold *scientific* medicine to the
public as a counter to the prevailing empiricism of the day. That

is, rigorous scientific method and underlying theory were to replace ad hoc, trial-and-error methods of diagnosis and treatment. Research, logical thought, and other "scientific" practices have by now become well entrenched in the profession as a result of what were, in their time, significant educational reforms. Another virtue of this curricular orientation was, as the public suspected, the suitability of science as a screen for undesirable applicants to the medical schools. Those, it was believed, would be intimidated by the rigorous scientific subject matter. Thus, the ideology of science was intended to increase the competence, confidence, and respect of the medical profession.

Yet not all the consequences of this educational ideology have been beneficial. Education for scientific medicine is internally directed, seeking to explain the biological basis of disease and the effects of medical intervention. It is not useful for medical tasks other than those of diagnosis and treatment. The other tasks of care require special skills and behaviors that are not considered part of the scientific paradigm. Knowledge about the behaviors that make up the care of patients may be viewed as logical or experiential, but not scientific. As a result, the learning of these behaviors is not viewed as relevant in most existing medical education. In effect, since medical education is not typically organized for the tasks of care, these tasks are rarely examined systematically in education or practice.

Other factors to influence the content of learning are institutions for education. Medical education has been located in the science classroom, the research laboratory, and the hospital. In the case of the teaching hospital, where clinical education is located, the emphasis is on medical diagnosis and treatment, and on reliance on technology and laboratory science that are ready at hand. As a result, less emphasis is given to learning the other tasks of care that have greater importance in practice outside.

Finally, education has derived much of its financial support not through educational funds per se, but through medical research organized at medical schools and hospitals. The values and directions of research exert considerable influence on the content and atmosphere of education—a situation common, indeed, to all academic areas, in which didactic energies are stimulated largely by research interests. Other humanistic concerns, even if appreciated in practice, rarely receive formal instructional attention or support. One justification for continuing the research grant as an avenue of fiscal support in medical education as opposed to direct educational grants is that the schools and their students do not warrant education subsidies when future earnings are bound to be so high. The nature of research may define the problems that are considered important within medical schools and, indirectly, the medical tasks that are considered necessary in clinical situations. Much research has been directed at elaborating the technology of hospital medicine, reinforcing the existing emphasis on medical diagnosis and treatment in the hospital.

The structure, ideology, organization, and support of medical education socialize the student to the technical work of the hospital, to the task of medical diagnosis and treatment almost exclusively, and to valuing medicine only if it is "scientific." Moreover, education is falsely rationalized as scientific when it is only technological. The genuinely "scientific" includes modes of investigation where hunches and gaps in existing knowledge lead to the generation and testing of hypotheses, including forms of prediction, replication, and validation. Although "technological" procedures of monitoring do work and *may* be very helpful, they are not, in any sense, science; moreover, they may become forms of distancing that keep the patient from experiencing the genuine presence and care of the doctor. Given this educational context, humanistic concerns will need to be represented by a countervailing force made up of new pressure groups capable of articulating the need for alternative goals and principles in education, and for emphasis on the other tasks of care. The primary-care movement is one significant vehicle for pressing these new claims.

The Evidence and the Critique

What has been argued here is that the professional tasks other than medical diagnosis and treatment are liable to be considered peripheral in the care of patients and in the preparation of the doctor. In the case of medical practice, such limited attention has been explained by several pressures on the doctor-patient relation where the caring acts are negotiated. Not all these pressures have been mentioned. For example, the social and economic determinants of access and of differential treatment are omitted. The argument has only been sketched; the evidence that documents diminished attention to caring tasks can be found in a variety of sources: anecdotal accounts of patients' experiences; official complaints against doctors; the writings of the new medical critics such as Illich, Carlson, Howard, and Strauss; malpractice claims; studies of the workload of medical practice; the work of medical sociologists on the profession and medical institutions; and the analysis of the outcomes of medical therapies.

In making these comments about care and education, one is easily open to criticism—in particular, for being too humanistic at the expense of science. One may be accused of being a card-carrying humanist, indifferent to medicine's technical interventions with the same narrowness of spirit that characterizes those out to "scientize" all of medicine by rejecting any knowledge or skill unless it has scientific provability. But such counterclaims against science are not being made here. Only a limited argument is proposed: A complementary emphasis on medicine's art *and* science, to use very old and familiar terms, is needed. Today, this argument is not often made because of the risks that are thought to result when less than undivided attention is given to science. What are such risks? First, the risk of harming patients by not diagnosing their diseases while attending to their other concerns; second, the risk of failing to prove scientifically what one does so that others can be sure of the integrity of one's acts; third, the risk of losing the power and status derived from scientific knowledge by insufficient attention to it; and fourth, the risk of the uncertainty of medical "art" as compared to the supposed certainty of scientific knowledge. Despite these risks and their possible consequences, the importance of redressing the balance between art and science is very great. And steps in this direction may demand educational reform both within the medical schools and outside them in the reorganization of practice.

Reform

Can a prescription for reform be written to enhance the "human dimensions" of medicine and medical education? Some would reform the *doctors,* changing the human relations of medicine by applying behavioral science to the clinical and pedagogical situation. Others would reorganize *society,* because the root causes of distorted patient care are political, social, and economic. Between these two positions are intermediate reforms that deal with medicine's *institutions.* One such intermediate reform is the primary-care movement. It promises the renewal of medical practice and perhaps medical education because it contains new ideologies, organizations, goals, priorities, and content. The elements of the primary-care movement are:

1. A preventive and rehabilitative (instead of curative) orientation of medicine
2. A content that emphasizes low- rather than high-technology medicine, basic rather than contrived medical services; and attention to all the caring tasks instead of medical diagnosis and treatment alone
3. A location of practice that emphasizes out-of-hospital care
4. A group organization of practice with primary care as much a priority as specialty care
5. A research direction that is concerned with the efficacy of technology, the caring process, and small organizations
6. A function within the health system that provides continuity and integration of services in order to promote the autonomy of the patient

1. New goals: prevention. Prevention is a goal of primary care. Medicine's traditional goal has been to "cure" disease, hoping to remove it from the community by treating it in the hospital. The result has been that more chronic illness and disability have been added to the community. With primary care, medicine's new goals are to prevent disease and disability and to provide optimal maintenance of patients. Such goals are more realistic, since "cure" is not accomplished by medical treatment; the prevention of disability and disease and the optimal maintenance of patients are, in fact, the functions of medical care.

2. *New content: low technology, basic services, caring tasks.* The content of primary care consists of low-technology interventions, basic medical services, and the several caring tasks. Low- as distinct from the high-technology medicine of the modern hospital is emphasized; basic rather than contrived services are provided. Thus, for example, the prevention and control of hypertension might take precedence over the surgical relief of coronary heart disease. Finally, the tasks of care are the explicit content of primary care rather than merely instrumental in facilitating technical treatment. Not only are medicine's caring tasks, both technical and psychosocial, important in an immediate sense, but they also hold promise for improving the course of chronic illness. The implication of this content for medical education is that learning should be for the tasks of care. Thus, the elements of medical education would be not only the basic sciences of medicine, the content of medicine and the clinical method, but also the medical tasks.

3 and 4. New locations and organizations; group practices and teaching group practices outside the hospital. The major, but not exclusive, site of primary care is an ambulatory practice. Its major organization is a group—not a solo—practice. Low-technology medicine, basic medical services, and the caring tasks are concentrated in ambulatory rather than hospital practices. Group practices, historically organized to integrate the work of specialists, now have new goals and purposes: the provision of primary care. The implication for medical education is that more training experience should be focused on basic outpatient medical practice rather than on hospital work alone. More of it should be related to service rather than to research. Thus new organizations, especially teaching group practices, will be needed to complement the teaching hospital. In effect, more of education will be decentralized to medical practices.

5. New research directions: technology, caring process, and organization. The research implications of primary care are three:

technology, the caring process, and organization. With primary care promising more benefits (prevention) for less cost, more research will have to be directed to the assessment of medical technology and to the applicability of available medical knowledge. With an emphasis on care rather than technique, the caring process, inside and outside the professional health care system, needs study in itself and for its effect on chronic illness. With primary care depending on small organizations, studies of the dynamics and performance of health care teams, group practices, and interprofessional systems will be important.

The assessment of technology that is part of this renewed emphasis on patient care actually dovetails with the question of how to pay for medical services. At the present time there is a greater financial incentive for a physician to perform a technical procedure than to spend time in conversation with a patient—whether this time is spent in history-taking, psychological comfort, or preventive education. Conceptual and educational reforms are likely to be frustrated as long as the person in the field expects to be reimbursed for the procedure and not for the time. The present pattern of payment suggests that, at least to the payors, the curative powers lie in techniques, not in caring behaviors. The question of what behaviors to teach in the schools thus becomes at the same time that of how to change the reward system so that tasks of primary care will be rewarded equally with technical tasks.

6. New relations and values. Among the fuctions primary care is to provide are the first contact with the professional system, continuity for the patient, and integration of services. These functions are to be explicit. They are not only administrative functions; they also renew values about *personal long-term relations* with patients.

The purpose of providing patients with continuity and integration is not merely to "broker" services for some but to provide *coherence* to care. Another important, but latent, purpose of long-term relations is to give the patient an ally or a therapeutic alliance within the system—in effect, more power than the patients might have on their own. Finally, there is great value in long-term relationships in which the psychosocial and educational functions of practice can have direct benefits toward the goal of increasing the autonomy of patients.

When one considers these several elements of the primary-care movement, it is clear that most of them, except for research, lie outside the domain of the medical school. The direction of reforms suggested here thus moves from the reorganization of practice toward renewal of medical education and the school. This is an opposite direction to that which medical schools have taken over the past fifty years, when they have intended to reform medical practice by introducing new technologies. Now, as practice changes with the primary-care movement, we can hope that new values will be infused into medical schools because they are supported by new organizations, financing, and content.

NOTES

1. T. McKeown, "A Historical Appraisal of the Medical Task," in *Medical History and Medical Care: A Symposium of Perspectives* (London: Oxford University Press, 1971).

2. Illich, *Medical Nemesis* (New York: Pantheon, 1971); Howard and Strauss, eds., *Humanizing Health Care* (New York: John Wiley and Sons, 1975); Carlson, *The End of Medicine* (New York: John Wiley and Sons, 1975).

CHAPTER 12

The Doctor's Dilemma:
Social Sciences and Emerging
Needs in Medical Education

Samuel A. Banks

John Stoeckle began some specific reflections on possible changes in medical educa-
tion, particularly regarding setting, content, funding, and clinical expectations,
and Samuel Banks expands this discussion. He looks directly at the changing and
complex challenges confronting the doctor, and he develops suggestions regarding
both educational policy and practical strategy for improvement.

Central to these suggestions are ideas about the explicit incorporation of social
scientific content in medical education. In many ways, this chapter looks back on the
variety of insights from the humanistic social sciences represented by the preceding
writers, and points to the problems and possibilities of including such perspectives in
the medical school. This could affect not only curriculum but also the structure and
ethos of medical work.

Of course the social sciences are hardly free of the same tensions between "art"
and "science" that earlier writers have suggested are problematic in medicine. If
anything, some of the humanistic and social studies of these fields have been
plagued even more painfully by obsessiveness in trying to prove their "scientific"
character. Yet there are both scientific and humanistic elements from the social
sciences that should be incorporated into the education of effective caretakers. To
achieve this, both medical educators and social scientists will need to listen more
carefully and sympathetically to each other's concerns. Banks helps to bring this
exchange into clear focus.

As the title suggests, this chapter reflects a perspective and addresses itself to a problem. It may be helpful to delineate both at
the outset.

The particular viewpoint of the author stems from an academic
odyssey of thirteen years as a psychologist on a medical school
faculty. The following assessment of medical education and its

need for engagement with the social sciences finds its roots in my experiences as a professor in departments of psychiatry, community health, and family medicine, and later as chief of a division of social sciences and humanities within a college of medicine. My current activities as president and teacher in a liberal arts college have offered me the opportunity to extend these medical school experiences to a broader spectrum of institutions of higher education.

This analysis of actual and potential relationships between social science and medicine, therefore, reflects a specific point of view and a concrete personal and professional history. That viewpoint rests on a persistent methodological assertion that the perceived problems and obstacles confronting an institution constitute the only gateways to growth. In James Russell Lowell's phrase, "new occasions teach new duties," but the demands of change are more often experienced as galling threats than as stimuli to expanded effectiveness.

Similarly, the resources for meeting the demands of an emerging future are often treated as alien and threatening. Specifically, those academic disciplines offering medical students new and vital assistance enter the Hippocratic halls as strangers in a strange land. Helpers in educational crises, they are seen as bringing both opportunity and hazard. On the one hand, the introduction of new faculties and studies into established curricula provides the chance for deeper freedom and creativity through the acquisition of new perceptions, attitudes, and actions. Archibald MacLeish puts it succinctly, "The gift that I have to give you is the gift of my difference from you." On the other hand, such opportunity constitutes a demand on overtaxed faculty time and energies and the risk of losing old, secure ways. Olmsted and Kennedy (1972) suggest:

The behavioral scientist in the medical school is in somewhat the same position as the house painter who comes in to decorate an apartment. . . . For months housewives beg and plead with the decorator, and he feels very wanted because all these lovely ladies keep asking him to come in and paint their homes. Finally he arrives—much invited, much welcomed. But the very nature of his activities is disruptive. He lifts up the carpets and forces the house into disarray. He becomes an invader, a nuisance. (pp. 12–13)

This chapter presents an argument in three stages. The first section, referring to trends in the nation and in medical practice and education, suggests that both the physician and the medical student are faced with a radically and rapidly changing world; that these changes constitute a "medical menopause," placing persistent and significant demands on doctors to alter their life-style and world view; and that the social sciences represent a potentially valuable but little used resource in the formation of the new physician.

The second portion of the chapter reflects a recognition that the social sciences (together with such other "new fields" in medical education as medical humanities, medical jurisprudence, and the management sciences) are the "new kids on the block." The rhetoric of conference proceedings and journal articles indicates a growing realization of new demands on doctors and the place of these new disciplines in assisting them to meet these challenges. Further, departments and divisions of behavioral sciences already have been established in many medical schools. Still, the social sciences are newcomers that must recognize the established histories and entrenched values of clinicians and biological scientists, older acquaintances of Aesclepius. This is not to say that the newcomers are second-class citizens. It is simply essential to know the soil into which one attempts to plant social science perspectives.

As in clinical practice, the needs of medical students and faculty members are more easily diagnosed than treated. The envisioning of a fruitful engagement between teachers of medicine and social science is only a first step. The establishing of ground rules and working relationships is an equally significant and much lengthier task. In "The Hollow Men," T. S. Eliot portrays the anxiety entailed in undertaking such an endeavor: "Between the idea and the reality . . . falls the Shadow . . . between the conception and the creation . . . falls the Shadow"

The social sciences, still relative strangers, offer assistance in solving the problems of the health care revolution. Of course, as Eric Sevareid remarked insightfully, "the cause of problems *is* solutions." Faculty and student resistance to the introduction of new courses and research may be grounded in the apprehension that new problems will arise in the use of new perspectives.

It is understandable and fitting that the newcomers be met with caution and questioning. Therefore, the concluding portion of the chapter is devoted to a discussion of the strategies for effective engagement. Questions abound: How can social scientists most effectively envision the resources they bring and the needs they meet? In translating their concepts into programs, how can they deal creatively with the constraints imposed by the institutional history they enter? What political decisions are entailed in the development and maintenance of these programs? What problems will subsequently emerge?

The Changing Shape of Medical Practice and Education

Social, political, and economic trends since World War II have had a strong and sustained influence on the lives of medical practitioners. They in turn have responded at times with an increasing awareness of the need for enlarged perspectives, more flexible attitudes, and more adequate concepts. Many recognize that the curricular and clinical experiences of today's medical students will require increasing enrichment as preparation for a more excellent professional life.

Of course, excellence as a physician has always required awareness of the myriad biological, personal, and social considerations that shape decisions regarding diagnosis, prognosis, and care. Now there is increasing acknowledgment that the medical student needs sustained help in learning to be a master juggler, balancing a precarious array of understandings. Courses and patients confront medical students with a range of phenomena from submolecular functions to the structure of neighborhoods. They must learn to cope daily with the polar pulls between social and individual needs, abstract theories and concrete choices, qualitative and quantitative evaluations, observer and participant roles. They feel the two-way stretch between concepts of medicine as an art and as an applied science, between the sharp crises of acute illness and the marathon continuity of chronicity. These polar demands are inherent in the medical endeavor. Events during the last three decades have created even greater pressures on the doctor's understanding. Let us examine some of these.

The first half of this century was marked by stunning discoveries and advances in the treatment of infectious diseases. These scourges of mankind yielded to the post–Flexner report emphasis on specialization and laboratory research. "Miracle drugs" and immunizations significantly reduced the impact of acute illness on human life. Consequently, attention has been shifted to the degenerative diseases such as heart disease, stroke, and cancer now afflicting those who would have fallen victim to fatal infections in an earlier time. Further, these long-term, progressive illnesses have led clinicians to emphasize preventive measures and the need for maintenance where cures are not available.

Such illnesses require a more active, self-supervising role on the part of the patient. Doctors cannot autocratically control patient's responses to their "orders" regarding medication or a dietary regimen. They must instead understand the patient's motives and attitudes, as well as the family and societal influences that will shape the way the patient treats himself or herself.

Patients have also broadened the range of reasons for visiting their doctors. Many in the past delayed until they were driven to seek help by intense discomfort or dysfunction. Current magazine articles and television shows portray the physician in the additional role of counselor, one to be sought out when questions of life's meaning arise. Although their requests may be couched in somatic terms, patients lacking other support systems turn increasingly to their doctors for understanding and support. In other words, practitioners must cope with culturally conditioned expressions of illness and with the need for socially shaped treatment plans.

To complicate matters further, our systems for providing care

are markedly more complex than they used to be. Educators recall with nostalgia the image of the school as a log with the student on one end and a teacher on the other. Such a model bears little resemblance to modern educational institutions. The network of health care is similarly intricate. The triad of doctor, nurse, and patient has enlarged to include medical technicians; occupational, physical, and recreational therapists; operating-room technologists; and a variety of denizens bearing other labels.

As the members of health care teams face the patient, they must also face each other, constantly clarifying questions of communication, decision-making, and evaluation. It is no longer a simple matter for the doctor merely to *tell* either the paraprofessional or the patient what to do. New helpers demand from the physician new skills in supervision. To utilize the talents of the physician's assistant and the nurse practitioner, the doctor must understand their education, goals, capacities, limits, and approaches to the patient.

One should note that medical students themselves have changed in recent years. During the first half of the century, doctors-to-be in the United States were largely white and male. The enlarging proportion of women and minority-group members in entering classes offers a richer mix with a broader repertoire of responses. For example, it was rare, if not unheard of, for the male medical student in the old days to cry when deeply moved by the loss of a patient. He had not regarded either his peers or his clinical professors as able to participate in such an openly emotional way. The urge to weep was perceived as a threat, not a resource. I have noted that women medical students have been able to assist their masculine colleagues to behave more fully as persons.

It appears that alterations in admissions policies are allowing, even encouraging, a broader range of students to enter medical colleges. Successful applicants include not only the traditional science major but also those engaged in humanities, social sciences, and fine arts. Students earlier acquainted with the full range of the liberal arts seem to be more receptive to social science emphases in the medical curriculum. In attitude, the medical students of the seventies are the children of their times: more tolerant of complex issues, cognizant that many problems must be lived with rather than fully solved, impatient with overfacile explanations, and wary of arbitrary and unreasoning authority.

Medical education itself is marked by two profound changes demanding increased social understanding. During the last decade, questioning of the Flexnerian emphases on medical research and specialization has led to increased demand for comprehensive approaches to patient care. Medical schools are incorporating required and elective courses in primary care and family medicine (Falk, Page, and Vesper, 1973). Studies of such programs reveal positive student and faculty evaluations of these experiences in primary care (Banks, Murphee, and Reynolds, 1973). As these programs develop, systematic teaching about the physician-patient relationship has impact on other portions of the curriculum (Kane, Wooley, and Kane, 1973).

There is, in summary, a trend from emphasis upon specialization and subspecialties to a more balanced provision of early and holistically oriented screening and treatment. In stressing the doctor's understanding of health care transactions, medical schools reflect society's increasing concern for more effective *delivery* of the knowledge and skills we have already attained. Stevens (1971) says, "The problems lie not in the lack of achievements but in the widening gap between what *can* be done for an individual under optimal conditions and what *is* being done for the individual under average and minimal conditions. The crisis is in the delivery, not in the potential of care" (p. 2).

Federal capitation grants and other incentives have been provided to induce medical schools to alter their curricula to include a greater emphasis on comprehensive care. Such changes are much more easily attained, of course, in new institutions. Since 1960, sixteen four-year medical schools have been established, and twelve more are planned. Stevens (1971) comments again:

The new schools are freer to develop new curricula; the new University of Arizona College of Medicine; the Milton S. Hershey Medical Center at Hershey, Pennsylvania; and the School of Medicine of the State University of New York at Stony Brook are three notable examples. These schools are seizing the opportunity for teaching first year students by contact with patients; for emphasizing patient care with research as an adjunct (rather than vice versa); for developing medicine as a humanity as well as a science. (p. 375)

A second trend in medical education deserves attention. The walls of the health center classroom have expanded to include inner-city storefront clinics, preceptorships in physicians' offices, and rural health care outposts (Murphree, Banks, and Reynolds, 1972). Students are no longer restricted to learning from a narrow range of patients in an artificially contrived hospital environment. This shift of setting has profound effects on the cast of characters and plot in the drama of medical education. The community, as a new and extended arena, offers an opportunity to question old ground rules, broadening the range of physician activity (Weinerman, 1970).

These changes also invite the participation of the social sciences as "basic sciences of the community." Physicians cannot limit themselves to the role of technician. The medical colleges of the early 1900s, fashioned on the German university pattern, required that a medical student pursue the functions of scholar and researcher as well. More recently, it has become apparent that physicians must also assume the mantle of citizen-leader if they are to affect the conditions that shape the lives of their patients and their relationships with them. Wray (1970) affirms the view as follows:

It is almost universally accepted that the medical student must have a working knowledge of certain "basic sciences" before he can begin to master clinical medicine. A comparable set of "basic sciences" exists for the student who is learning to practice community medicine on a scientific basis. . . . The physician practicing community medicine must act as a "social change agent," stimulating and leading the population to alter their behavior in ways that will foster better health. Obviously, then, he must understand how health behavior is determined by cultural patterns, how these patterns came into being, the value systems on which they are based, and the motivations that sustain them. Furthermore, if he is to mobilize individual and community resources to produce the required changes, he must understand the interaction between the individual and the social group. (pp. 160-61)

Anthropologists, sociologists, economists, and other representatives of the social sciences can offer the student increased awareness of the individual and cultural meanings underlying clinical skills and biological concepts—meanings that demand physicians' systematic attention if they are to provide effective care for the person in society. The social sciences can further students' development in the following areas:

1. Deepening understanding of patients' views of illness and health, their attitudes toward health care, and responses to health care personnel and organizations.

2. Recognition of patients' social, psychological, and cultural characteristics affecting their accessibility and participation.

3. Acquaintance with patients' and physicians' ways of understanding and living with the life crises, developmental tasks, significant relationships, and self-understanding arising in health care settings.

4. Enhanced awareness by students of their own particular values, motives, ways of learning, and style of life as developing physicians.

5. Clarity in identifying and responding to social problems linked with the health of individuals and populations (such as race, poverty, and aging).

6. Acquaintance with factors that shape the transactions between physician and patient: communication and behavior patterns, decision-making processes, and expectations regarding specific responses and outcomes.

7. Consideration of the physician's personal identity and professional roles in the community. Experience in relationships with

other personnel on the health team. Understanding of the complex social matrix of systems and services underlying health maintenance.

8. Exploration of cultural factors (religious, economic, political, family) determining the organization of health care and the allocation of scarce health resources. Evaluating the effect of individual and social values on the formation of goals and priorities in health care.

The social sciences thus give students a chance to examine intensively the possibilities, problems, and solutions thrust at them by the human condition. The emerging profile of the physician as health planner will demand such learning as never before.

The Shape of the Encounter

In childhood play or athletic contests, understanding and agreement regarding the ground rules is a precondition for free and satisfying activity. The serious development of medical courses and programs has a gamelike quality too. That is, the interplay of committees and courses, professors and plans, depends on a history of informal rules. A new player will be far more effective if she or he understands the moves, the boundaries. and the methods of scoring. The following paragraphs provide a sample of such shaping factors.

The average citizen is familiar with the national occurrences molding medical education, but the detailed analysis of their specific impact is an intricate task beyond the purview of this chapter. A few examples must suffice. The many expressions of heightened consumerism reflect the general rise in expectations regarding what benefits constitute the necessities of life. Our century has witnessed demands for univeral suffrage, a minimum wage, provision of elementary and secondary education for all citizens, tax subsidies for state higher education, and equal opportunities for employment. Most citizens expect to receive retirement benefits, unemployment compensation, and federal health insurance for catastrophic illnesses.

The last quarter-century has been one of great expectations, an expanding economy, and the transformation of perceived luxuries into virtual necessities. In the last decade, similar expectations have begun to center on the standards and styles of medical care. The proposal of peer review procedures, the plethora of malpractice suits, and even the prevalent "delivery" model of health care all indicate vividly the accent on rights, accountability, and evaluation.

Medical educators are realizing that the acceleration of our desires and dreams for better health care is not matched by predictions for a comparable increase in the resources necessary for the expensive education of physicians. Inflation erodes the power of medical schools and teaching hospitals to purchase expensive equipment and to attract highly educated and salaried faculty and staff. An unstable economy inhibits foundation and donor giving and legislative action for adequate tax support. Institutions have leveled off the growth of their students, faculty, and budgets, abandoning "add-on" management styles for careful priority-setting.

Recent years have witnessed a general rise in criticism of the doctor. Charges of inaccessibility, exorbitant fees, geographical maldistribution, and overpopulation of some specialties are an easily recognizable refrain. In short, both doctors and their alma maters are suffering from alienation of societal affections and resulting fiscal constraints. Such conditions usually lead to narrowed vision and a diminished receptivity to important but costly innovations.

Medical education bears the mark of these and other national influences. It is shaped even more strongly by the responses of its own participants. For example, the difficulties that arise in selecting an entering class result both from pressures beyond the school and from the values within it. It is common knowledge that the demands of applicants far exceed the supply of places available in first-year classes. In such a seller's market, the criteria and methods of selection are easily overmagnified and distorted. Small differences on admissions tests may be given undue weight. Hurried interviews may be assigned greater significance than they deserve. Essays on application forms may receive inadequate attention.

Of greater importance, admissions committees can become uncritical of their own biases and assumptions. In past decades, applicants majoring in the natural sciences and in quantitative courses received the greatest approbation. In contrast, strong scholarship in philosophy, history, or anthropology was ignored or considered detrimental to the applicant's chances. This imbalance was partially corrected in the late sixties and early seventies. However, regression is a constant and disturbing possibility. The experimental Medical College Admissions Test (spring 1977) omitted questions and scores regarding general knowledge, drew its reading materials (testing verbal skills) from science materials only, and expanded threefold the number of sections devoted to knowledge of science! A biased selection process resulting in a generation of culturally illiterate medical students would be a tragedy.

The entering medical student is confronted with a crowded curriculum resulting from the balancing of basic science and clinical department territorial demands. Innovators requiring additional course time are often regarded as unwelcome by faculty colleagues in well-entrenched, traditional fields.

Aware of the need for more physicians, a number of medical colleges tried to reduce the years required for study by early admissions procedures and by compression of the traditional four-year programs. These attempts produced a painful curricular squeeze and, in a number of cases, resulted in a return to former practices. Such academic volatility, characterized by unimaginative and uncritical contraction and expansion, makes clinicians and basic scientists wary of new courses and perspectives, identifying them with irresponsible innovation.

This suspicion is rooted in the unquestioning and unquestioned style of much clinical teaching, a tight, exclusive triangle composed of patient, medical student, and attending physician. Both student and teacher find security at the expense of optimal learning in such a potentially uncriticized apprenticeship. It is not surprising that attempts to transform the triangle into a square by introducing nonphysicians as resource faculty are often met with resistance. Nevertheless, this guild mentality has been a widespread, weakening characteristic of medical education.

This traditional insularity is changing. Behavioral science departments are no longer considered transient or startling phenomena. There are over forty humanities programs in U.S. medical colleges (Banks and Vastyan, 1973). However, crossfertilization between medical and other university faculties is restricted by the time-honored segmenting of the medical student's career into three "knowledge-tight" boxes: baccalaureate studies, the professional school program, and the post-M.D. "house staff" experiences of internship and residency.

These divisions are appropriate and helpful, perhaps, but the barriers between them are too often impermeable, blocking the creative flow of teachers, insights, methods, and materials that can broaden a student's horizons. The student preparing for medical school turns to professors in colleges of arts and sciences. The resident and intern take their cues from specialty boards. Within the medical curriculum, basic scientists and clinicians often structure and teach their courses without consulting premedical professors or teachers in postgraduate medicine.

Although this is still the dominant state of affairs, one senses a changing climate. The intermingling of clinicians and biologists in team-taught courses is much more common. The report of the Citizens' Commission on Graduate Medical Education (1966) is an eloquent plea for the integration of undergraduate and graduate medical education (Stevens, 1971). Matlack (1972) indicates the increase in integrated premedical programs during the last five years. The Commonwealth Fund and the National Endowment for the Humanities have provided grants to build bridges between premedical and medical school programs.

If social science perspectives are to affect the life and work of the young physician, then teaching in these areas cannot be confined to sporadic, one-shot faculty encounters or encapsulated courses. There must be continuity and coherence throughout the student's ten-to-twelve-year journey.

We have focused attention on the ground rules embedded in

the traditions of medical education. Social scientists possess some of their own. They share with medical professors an appreciation for clinical modes of learning. Development of the case-study approach is not unique to medicine. Anthropologists, clinical psychologists, and sociologists have used the method regularly in relation to individuals, societal groups, and civilizations.

Moreover, social scientists share with clinicians the tensions experienced in striving to embody the elements of "art" and "science" in some unified way. Since human beings are both persistently physical and stubbornly symbolic in nature, it follows that studies of humans must struggle constantly to balance biological and social perspectives. It is not easy to integrate the results of laboratory experimentation, attitudinal surveys, field studies, and phenomenological investigations. The danger lies in social scientists' temptation to impoverish their field by constricting their methods and models to gain entrée into the medical school and secure support from newfound colleagues.

Since the turn of the century, the social sciences have narrowed their focus from panoramic theoretical constructions to sharper empirical data-gathering concerning specific social functions. In the analysis of our increasingly complex society, new specialties have arisen (for example, applied sociology and anthropology, social and community psychology). However, the intricacy of the problems faced has required the breaching of specialist barriers in new attempts at synthesis, as in the work of Talcott Parsons. Refined methods of measurement have led to the growth of econometrics, new sampling approaches, and the use of factor and multivariate analyses. Increasing emphases on experimentation and quantification have narrowed the horizons of a number of social scientists to events that can be easily replicated and measured. The tendency to substitute statistical for human significance has enhanced the status of social studies as sciences at the expense of recognized relevance (Sorokin, 1965).

This trend is amplified in the recent movement of the social sciences into medical education as "behavioral sciences." Prior to World War II, very few nonphysicians other than biologists taught in colleges of medicine. During the 1940s, some medical educators became aware of the potential contributions of social scientists to the understanding of patient and physician behavior. These disciplines were introduced into the medical curriculum during that decade on a sporadic, ad hoc basis by visiting professors and imported consultants. Through support by the Russell Sage Foundation residency programs and through other sources, faculty positions emerged during the 1950s, followed by the establishment of a number of divisions and departments of behavioral sciences.

In the main, these groups tended to attach themselves to departments of psychiatry. The result has been a double problem: difficulty in gaining psychiatrists' acceptance as significant partners in teaching and research, and avoidance of the stereotypes and negative attitudes directed by other medical faculty members toward psychiatrists.

Further, some behavioral scientists overemphasized their similarity to colleagues in the biological sciences in order to obtain acceptance in their new neighborhood. In so doing, they unnecessarily constricted their contributions to studies of easily discerned and measured behavioral functions, neglecting the broader ranges of patient-doctor experiences that do not lend themselves to repetition and measurement in the laboratory.

Social scientists have distinctive values that can arm medical students for effective life and work. Students can only come to know that they hold a perspective by recognizing the existence of other perspectives than their own. Doctors' responses to their patients will be far more flexible and profound if they can grasp the relativity of time described in historical studies, the effects of class and caste participation examined by the sociologist, the impact of culture seen by the anthropologist, and the intricacy of interpersonal and intrapsychic forces in psychology. Through these disciplines, physicians can become freer from the tyranny of the single view without descending into the chaos of complete relativity.

This enrichment cannot take place if the social sciences lose their distinctive integrity through shallow attempts at rapprochement. However, the fear of seduction can lead to academic impotence through sheer avoidance of significant encounters between social and medical studies.

Guidelines and Strategies

Since the history of relationship between social sciences and medical education has been brief, conclusions drawn regarding the rules of the relationship must necessarily be few and tentative. It is useful to take inventory and share my insights, testing their validity against the reader's experiences and viewpoints.

A new faculty member can be caught in the crack formed by the classic dichotomies posed by medical education: Should social scientists focus on the attitudes and behaviors of the doctor or the patient? Should their teaching take place in clinical or basic science programs? For that matter, should they give their time and energies primarily to the medical school or to schools of allied health and nursing? Should they attempt to provide "hard data" similar to and respected by biological and physical scientists, or should they offer less quantitative "soft data," open to criticism as "unscientific"?

Answers to these questions as they are posed fall into the traps that have diminished the creativity of medical educators in the past. The best answer may be that an adequate social science faculty can provide a range of data and perspectives, span between the medical school and other programs, relate to both the clinical and basic science offerings, and study the experience and behavior of both doctor and patient. Nevertheless, successful programs cannot begin everywhere at once. Priorities of timing and energy outlay must be considered.

Experience indicates, for instance, that programs which begin in colleges of medicine can be extended to other health science schools. On the other hand, it is difficult to swim upstream from those curricula with less academic prestige to the medical school program.

In like fashion, it seems to be more effective to ground social science teaching and research in the four-year medical school program (preferably beginning at the point of the student's first contacts with patients), carefully and tenaciously expanding to the residency and premedical programs that bracket these years.

It seems to be more effective in the long run, if not easier in the beginning, to initiate social science programs in close relationship with "mainline" clinical courses, clerkships, and departmental structures such as internal medicine, pediatrics, and family medicine. From such a beachhead, one can move beyond to the tightly packed hours of the basic sciences and the limited academic territory of the specialities. Although programs may be initiated successfully in basic science areas, medical students seem to move most easily in their learning from their activity in clinical events to the theoretical constructs and basic values examined by the social sciences.

For many years, medical schools engaged in a form of academic tokenism by offering sporadic, occasional lectures by a visiting anthropologist, an adjunct professor of psychology, or a clinician with a tangential interest in history. These gambits forestall criticism and allow administrators to point with pride, without making any lasting impact on students or faculty. Substantial enrichment of the program requires continuous impact through required and elective courses in all phases of the curriculum by a number of social scientists representing the varied fields. Further, these teachers should occupy tenure-track positions with salaries comparable to those of basic scientists. They should be full participants in committee and governance activities of the college, carrying their weight as colleagues.

To ensure stability, the primary sources of support for the social science programs must be found within the political and budgetary structures of the medical school rather than beyond it. Behavioral science departments founded predominantly on "soft money" from foundations or outside agencies tend to have a precarious and brief existence.

It is important, too, to have the strong support of the chief executive and the executive committee for the program. Students, house staff, and other faculty can inhibit a new program if they are opposed to it. Therefore, it is necessary to build strong relationships with these constituencies. However, they cannot enable these programs to exist. Such power is found at upper administrative levels. Without a genuine commitment from the sources of decision and funding, the prognosis for a social science program must be considered grave. In any event, an effective social science faculty will turn outward toward the major medical school constituencies in a systematic way. They will relate to the student through teaching, to other faculty through research and planning, to administrators through grant proposals and committee activity.

Like tourists in a foreign country, some behavioral scientists have tended to talk and work in ingrown fashion, avoiding creative contact with the medical "natives." Although unpleasant differences of viewpoint and limitations of knowledge can be dismissed by this tactic, social scientists need to be deeply related to the activities of clinical and basic science departments, where the "action" is. The formation of academic ghettoes begins with the understandable but lethal desire to talk only to one's own kind.

The strategies outlined here require careful selection and development of these new teachers. They should be characterized by unusual energy, strong motivation to bridge between academic disciplines, clear competence in their fields, and security in the teaching setting. Even then, it will require several years for a social scientist to become fully at home with the issues, rhythms, and climate of medical education.

In relatively new fields, confidence cannot be built in isolated activity. Whether gathered in separate departments, crossdepartmental divisions, or subdivisions of traditional clinical or basic science departments, social scientists become a creative "critical mass" through everyday working relationships with one another. Finally, it is essential that members of nonmedical fields teaching in medical schools continue to write for professional journals and participate in learned societies related to their primary disciplines. Such collegial support and professional recognition can protect against becoming marginal people. In essence, the double commitment to a scholarly field and to the medical milieu avoids a peripheral position by providing two central foci: a community of peers and a lively arena for teaching and study.

Conclusion

What is the future of the engagement I have described? This chapter is built on the assertion that a continued relationship between the social sciences and other areas of medical education is not only appropriate but necessary for the fulfillment of future physicians and patients. Whether this relationship will develop fully depends not only on the worth of the programs but also on such contingencies as tax and foundation support, shifts in social demands for comprehensive health care, and the specific attitudes of university and medical college administrators.

Whatever the structural means by which humanistic social perspectives are offered, two major risks must be avoided. First, the inertia of unquestioned academic goals and procedures can lead to the tacit decision *not* to decide what place these studies will have in the life of the student. Such academic minds have been described as similar to concrete—mixed up and permanently set! There is a twin danger of settling for pseudo-decision, offering the social sciences an ineffective place and unworkable relationships. Such abortive strategies offer immediate promise but diminishing returns. H. L. Mencken put it succinctly, "For every complex and difficult issue there is always an answer that is simple, easy, and wrong!"

REFERENCES

Banks, S. A.; Murphree, A. H.; and Reynolds, R. C. "The Community Health Clerkship: Evaluation of a Program." *Journal of Medical Education,* 48 (1973):560–64.

Banks, S. A., and Vastyan, E. A. "Humanistic Studies in Medical Education." *Journal of Medical Education,* 48 (1973):248–57.

Falk, L. A.; Page, B.; Vesper, W. "Human Values and Medical Education from the Perspectives of Health Care Delivery." *Journal of Medical Education,* 48 (1973):152–57.

Kane, R; Wooley, F. R.; and Kane, R. "Toward Defining the End Product in Medical Education." *Journal of Medical Education,* 48 (1973):615–24.

Matlack, D. R. "Changes and Trends in Medical Education." *Journal of Medical Education,* 47 (1972):612–19.

Murphree, A. H.; Banks, S. A.; and Reynolds, R. C. "The Community Health Clerkship: Profile of a Program." *Journal of Medical Education*, 47 (1972):925–30.

Olmsted, R. W., and Kennedy, D. A. *Behavioral Sciences and Medical Education.* Washington, D.C.: U.S. Department of Health, Education, and Welfare, 1972.

Sorokin, P. A. *Fads and Foibles in Modern Sociology and Related Sciences.* New York: Regnery, 1965.

Stevens, R. *American Medicine and Public Interest.* New Haven: Yale University Press, 1971.

Weinerman, E. R. "The Response of the University Medical Center to Social Demands." *Journal of Medical Education,* 45, pt. 2 (1970):69–77.

Wray, J. D. "Undergraduate and Graduate Education in Community Medicine." In *Community Medicine: Teaching, Research, and Health Care,* ed. W. Lathan and A. Newberry. New York: Appleton-Century-Crofts, 1970.

CHAPTER 13

Some Policy Implications and Recommendations

William R. Rogers and David Barnard

The diversity of the social science disciplines that have collaborated in this effort to articulate the human values in medicine and medical education appears to result in divergent recommendations for future research and policy change. At least two arenas seem to compete for the energies of investigators and reformers, and it is not immediately clear that they are thoroughly compatible. On the one hand, much insight is gained regarding the emotional, intellectual, and moral issues that affect the intimate *personal* relationships of medical care: the negotiations between individual doctors and patients; the tender or callous, sensitive or detached ministrations of doctors, nurses, and technicians; the private self-understanding of patients and doctors as they come to grips with the limitations and negativities imposed by disease, weakness, and death.

On the other hand, a range of problems and issues concerning *economic and public* accountability are illuminated that appear to be of wholly different proportions. These problems are related to what William R. Roy characterized in his 1976 Shattuck Lecture to the Massachusetts Medical Society as "three medical facts of life": "that we cannot do everything that is scientifically possible for everyone everywhere; that if we cannot do everything for everyone everywhere, we must decide what we are going to do for whom where; and that personal health care is only one of the determinants of health."[1] It is Roy's conviction that physicians who attend to social scientific investigations will discover that their agenda for the future centers on determining total national expenditures for health, on assuring adequate money for initiatives in areas other than personal health services, and on means of rationing health services. The intense efforts aimed in these directions will have to be made in the legislatures and the Congress rather than in physicians' consulting rooms; what is apparently called for is increased political and financial acumen on the part of the medical community, and not so much the deepening of psychological and moral sensitivities. In fact, the question arises as to whether the issues and goals of the first type, concentrated as they are in the area of more "humane," *personalized* health services, are not actually contradicted or superseded by the issues of the second type.

The seeming tension between these perspectives is partly due, no doubt, to the lack of consensus among the disciplines as to what constitutes a humanistic value. Psychologists, ethicists, economists, historians, and physicians will propose as great a variety of candidates as there are notions of health within the medical, psychiatric, and philosophical communities. And each conception of a human value worthy of affirmation and pursuit will entail certain types of action or commitment for its realization. A further explanation may lie in the sources of leverage or power that are associated with various forms of participation in the health care system. Thus, those who control and distribute the billions of dollars' worth of insurance reimbursements, construction costs, and research grants that finance the system can be expected to express value judgments in a form quite different from that which guides the genetic counselor or the physician who agonizes over whether to communicate or withhold a diagnosis from a dying patient.

Yet the most cogent explanation may simply be that social scientific reflection on medicine encounters a malaise on the part of many people that is at least doubly determined, both personal and public. Something is out of joint in the intimate interactions between providers and patients; and several of the essays presented here reinforce an increasingly published awareness of—and progressively richer vocabulary for—the personal dynamics of these problems. At the same time, the sheer size of the medical enterprise in its educational, political, and cultural aspects provokes a set of urgent questions of an institutional, legislative, and even international character that are also represented in this volume. In this sense, then, the exchange reported here may be representative in its diversity of methods and conclusions. The question remains, however, of the possibility for any unified value commitment when these approaches, each sensitive to matters of genuine concern, are brought together.

Three salient themes decide firmly in favor of such a unity. The themes, sounded consistently within these essays, are, first, the *respect and nurturance of individual autonomy* complementing the value of medical support and intervention; second, a commitment to the *empowerment of persons and groups* with respect to self-determination in treatment programs, the achievement of life-styles and life opportunities propitious for health, and dignified experiencing of treatment settings; and third, *aggressive, benevolent professional action* accompanied by full recognition of fundamental and certain *human limitations,* the most crucial of which is our mortality.

The power of these conceptions to unify the approaches and recommendations involved here lies in the fact that the difficult political and financial decisions affecting national health care structures and goals depend largely on informed, thoughtful, and responsible judgments made by individual citizens. Although these judgments will ultimately involve actions taken at distant levels of government, the judgments themselves will be formed at least in part on the basis of the quality and tone of private experiences with particular medical professionals and treatment settings. Individuals' ability to think clearly about the value they place on health, the measure of personal responsibility they are prepared to assume for treatment or life-style, and the spirit in which they respond to limitations and even failures in care will depend substantially on their experiences of autonomy, empowerment, and professional actions performed with humility. There is no final conflict, then, between the levels of discourse carried on in these essays; they emphasize, rather, a singular interpenetration of personal values, interpersonal relationships, and socially responsible corporate actions.

Accordingly, the specific recommendations that follow reflect these several levels of concern, from relations between individual practitioners and patients, through the educational policies that prepare physicians to participate in those relationships, to broader policy issues that set the political and social context for both medical education and practice. In addition, there are some suggestions for further research along the lines generated by this effort.

Relationships in Medical Practice

1. Patients should be included as full participants in diagnostic efforts and discussions, with significant sharing of information relevant to an individual's condition and prognosis.

2. An essential component of diagnostic and therapeutic interactions should be the attempt to assist patients in interpreting the meaning of their situation, in terms of both the technical and scientific dimensions of their participation in the medical system, and the implications of their condition for their future life prospects, self-image, and social status.

3. A dialogue should be fostered between physicians and patients concerning philosophies of terminal care to facilitate a matching of sufferers and healers on the basis of fundamental beliefs and expectations, including the possibility of a patient's transferring to another physician when philosophies are incompatible.

These recommendations address the need to nourish patients' autonomy and self-determination to the greatest extent that is compatible with the physician's exercise of professional wisdom and expertise. They call attention to the critical role played by information in assigning power in relationships, and to the desirability of making the doctor-patient relationship a setting in which both parties are comfortable in acknowledging genuine limitations. At the same time, the relationship can be an occasion for mutual clarification of values and for an appreciation of each participant's strengths. The honest disclosure of the serious implications of illness is thus a paradigm for acknowledging limits *and* for appreciating courage, but it is clearly not the only example of such mutuality in medical practice. The principles of patient participation and collaborative diagnostic procedures refer to the everyday aspects of routine medical care, which offer just as many opportunities for upholding these values.

Educational Curriculum

1. Advising and seminar systems should be devised to deal with the personal responses of medical students to both laboratory and clinical material that could otherwise be brutalizing and numbing.

2. Value issues should be explicitly explored within the curriculum with particular attention to the questions of personal accountability, social responsibility, and the influence of cultural values on the role of medicine in society and on doctor-patient relationships.

3. Coursework should be provided in the history of medicine, emphasizing especially the emerging images of the role of the physician, coupling humanistic care-giving with the scientific technology of treatment and research.

4. Coursework should be offered in areas such as economics, social psychology, social ethics, and public policy, examining questions of the social matrix of health care, theories of health and personhood that medical systems serve, and the interpersonal and socioeconomic dimensions of specific medical interventions.

5. Interdisciplinary coursework should be introduced, preferably drawing on the resources of other professional schools and caring institutions, in the processes and implications of death, dying, and bereavement, with attention to the physiology and psychodynamics of terminal experiences, legal and religious contexts for viewing death, and modes of humane care for the dying and the bereaved.

6. Workshops, training groups, and audiovisual techniques should be employed to increase sensitivity in interpersonal relations, and enhance effective history-taking and professional consultation. They should include accurate listening for the vagaries

of feelings and attitudes that may be unique in each case, and help combine respect for persons with accuracy of understanding and effective counseling.

7. Clinical rotations and assignments should include community health services as well as major urban medical centers to bring some balance to students' exposure to patients, complaints, and uses of various mixtures of technological and personal competence.

These recommendations call particular attention to the impact of setting and set in both medical practice and education. To take the issue of setting in practice first, it is important to develop students' familiarity with a variety of professional roles, and with the different expectations and demands of patients that can arise in neighborhood clinics as compared with hospital centers. This variation in setting also makes possible greater experience with family and community networks that can be relied on to improve self-care, continuing care, and compliance with treatment plans, so that the caring tasks can root themselves in patients' ongoing patterns of living and adapting, rather than existing in the isolation of more impersonal, intimidating bastions of medical technology. The question of setting arises in the educational process in connection with opportunities for reflection and honest dealing with the traumatic aspects of clinical medicine in a supportive, accepting atmosphere. The goal here is to neutralize pressures toward conforming with images of complete stoicism and impersonal detachment that represent the numbing aspect of students' confrontation with helplessness and death, to make it easier to incorporate a sense of limitation complemented by the sense of confidence that comes with feelings of collegiality and personal bonding with others who are encountering the same experiences.

The recommended coursework addresses the issue of the intellectual set with which a student assumes clinical responsibilities. This set includes frameworks for interpreting behaviors and attitudes of patients and colleagues in the stressful circumstances of illness. It includes awareness of the personal stakes involved in particular clinical encounters, as well as the implications of institutional arrangements, social conditioning, and moral considerations. Finally, it is to be hoped that this type of intellectual work will, in a reflexive way, throw light on the educational process itself, uncovering value assumptions and intellectual methods that affect the medical profession as a whole. In this way, medical education can increase its potential for contributing to the profession's ongoing process of internal control, including the identification, defense, and enforcement of professional norms that are in accord with the role of the profession in the society at large.

Social Policy

1. Substantial public funds, especially "seed money," should be committed to developing and strengthening ambulatory care services, and medical education programs connected to such services, which stand outside the traditional system of rewards for high-technology apparatus.
2. Medical schools should continue to be encouraged to increase residency positions in primary care and family medicine.
3. Modes of support should be explored for students interested in rural medicine, coupled with new incentives for physicians to choose rural practice. These efforts should include investigation of the application of modern telecommunications and information-processing to increase rural practitioners' participation in and follow-through on all levels of care for their patients, and to enhance the intellectual satisfactions of participation in the general medical community.
4. Medical ethics, human values, and humanistic medicine should be recognized as an integral part of the federal health manpower policy as it relates to the funding of medical education, as a necessary complement to federal support of research and development in the biomedical sciences.

These recommendations reflect the awareness that intellectual and moral commitments by themselves cannot accomplish major reforms within medicine and medical education without significant restructuring of organizational, institutional, and financial arrangements. Indeed, a social scientific perspective on human values in medicine ought to be particularly sensitive to the social and political dynamics of proposals for significant change. Although the more personal commitments can, at their best, stimulate desires for change or prepare individuals better to fulfill the potentials of renewed organizations and institutions, those larger structures have the power to mold new concepts into old patterns of professional behavior; similarly, the availability or lack of funding can determine the fate of innovative programs in education or practice that are outside conventional reward systems. This is, then, a critical point of intersection between the levels of personal and intellectual reform, and political and legislative tactics.

Further Research in Social Science and Medicine

1. More research and experimentation are needed into the effects of varying fee structures and modes of reimbursement and insurance on the behavior of physicians, particularly in the proportion of time spent in technical operations and procedures as opposed to history-taking, effective listening, or explanation of disease processes and treatment plans, and into the effects of directing insurance coverage to catastrophic, hospital-centered care compared to routine, preventive care.

2. More research is needed on the effects of various forms of national health insurance on access to health services, quality of care, the qualilty of life for physicians and other health professionals, and control of costs. Particular attention should be paid to comparative studies of other countries' systems and the applicability of their experience to the U.S. situation.

3. There should be more emphasis on opportunities for practicing physicians to continue self-learning and personal growth, with specific attention to the applicability of educational structure and content to the nature of medical practice. Such opportunities should combine the functions of professional self-renewal and research into the real demands of everyday life in the profession, with direct input into curriculum planning in the medical schools.

4. The exchange of ideas between social scientists and physicians that produced this book should be considered as a potentially significant model for the type of self-learning and research opportunities just described.

These final recommendations, which are both substantive and procedural, and which touch on both research and self-renewal, aptly characterize the process that was described in the introduction to this volume. Just as one of the major themes of the foregoing essays was the special link between the scientific and the personal dimensions of medicine, so does the search for points of fruitful contact between social science and medical education become itself an occasion for furthering both scientific and personal integrity.

The formation of this integrity is in one sense an awesome task, for there is implied within it a patient and profound expression of the resources of human compassion coupled with enormous demands for the growth of knowledge and the refinement of skills. Yet, at the same time, the interplay of scientific and humane engagement can be invigorating and refreshing, if not downright fun. Far from the depressingly obsessive and lonely existence of a humorless dedication to some sterile norms in either social science or medical research, the style of work and life that inspires the insights and recommendations of this book reflects something of the joy of a genuinely open and caring human community. As we share our questions, our hopes, our enthusiasm, our pain, our ideas, our wonder, we may move closer to the integrity of truth and personhood. And from that should stem a more whole and life-giving vision of health and health care.

NOTE

1. *New England Journal of Medicine*, 295, no. 11 (September 9, 1976):589.

Notes on Contributors

SAMUEL A. BANKS
President, Dickinson College
212 West High Street
Carlisle, Pennsylvania 17013

Formerly Chairman—Division of Humanities and Social Sciences, Department of Community Health, University of Florida College of Medicine, with interests in philosophy of medicine, ethics, and social psychology of health care.

DAVID BARNARD
Andover Hall 205
Harvard University
45 Francis Avenue
Cambridge, Massachusetts 02138

Doctoral candidate in religion and society, with special interests in psychology, history of medicine, ethics, and humanistic interdisciplinary research on competence.

ROBERT JAY LIFTON
Research Professor
Yale Medical School
25 Park Street
New Haven, Connecticut 06519

Psychiatrist and writer concerned with effects of war, nuclear weapons, and the psychology of the survivor, as well as broader symbolic and "formative" issues around death and the continuity of life.

THOMAS K. MCELHINNEY
Director of Programs
Institute on Human Values in Medicine
925 Chestnut Street
Philadelphia, Pennsylvania 19107

Ethicist, administrator, and consultant on human values issues in medical education curricula.

ANTHONY OLIVER-SMITH
Departments of Social Sciences and Anthropology
University of Florida
Gainesville, Florida 32611

Anthropologist and professor who has written in philosophy and social sciences on the dual functions of human compassion and research.

PAUL W. PRUYSER
Henry March Pfeiffer Professor
The Menninger Foundation
Topeka, Kansas 66601

Clinical psychologist, writer, and educational administrator with special interests in diagnosing, medical team dialogue, and belief systems.

WILLIAM R. ROGERS
Parkman Professor of Religion and Psychology
Andover Hall 406
Harvard University
Cambridge, Massachusetts 02138

Psychologist and theologian with research interests in values and health, psychotherapy and social change, and the construction of meaning.

BARBARA SICHERMAN
Radcliffe College
Editor, Notable American Women
10 Garden Street
Cambridge, Massachusetts 02138

Historian who specializes in medical and psychiatric history and in women's history; currently editor of *Notable American Women*.

Frank A. Sloan
Professor of Economics
Vanderbilt University
Nashville, Tennessee 37235

Economist with interests in crosscultural studies of urban and rural health care delivery systems, particularly their accessibility, and costs and benefits.

John D. Stoeckle
Massachusetts General Hospital
Fruit Street
Boston, Massachusetts 02114

Primary-care physician and outpatient clinic director at MGH, with responsibility in medical school curriculum development.

Ernest Wallwork
Department of Religious Studies
Yale University
New Haven, Connecticut 06515

Ethicist with interests in social psychology, especially the social psychological effects of institutional practices.

Selected and Annotated Bibliography

David Barnard

This selected bibliography is an opportunity to continue delineating the special nature of the humanistic dialogue between social science and medicine that has emerged from the preceding essays. The orienting focus of these essays is a mutual reflection upon the basic questions of value and human meaning that arise in the training and practice of physicians, and in the social sciences themselves, rather than the unidirectional application of social theory to medical problems. The intent of this bibliography is to call attention to works in the vast literature of social science and medicine that in one way or another speak to the main themes of this book, in the problems they address, the methods they employ, or the values they examine or espouse. It is thus intended not to be representative of medical social science as a whole, or to substitute for the many excellent bibliographic guides to that field, but to help readers whose interests have been sparked by this book to pursue their concerns further, or to assist those who are engaged in human values curriculum-building in the education of health professionals.

In order, however, to serve readers who wish to sample the field more broadly, this bibliography is divided into two parts. Part 1 is a listing of several general reference sources in medical social science. All of these works have further bibliographic information which will guide investigators to important sources in social science and medicine. Part 2 contains citations and brief descriptions of works in which the *humanistic* dimensions of the social sciences' interaction with medicine seem to be especially prominent.

Once again, the themes and interests of the foregoing chapters must be relied on to supply more precise meaning to the notion of the humanistic as a principle of selection. Nevertheless, the works that follow have certain qualities in common. First, they focus specifically on value questions, or on the implications for the kinds of people we become as we assume our professional identities and roles. They reflect a concern for the survival of respect for persons and commitment to ideals in the medical tasks and the institutions in which those tasks are performed. And they represent, in many cases, a probing and questioning of assumptions within the disciplines of social science themselves, as well as within medicine or medical education. These are approaches in scholarship, education, and professional practice that this book hopes to encourage, and this selected and annotated bibliography is a chance to identify other voices speaking in the same tone.

1. General Reference Sources in Social Science and Medicine

A. Anthologies and Texts

Freeman, H. E.; Levine, S.; and Reeder, L. G., eds. *Handbook of Medical Sociology.* 3rd ed. Englewood Cliffs, N.J.: Prentice-Hall, 1979.
> Includes, in addition to fully referenced articles, a thorough bibliography, "Social Research in Health and Medicine."

Freidson, Eliot. *Profession of Medicine.* New York: Dodd, Mead, 1970.

Jaco, E. Gartly, ed. *Patients, Physicians, and Illness: A Sourcebook in Behavioral Science and Health.* 2nd ed. New York: Free Press, 1972.

Mechanic, David. *Medical Sociology.* 2nd ed. New York: Free Press, 1978.

Millon, Theodore, ed. *Medical Behavioral Science.* Philadelphia: Saunders, 1975.

B. Journals

Culture, Medicine, and Psychiatry
Death Education
Ethics in Science and Medicine
Hastings Center Report
Journal of Health and Social Behavior
Journal of Medical Education
Journal of Medicine and Philosophy
Man and Medicine
Medical Anthropology
Milbank Memorial Fund Quarterly
Social Science and Medicine

C. Specialized Bibliographies and Reference Sources

Clouser, K. Danner, and Zucker, Arthur. *Abortion and Euthanasia: An Annotated Bibliography.* Philadelphia: Society for Health and Human Values, 1974.

Foundation of Thanatology. 630 W. 168th Street, New York, NY 10032.
> Research, education, and publications on psychosocial aspects of death, loss, bereavement, and grief.

Institute of Society, Ethics, and the Life Sciences. *Bibliography of Society, Ethics, and the Life Sciences.* The Hastings Center, 360 Broadway, Hastings-on-Hudson, NY 10706. Issued annually.

Society for Health and Human Values. 1100 Witherspoon Building, Philadelphia, PA 19107. Various publications on human values, medicine, and medical education.

2. Humanistic Dimensions in Social Science, Medicine, and Medical Education

Alpert, Joel J., and Charney, Evan. *The Education of Physicians for Primary Care.* Washington, D.C.: U.S. Department of Health, Education, and Welfare, Health Resources Administration, 1973. Pub. no. HRA-74-3113.

A concise monograph addressed to two problems: Not enough physicians enter primary-care practice, and those who do are inadequately prepared. Discusses problems encountered in primary care, aspects of present educational structure that compromise education for primary care, and the potential of every level of medical education to contribute to improved preparation. Specific recommendations for a successful program in admissions policies, faculty, patients, curriculum time, and setting. Each section is accompanied by an extensive bibliography.

Ashley, Jo Ann. *Hospitals, Paternalism, and the Role of the Nurse.* New York: Teachers College Press, 1976.

A feminist perspective on nursing education, the professional status of nurses, and the role of nursing in U.S. hospitals. Particularly valuable for its documentation of the experience of being a student nurse and the relation of nursing issues to feminism in general.

Balint, Michael. *The Doctor, His Patient, and the Illness.* New York: International Universities Press, 1957.

The psychological aspects of general medicine. The basic premise is that the doctor as a person is always potentially the most effective therapeutic agent, but to maximize this effectiveness requires awareness of interpersonal and internal dynamics in the medical encounter. Reports on groups of general practitioners in which psychological issues in daily practice were analyzed, both for research purposes and for the doctors' personal growth. Physicians' groups after the Balint model are increasingly common in this country.

Becker, Ernest. *The Denial of Death.* New York: Free Press, 1973.

Death and finitude as the animating structures of human life, character, and culture. The need to deny death is seen as the basis for both constricting, depersonalizing repression and creative, immortalizing "heroism." Implications for theories of mental illness and personal creativity, as well as for the cultural and symbolic aspects of medical care.

Bier, William C., ed. *Human Life: Problems of Birth, of Living, and of Dying.* New York: Fordham University Press, 1977.

Perspectives from psychiatry, clinical medicine, theology, and pastoral care on questions raised by new medical technology. Topics include the value of human life, eugenics and population issues, the experience of handicapped and disabled persons, artificial life support, and religious views of immortality.

Blanpain, Jan; Delesie, Luc; and Nys, Herman. *National Health Insurance and Health Resources: The European Experience.* Cambridge: Harvard University Press, 1978.

A timely, comparative analysis of the development and implementation of compulsory health insurance in West Germany, England and Wales, France, the Netherlands, and Sweden. Discussion of the phases in governmental policy, from the goal of equal access to physicians' services to the development of hospitals and specialized institutions, and the dangers of expecting unlimited health services to result in unlimited health. The roles of physicians, insurance companies, labor unions, and legislators in developing health policy in these countries.

Cabot, Richard C. *Social Service and the Art of Healing.* Washington, D.C.: National Association of Social Workers, 1973.

Originally published in 1909, this book remains a moving, classic statement of the human, social, and moral contexts of medical work. Cabot utilizes the concept of "medical teamwork" to describe the essential sharing of responsibility for health among doctors, patients, social service workers, and social and behavioral scientists. Argues for intimate cooperation of medicine and social science, theoretically in the education of physicians and in research on etiology of disease, and practically in the clinical interview and in assuring meaningful, understandable treatment regimens. Included is Cabot's profound essay, "The Use of Truth and Falsehood in Medicine."

Cassell, Eric J. *The Healer's Art: A New Approach to the Doctor-Patient Relationship.* Philadelphia: Lippincott, 1976.

An attempt to define the essential, personal features of medical care apart from modern technological trappings. Based on the author's earlier work on language in medicine and the distinction between the technological and moral order. Free of jargon, this book is a humane, reflective look at doctors and patients, their ways of perceiving, their fears, and their strengths. Special attention to professional omnipotence in confrontation with chronic illness and death.

Coles, Robert. *Children of Crisis, Volume II: Migrants, Sharecroppers, and Mountaineers.* Boston: Little, Brown, 1971.

The life experience of children and their families in the rural United States, primarily told by the people themselves in open-hearted dialogue with the author. An attempt to transcend the distancing and objectifying aspects of sociological and psychological research, Coles's method incorporates elements of therapy and moral commitment. The subjects emerge on their own terms—with their aspirations and values, hopes and despair. The many references to rural health and health care take on fuller meaning in the context of Coles's sensitive, humane approach.

_____. *The Mind's Fate.* Boston: Atlantic–Little, Brown, 1975.

Essays on psychiatry, psychoanalysis, and the relationship of professionals to social and political conflict. Special emphasis on responsibilities to children in times of social upheaval.

Davis, Alan, and Horobin, Gordon, eds. *Medical Encounters: The Experience of Illness and Treatment.* London: Croom Helm, 1977.

Essays by British medical sociologists based on their own experiences of illness, combining personal narration with sociological theory and interpretation. Attempting to correct what is perceived as a defect in much medical social science that ignores the unique, particular human encounter in favor of abstraction and theory-building, these essays try to make constructive use of participant observation, with all its biases and idiosyncrasies. Included are discussions of chronic illness, life and routines on the hospital ward, and the tasks, frustrations, and anxieties associated with learning to be a patient in the medical system.

Davis, Fred. *Passage Through Crisis: Polio Victims and Their Families.* New York: Bobbs-Merrill, 1963.

Social and psychological impact of polio on fourteen children and their families. An attempt at naturalistic description and theoretical analysis of the nature of the crisis experience from earliest warning signs to hospitalization and final return home. Discussion of the families' conceptions of the disease and recovery, and the clashes of their perspectives with those of the hospital personnel; effects of the child's illness on family functioning; problems of identity for both child and family in adapting to the status of handicapped person; clashes of interest between hospital and home.

Dingwall, Robert. *Aspects of Illness.* London: Martin Robertson, 1976.

An extended critique of fundamental assumptions and values in medical sociology, and an attempt to provide a theoretical framework for further research to answer the question, "How do people come to feel ill and what do they do about it?" rather than the more frequently asked question, "Who uses official medical services?" Criticism of "scientism" and "absolutism" in medical sociology, and a call for a major paradigm shift to construe illness as social action, and to see patients as purposive, rational actors rather than puppets moved by environmental stimuli or dominant attitudes and precepts. Analysis of ways in which sociologists' adoption of official medical concepts of illness and deviance ignores the social construction of medical knowledge and allows medical sociology itself to function as an agent of social control.

Ehrenreich, Barbara and John. "Health Care and Social Control." *Social Policy*, 5 (1974):26–40.

Disciplinary and cooptative social control as elements of the medical system, relying on the dynamics of intimacy and authority in the doctor-patient relationship. Class differences in the impact of social control in the system, with special focus on the "medical poor" in the United States and the phenomenon of underutilization of health services. An effort to move beyond the simple demand for "more" medical care to ask, More of what? For what purpose? To what effect?

Engelhardt, H. Tristram, and Spicker, Stuart F., eds. Series on *Philosophy and Medicine*, esp. Volume I, *Evaluation and Explanation in the Biomedical Sciences* (1974), and Volume IV, *Mental Health: Philosophical Perspectives* (1977). Dordrecht, Holland: D. Reidel.

Collaboration of philosophers, physicians, and social scientists to understand the principles and methods of medicine as a scientific and intellectual
discipline. Continual emphasis on medical ethics and human values.

Erikson, Erik H. *Insight and Responsibility.* New York: Norton, 1964.

The ethical implications of psychoanalytic insight, and the intersection of
clinical, moral, and historical perspectives on human relationships, the
transmission of values across the generations, and the growth of a moral—as
well as a psychological—identity. An example of criticism and reevaluation
within social scientific theory itself, and not merely its application to value
questions in other fields.

Feifel, Herman, ed. *The Meaning of Death.* New York: McGraw-Hill, 1959. *New
Meanings of Death.* New York: McGraw-Hill, 1977.

The original version of this book drew on theological and philosophical
perspectives on death and supplemented these with clinical and empirical
research. The updated version has a stronger clinical and empirical slant,
with more attention to patient management, the impact of death on the
values, attitudes, and emotions of health professionals, and the family as
survivors of death. The philosophical dimension is still present, particularly
in introductory and concluding essays by the editor.

Fine, Virginia, and Therrien, Mark. "Empathy in the Doctor-Patient Relationship: Skill Training for Medical Students." *Journal of Medical Education,* 52
(1977):752–57.

Empirical evaluation of teaching methods designed to increase empathic
responses of medical students to patients as individuals and to presentations
of disease symptoms. Results demonstrate a higher level of empathy and
greater initial rapport with patients on the part of the experimental group
following training, as compared with a control group.

Fox, Renee C. "Training for Uncertainty." In *The Student Physician,* ed. R. K.
Merton, and P. L. Kendall. Cambridge: Harvard University Press, 1957.

The student's experience of medical education from the point of view of the
need to incorporate several types of uncertainty: imperfect mastery of available knowledge, awareness of the limits of knowledge, and difficulty in
differentiating between poor mastery of what is known and true limits to
knowledge. Discusses the progressive exposure to and assimilation of uncertainty through the course of medical school, and emphasizes death and the
autopsy as paradigms of uncertainty. The difficulties of first trying to establish long-term relationships with patients in this atmosphere. Suggestions
for restructuring the educational process to take these problems into account.

Fox, Renee C., and Swazey, Judith P. *The Courage to Fail: A Social View of Organ
Transplants and Dialysis.* Chicago: University of Chicago Press, 1974.

Existential, social, psychological, and religious elements in experimental
medicine. Courage under uncertainty and the dynamics of gift exchange,

with the physician as gatekeeper, as the dominant aspects in these interventions, in addition to the technical difficulties. Extended case histories, and a bibliography of medical experimentation.

Fox, T. F. "The Personal Doctor and His Relation to the Hospital." *Lancet,* 1 (1960):743–60.

Reflections on general practice, and the status of the independent practitioner amid pressures for specialization and hospital-based medical care. Stimulated by the author's visit to the United States, the essay compares British and U.S. health systems from the perspective of the availability of "personal medicine" in an age of technical sophistication. A portrait of the "personal doctor" as a faithful, dependable ally for the patient—especially during hospitalization—as well as a thorough analysis of the depersonalizing aspects of even the most well-intentioned hospital-based group practices. An essay that balances forceful statements of ideals and values with sensitivity to educational, institutional, and social barriers to their realization.

Freidson, Eliot. *Doctoring Together: A Study of Professional Social Control.* New York: Elsevier, 1975.

Social control, professional relationships, and the organization of work in a group medical practice. Physicians discuss themselves, their work, their patients, and their colleagues. The concrete operations of physicians in their workplace below the level of formal administrative planning. Especially valuable for insights into the relations between primary practitioners and specialist-consultants, and the informal mechanisms for enforcing professional norms. Considerable attention to the distinctive nature of human services organizations as objects of social research.

––––––––. *Patients' Views of Medical Practice.* New York: Russell Sage Foundation, 1961.

A study of subscribers to a prepaid medical plan in the Bronx. Patients' expectations of physicians and standards of "personal interest" and "competent care." Dilemmas in the doctor-patient relationship and various levels of conflict are seen as arising out of clashes between the separate worlds of experience on the part of lay people and professionals.

Fuchs, Victor. *Who Shall Live?* New York: Basic Books, 1974.

Problems of cost and access in medical care in the context of an analysis of the actual contributions to the state of health from the health system. Economic aspects of medical education, physician supply, hospital services, drugs, and insurance plans. Emphasis on income, education, and life-style as significant determinants of mortality and morbidity. Also includes a critique of the limits of economic analyses and the need for value choices regarding costs, access, and the shape of future health systems.

Gold, Margaret. "A Crisis of Identity: The Case of Medical Sociology." *Journal of Health and Social Behavior,* 18 (1976):160–68.

An analysis of the value orientations of all research articles published in the *Journal of Health and Social Behavior* suggests that social research is profoundly influenced at all stages by medical values and reveals a distinct "medical bias" in collaborative research between sociology and medicine when medicine sponsors and defines the research situation. A call for more self-consciousness on the part of medical sociologists about their own needs for professional integrity in order to maximize possibilities for critical examination of medical values as they affect actual medical care.

Gray, Bradford. *Human Subjects of Medical Experimentation.* New York: John Wiley, 1975.

Empirical sociological study of medical research with human subjects, with particular emphasis on the experience of the subject, beginning with the process of entry into the experiment. Difficulties with informed consent are examined in terms of barriers to comprehension due to personal, social, and institutional factors.

Howard, Jan, and Strauss, Anselm, eds. *Humanizing Health Care.* New York: John Wiley, 1975.

Papers and commentaries on the theme of "dehumanization" in medical care, organized around causes of dehumanization, definition of the concept, consequences, and strategies for change. A final section discusses issues and problems in future research on dehumanization from the perspectives of medicine, anthropology, sociology, and architecture.

Katz, Jay. "The Education of the Physician-Investigator." In *Experimentation with Human Subjects,* ed. Paul Freund. New York: Braziller, 1970.

Beginning with the comment that most arguments concerning the protection of human subjects rely heavily on the ethical sensitivity and personal responsibility of the physician-investigator, Katz asks whether the medical curriculum actually prepares students for this type of decision-making. Conflicting values in the clinical and research roles are discussed in relation to medical education. Recommendations are illustrated by a description of a seminar on the ethics of experimentation at the Yale Law School.

_____. *Experimentation with Human Beings.* New York: Russell Sage Foundation, 1972.

The basic sourcebook for legal, ethical, philosophical, social, and psychological issues in human experimentation. Includes legal opinions, codes of ethics and conduct governing research and medical practice, analyses of problems of informed consent, freedom of choice, and the definition of harms. Decision-making procedures, and responsibilities to persons, to science, and to society are described and analyzed.

Koos, Earl L. *The Health of Regionville.* New York: Hafner, 1967.

Portrait of the state of public health, the functioning of medical services, and people's perceptions of medical care in a rural community. Social factors in illness, how values in health matters are established and maintained, and how health patterns accept or resist change. Analysis of class and economic factors in recognition and acceptance of disability, and the use of health professionals. A picture of the physician and his roles in the community.

Krause, Elliot A. *Power and Illness: The Political Sociology of Health and Medical Care*. New York: Elsevier, 1977.

Marxist and liberal sociological analysis of political, economic, and social power struggles which have shaped the current U.S. health system. Relation of the labor movement to health organizations, social and political aspects of health planning, assessment, and regulation, with special attention to occupational health and possibe future health systems.

Kübler-Ross, Elizabeth. *On Death and Dying*. New York: Macmillan, 1969.

An important step in the movement to make a frank confrontation with death an acceptable part of medical professionals' identity and purpose. Although there is a danger in taking the author's stages for the dying process too rigidly, the case material is valuable evidence that strivings for meaning and hope continue to the very end of life. Also, emphasis is placed on strategies of distancing and denial on the part of physicians, nurses, families, and patients.

Lain Entralgo, Pedro. *Doctor and Patient*. New York: McGraw-Hill, 1969.

Historical and social treatment of the medical encounter as a meeting between two persons. Four aspects of the encounter are followed: the cognitive, the operative, the affective, and the ethico-religious. The doctor-patient relationship in Greek antiquity, the Middle Ages, the nineteenth century, and the present.

McDermott, Walsh; Deuschle, Kurt; and Barnett, Clifford. "Health Care Experiment at Many Farms." *Science,* 175 (1972):23-31.

Collaboration of medicine, public health, and anthropology in evaluating the "technological misfit" of modern health care and the disease patterns of a Navajo community. Report of mortality and morbidity for several diseases and conditions before, during, and after the establishment of a primary-care facility. Relations between the cultural setting and Western medical technology, with attention to the positive as well as negative aspects of the encounter.

McKeown, Thomas. *The Role of Medicine: Dream, Mirage, or Nemesis?* London: Nuffield Provincial Hospitals Trust, 1976.

Important and lucid attempt to assess modern medicine amid the competing philosophies of therapeutic nihilism and grandiose claims for advancing technology. Examines the validity of the concept that human health depends on a mechanistic approach based on the functions of the body and its diseases, and the implications of this discussion for medicine in terms of health services, medical education, and medical research. Includes historical and social perspectives on the determinants of health, and a view of the role of medicine that can stand up to both its intense critics and its zealots. Special attention to the effects of concentrating medical teaching in major hospital centers.

Miller, Jean Baker. *Toward a New Psychology of Women*. Boston: Beacon Press, 1976.

A major reexamination of assumptions and values in the psychology of women that has profound implications for issues of personal identity, control, and authority in the helping professions. An analysis of the roles of nurturer and care giver, and the possibilities for integrating them with traditionally opposed values of autonomy, assertiveness, and power.

Navarro, Vicente. "Social Policy Issues: An Explanation of the Composition, Nature, and Functions of the Present Health Sector of the United States." *Bulletin of the New York Academy of Medicine,* 51 (1975):199–234.

Economic and political forces determining the U.S. class structure and their decisive impact on the nature and function of the health system. Special emphasis on financing and delivery of care in health institutions, relationships between the public and private health sectors, and the reflection of class and economic differences in the stratification of the various health professions.

Noble, John, ed. *Primary Care and the Practice of Medicine.* Boston: Little, Brown, 1976.

Collection of essays analyzing primary care both as a patient service and as a medical discipline. Includes discussions of the views of disease and the person which underlie the practice of family medicine, legal and psychological aspects of doctor-patient relationships, physicians' relationships to institutions, specialists, and midlevel practitioners, continuing care, and the role of the physician in community medicine. Each essay includes a substantial bibliography.

Ramsey, Paul. *Ethics at the Edges of Life: Medical and Legal Intersections.* New Haven: Yale University Press, 1978.

Dilemmas concerning abortion, euthanasia, and the care of defective newborns are discussed from three perspectives: medical practice, public policy as expressed in law and judicial opinion, and ethics. Compassionate—and impassioned—medical, legal, and ethical arguments evaluate current public discourse and moral reasoning on these issues while seeking to raise the level of policy-making and to ground institutions and practices on the principle that the individual human life is unique, inviolable, and irreplaceable. Detailed analysis of the U.S. Supreme Court's abortion decisions, the case of Karen Ann Quinlan, and the California Natural Death Act, as well as extended replies to ethicists' criticisms of the author's previous work in medical ethics, especially *The Patient as Person* (1970).

Reiser, Stanley J. *Medicine and the Reign of Technology.* New York: Cambridge University Press, 1978.

Major technological innovations of the last four centuries for diagnosing illness, from the microscope and stethoscope to the electrocardiograph, the computer, and new techniques of telecommunications. The circumstances influencing the adoption of these and other innovations, along with their influence on the physician and patient, particularly the way in which they have changed the way the physician perceives and comprehends illness, the physician's self-image and values, and his or her ability and role as a decision maker.

Reiser, Stanley J.; Dyck, Arthur J.; and Curran, William J., eds. *Ethics in Medicine.* Cambridge: MIT Press, 1977.

Comprehensive sourcebook in medical ethics, drawing on historical, philosophical, legal, and social science contributions. Ethical aspects of doctor-patient relationships and broader questions of the role of medicine in society are illustrated by primary documents, organized historically and thematically. Each section contains extensive bibliographic material and illustrative cases.

Robertson, James. "A Two-Year-Old Goes to Hospital." London: Tavistock Child Development Research Unit; New York: New York University Film Library, 1952 (film); and *Hospitals and Children: A Parents'-Eye View.* New York: International Universities Press, 1963.

The human situation of young children and their families during the child's hospitalization. The book consists primarily of letters from parents to Robertson, written after the showing of the film on British television, describing their own and their children's experiences. Vivid and personal accounts of the impact of separation, isolation, admissions procedures, surgery, and the return home. Includes one complete "case history" and a discussion of visiting privileges in various British hospitals, many of which have been reformed partly as a result of Robertson's work, which is related to John Bowlby's research on attachment and separation.

Roth, Julius A. "Care of the Sick: Professionalism vs. Love." *Science, Medicine, and Man,* 1 (1973):173–80.

Analyzes the role of the caretaker as combining love and competence, and compares the alternatives of teaching love to trained hired hands or teaching skills and information to those who already have a bond of relationship and affection to the patient. Roth argues that it is easier to achieve the latter than to exhort professionals to love more. He emphasizes heavier reliance on a person's network of nonprofessional loved ones and increasing the level of health knowledge in the population at large.

Saunders, Lyle. *Cultural Difference and Medical Care.* New York: Russell Sage Foundation, 1954.

The impact of cultural values on the acceptance or rejection of Western medical care among Spanish-speaking Americans in the Southwest. The clash of fundamental value orientations and life-styles between the medical system and its prospective clientele.

Stimson, Gerry, and Webb, Barbara. *Going to See the Doctor: The Consultation Process in General Practice.* London: Routledge and Kegan Paul, 1975.

An attempt to depict the process of consultation with the general practitioner in England from the patient's perspective. Emphasis on patients' expectations of physicians, the nature of the face-to-face interaction, and the aftermath of consultation, including the continuous process of reinterpreting subjective feelings, reevaluating the doctor, and changing attitudes toward ongoing treatment. A discussion of the physician's power to control time, his or her availability, and information leads to reflection on the nature and limits of both professionals' *and* patients' autonomy in medical treatment. Includes methodological criticism of research on consultation that too often views the patient through the eyes of the doctor, perpetuating institutional and professional images of model patients as compliant or naive.

Strauss, Anselm, and Glaser, Barney. *Anguish: A Case History of a Dying Trajectory.* London: Martin Robertson, 1977.

An intense account of one woman's long-term course of dying in a hospital, an extension of the authors' previous theoretical work on the process of dying, from the point of view of both the dying person and the nursing staff and physicians. Theoretical commentary is secondary in this book, as the main people involved, the dying woman and her care givers, speak dramatically and personally of their reactions to the day-by-day progress toward death. Discussion of the implications of this case for sociological method and for terminal care.

Taylor, Shelley, and Levin, Smadar. "The Psychological Impact of Breast Cancer: Theory and Practice." In *Psychological Aspects of Breast Cancer,* ed. Allen Enelow. Oxford: Oxford University Press, 1977.

Review of the literature on breast cancer, particularly its psychological impact in all phases of symptomatology, diagnosis, treatment, and postmastectomy recovery. The authors' goals are policy formulation and the advancement of social science research methodology. Major emphasis is on the elaboration of a "patient -participation model" for intervention in treatment of breast cancer, in which the patient is neither a passive recipient of services nor fully in charge of medical decisions, but an informed, active member of the team responsible for her health.

Titmuss, Richard M. *The Gift Relationship: From Human Blood to Social Policy.* New York: Random House, 1971.

Fundamental questions of human relationships, social bondedness, and the possibilities for altruism in the modern welfare state are approached from the starting point of human blood. The scientific, social, economic, and ethical issues involved in the procurement, processing, distribution, and use of blood in Britain, the United States, the Soviet Union, South Africa, and other countries. The personal, national, and international consequences of treating blood as a commercial commodity, morally sanctioned to be bought and sold in the marketplace, and the symbolic as well as economic differences between voluntary and commercial programs for blood donation and supply. Consideration of blood policy as a metaphor for contrasting images of "economic" and "social" man emerging from different policies regarding all human services, and attention to the dangers of economists' claims to ethical neutrality in their cost-benefit computations.

Veatch, Robert M. *Death, Dying, and the Biological Revolution.* New Haven: Yale University Press, 1976.

Analysis of the options for a workable public policy in care for the dying. Technical, moral, political, and psychological aspects of the definition of death, problems posed by organ transplantation and artificial life support, and the ethical arguments for and against the disclosure to the patient of a terminal diagnosis. Useful bibliographical materials.

Veatch, Robert M., and Branson, Roy, eds. *Ethics and Health Policy.* Cambridge, Mass.: Ballinger, 1976.

An effort to broaden the concerns of medical ethics to complement the more individualized problems such as abortion, euthanasia, and truth-telling. This book is a running discussion among philosophers, social ethicists, and people involved in health policy and planning. Major topics include the allocation of scarce resources, decision-making as a function of local communities, the right to health care, justice and health care delivery, genetics, and technology assessment. Attention is also paid to the possible limitations of ethics as a discipline when applied to these aspects of medicine.

Wadsworth, Michael, and Robinson, David, eds. *Studies in Everyday Medical Life.* London: Martin Robertson, 1976.

A collection of papers attempting to capture and understand "the nitty-gritty of everyday life" in medical practice. Sociological analysis of the nature of communication and negotiation between doctors and patients, and the role of the physician as an agent of social control. Verbatim reports of medical encounters reveal the hierarchical nature of most interactions and the need to increase communication and compassion in the relationship. Attention to methodological issues, suggestions for more empirical study of doctors and patients interacting, and an extensive bibliography.

Waitzkin, Howard, and Stoeckle, John D. "The Communication of Information About Illness." *Advances in Psychosomatic Medicine,* 8 (1972):180–215.

Theory in sociology and social psychology applied to the dynamics of power and control in the doctor-patient relationship. Uncertainty in diagnosis as a source of asymmetry and power differentials, and the responsibility of the physician to compensate with special efforts to include the patient in the decision-making process.

White, Robert W. "Hartley Hale, Physician and Scientist." In his *Lives in Progress.* 3rd ed. New York: Holt, Rinehart and Winston, 1975.

A case study of the personal growth of a physician, part of White's study of psychodynamic, social, and cultural influences on individual development. Special focus on the tension between professional achievement and the capacity for intimacy in personal relationships, and the potential for the social rewards of success in a medical career to mask failures and difficulties in other aspects of living.

Index

Index

Contemporary Community Health Series

HEALTH CARE IN THE EUROPEAN COMMUNITY
Alan Maynard

HOME TREATMENT
Spearhead of Community Psychiatry
Leonard Weiner, Alvin Becker, and Tobias T. Friedman

LONG-TERM CHILDHOOD ILLNESS
Harry A. Sultz, Edward R. Schlesinger, William E. Mosher, and Joseph G. Feldman

MARRIAGE AND MENTAL HANDICAP
A Study of Subnormality in Marriage
Janet Mattinson

THE PSYCHIATRIC HALFWAY HOUSE
A Handbook of Theory and Practice
Richard D. Budson

A PSYCHIATRIC RECORD MANUAL FOR THE HOSPITAL
Dorothy Smith Keller

RACISM AND MENTAL HEALTH
Essays
Charles V. Willie, Bernard M. Kramer, and Bertram S. Brown, Editors

SOCIAL SKILLS AND MENTAL HEALTH
Peter Trower, Bridget Bryant, and Michael Argyle

THE SOCIOLOGY OF PHYSICAL DISABILITY AND REHABILITATION
Gary L. Albrecht, Editor

THE STYLE AND MANAGEMENT OF A PEDIATRIC PRACTICE
Lee W. Bass and Jerome H. Wolfson

In cooperation with the Institute on Human Values in Medicine:

NOURISHING THE HUMANISTIC IN MEDICINE
Interactions with the Social Sciences
William R. Rogers and David Barnard, Editors